National Academy Press

The National Academy Press was created by the National Academy of
Sciences to publish the reports issued by the Academy and by the
National Academy of Engineering, the Institute of Medicine, and the
National Research Council, all operating under the charter granted to
the National Academy of Sciences by the Congress of the United States.

An Evaluation of the Role of Microbiological Criteria for Foods and Food Ingredients

Subcommittee on Microbiological Criteria
Committee on Food Protection
Food and Nutrition Board
National Research Council

NATIONAL ACADEMY PRESS
Washington, D.C. 1985

NATIONAL ACADEMY PRESS ● 2101 CONSTITUTION AVENUE, NW ● WASHINGTON, DC 20418

NOTICE: The project that is the subject of this report was approved by the Governing Board of the National Research Council, whose members are drawn from the councils of the National Academy of Sciences, the National Academy of Engineering, and the Institute of Medicine. The members of the committee responsible for the report were chosen for their special competences and with regard for appropriate balance.

This report has been reviewed by a group other than the authors according to procedures approved by a Report Review Committee consisting of members of the National Academy of Sciences, the National Academy of Engineering, and the Institute of Medicine.

The National Research Council was established by the National Academy of Sciences in 1916 to associate the broad community of science and technology with the Academy's purposes of furthering knowledge and of advising the federal government. The Council operates in accordance with general policies determined by the Academy under the authority of its congressional charter of 1863, which established the Academy as a private, nonprofit, self-governing membership corporation. The Council has become the principal operating agency for both the National Academy of Sciences and the National Academy of Engineering in the conduct of their services to the government, the public, and the scientific and engineering communities. It is administered jointly by both Academies and the Institute of Medicine. The National Academy of Engineering and the Institute of Medicine were established in 1964 and 1970, respectively, under the charter of the National Academy of Sciences.

The work on which this publication is based was performed pursuant to Contract No. Na80 GA-C-0060 from the Food and Drug Administration, the Department of the U.S. Army Natick Research and Development Center, the U.S. Department of Agriculture, and the National Marine Fisheries Service of the Department of Commerce, which served as administrator of the contract.

Library of Congress Cataloging in Publication Data

National Research Council (U.S.). Food Protection
    Committee. Subcommittee on Microbiological
    Criteria.
    An evaluation of the role of
microbiological criteria for foods
and food ingredients.

    Includes bibliographies and index.
    1. Food—Microbiology—Congresses. 2. Food
poisoning—Congresses. I. Title.
QR115.N37 1985   664'.028   84-25555
ISBN 0-309-03497-3

Printed in the United States of America

First Printing, May 1985
Second Printing, May 1988
Third Printing, October 1988

Subcommittee on Microbiological Criteria for Foods and Food Ingredients

CARL VANDERZANT, Department of Animal Science, Texas Agricultural Experiment Station, Texas A&M University, College Station, *Chairman*

DON F. SPLITTSTOESSER, Department of Food Science and Technology, Agricultural Experiment Station, Cornell University, Geneva, New York, *Vice-Chairman*

DAVID H. ASHTON, Hunt-Wesson Foods, Fullerton, California

FRANK L. BRYAN, Centers for Disease Control, Atlanta, Georgia

DAVID L. COLLINS-THOMPSON, Department of Environmental Biology, Ontario Agricultural College, University of Guelph, Guelph, Ontario, Canada

EDWIN M. FOSTER, Food Research Institute, University of Wisconsin, Madison

JAMES J. JEZESKI, Department of Food Science and Nutrition, University of Florida, Gainesville

RICHARD V. LECHOWICH, Technical Center, General Foods, Tarrytown, New York

RUSSELL J. MARINO, Corporate Quality Assurance, Ralston Purina Company, St. Louis, Missouri

JOSEPH C. OLSON, JR., Sun City Center, Florida

JOHN H. SILLIKER, Silliker Laboratories, Carson, California

MARGARET R. STEWART, Blacksburg, Virginia, *Staff Officer*

Committee on Food Protection

DON F. SPLITTSTOESSER, Department of Food Science and Technology, Agricultural Experiment Station, Cornell University, Geneva, New York, *Chairman*

ANDREW G. EBERT, Pet, Inc., St. Louis, Missouri

FREDERICK J. FRANCIS, Department of Food Science and Nutrition, University of Massachusetts, Amherst

JESSE F. GREGORY, III, Department of Food Science and Human Nutrition, IFAS, University of Florida, Gainesville

ALBERT C. KOLBYE, The Nutrition Foundation, Inc., Washington, D.C.

DAVID R. LINEBACK, North Carolina State University, Department of Food Science, Raleigh, North Carolina

RUSSELL J. MARINO, Corporate Quality Assurance, Ralston Purina Company, St. Louis, Missouri iv

Foreword

Over the last 20 years interest in and controversy over the application of microbiological criteria to classify foods as either microbiologically acceptable or microbiologically unacceptable have grown steadily. A 1964 report of the National Research Council, *An Evaluation of Public Health Hazards from Microbiological Contamination of Foods* made some early recommendations toward establishment of meaningful microbiological criteria.

In recent years food industry groups at the national and international levels have expressed concern that microbiological criteria for foods established by regulatory agencies often were not based on sound principles and for some foods were set without justifiable rationale. Regulatory agencies charged with enforcement of laws and regulations on safety and quality of foods must evaluate a myriad of complex production, processing, and distribution practices and must frequently do so with limited staff and an extremely tight budget. Microbiological criteria often provide a definitive figure on which a decision to classify a food as being microbiologically acceptable or unacceptable can be based.

When microbiological criteria for foods are not based on definite needs, sound principles, and statistically solid background information, they may become a burden to the food industry, give a false sense of security to the public and lessen confidence in the ability of regulatory agencies to regulate the food supply.

Lack of sound guiding principles for the establishment of microbiological criteria has, at least in part, been responsible for the large number of standards and guidelines (particularly at the state and local level) that are impractical, unenforceable, and without uniformity.

For these reasons, the National Research Council through a subcommittee of the Food and Nutrition Board's Committee on Food Protection initiated in 1980 a study to formulate general principles for the consideration and application of microbiological criteria for foods and food ingredients and to provide recommendations for a unified, coordinated approach. The study was to include (1) definitions, purposes, priorities, and evaluation of methods for microbiological criteria; (2) recommendations for sampling plans, collection locations, and interpretation of analytical results; and (3) evaluation of existing or proposed international and federal programs.

The subcommittee has sought the advice and counsel of representatives of the sponsoring agencies: the Food and Drug Administration, the U.S. Department of Agriculture, the National Marine Fisheries Service, and the U.S. Army Natick Research and Development Center. Meetings were held with members of the Food and Nutrition Board's Industry Liaison Panel and representatives of the Centers for Disease Control, the Canadian Bureau of Microbiological Hazards, and 15 industry and public health groups. The subcommittee has benefited from the assistance and advice of many colleagues in industry, government, and academia. The contribution of all these groups is gratefully acknowledged.

In this book, the subcommittee has tried to set forth the principles for establishment of *meaningful* microbiological criteria. Recommendations are given on the need for microbiological criteria for 22 "commodity" groups. In addition, plans of action are presented for implementation of the Hazard Analysis Critical Control Point (HACCP) system and of microbiological criteria for foods and food ingredients.

Acknowledgments

The Subcommittee on Microbiological Criteria for Foods and Food Ingredients wishes to acknowledge the valuable assistance of the following individuals on the staffs of the contracting agencies:

E. Spencer Garrett, National Marine Fisheries Service of the Department of Commerce, Project Officer for the study

R. B. Read, Jr., J. David Clem, Howard J. Pippin, Barry Wentz, Robert Weik, Robert Sanders, and Garrett Higginbotham of the Food and Drug Administration of the Department of Health and Human Services

Ralph W. Johnston, T. R. Murtishaw, W. H. Dubbert, Gerald Parlett, Eddie F. Kimbrell, George Fry, and Richard Webber of the Department of Agriculture

Durwood B. Rowley, Edmund Powers, and Gerald Silverman of the U.S. Army Natick Research and Development Center of the Department of the Army

The subcommittee also wishes to acknowledge the assistance and advice of the following individuals in the development of its report:

O. Brian Allen, Department of Mathematics and Statistics, University of Guelph, Ontario, Canada

Bruce Brown, Health Protection Branch, Health & Welfare, Canada

D. S. Clark, Bureau of Microbiological Hazards, Health Protection Branch, Health & Welfare, Canada

Donald A. Corlett, Jr., Corporate Quality Assurance, Del Monte Corporation, San Francisco, California

F. A. Gardner, Department of Poultry Science, Texas A&M University, College Station

Keith A. Ito, National Food Processors Association, Concord, California

G. Jarvis, Health Protection Branch, Health and Welfare, Canada

D. C. Kilsby, Unilever Research Laboratory, Colworth House, Sharnbrook, Bedford, United Kingdom

R. Nickelson, II, Seafood Technology Section, Department of Animal Science, Texas A&M University, College Station

A. Peterson, Campbell Soup Company, Camden, New Jersey

H. Michael Wehr, Oregon State Department of Agriculture, Salem

Roy Widdus, Institute of Medicine, Washington, D.C.

Contents

An Evaluation of the Role of the Role of Microbiological Criteria for Foods and Food Ingredients

Executive
Summary

In September 1980 four federal agencies[1] requested that the National Research Council convene a panel of experts to formulate general principles for the application of microbiological criteria to food and food ingredients and to provide recommendations for a unified, coordinated appproach to the subject by policy-setting agencies. This report has been prepared by the Food and Nutrition Board Subcommittee on Microbiological Criteria in response to that request. The summary presented here follows the structure of the report:

I. Introduction (Chapter 1)
II. Basic Considerations
    A. Definitions, Purposes, and Needs for Microbiological Criteria (Chapter 2)
    B. Selection of Foods for Criteria Related to Safety (Chapter 3)
    C. Selection of Pathogens as Components of Microbiological Criteria (Chapter 4)
    D. Selection of Indicator Organisms and Agents as Components of Microbiological Criteria (Chapter 5)
    E. Consideration of Sampling Associated with a Criterion (Chapter 6)
    F. Consideration of Decision (Action) to be taken when a Criterion (Limit) is Exceeded (Chapter 7)

---

[1]The National Marine Fisheries Service (NMFS), the U.S. Department of Agriculture (USDA), the Food and Drug Administration (FDA), and the U.S. Army Natick Research and Development Center.

G. Current Status of Microbiological Criteria and Legislative Bases (Chapter 8)
III. Application of Microbiological Criteria to Foods and Food Ingredients (Chapter 9)
IV. Expansion of the HACCP System in Food Protection Programs (Chapter 10)
V. Plans of Action for Implementation of the HACCP System and of Microbiological Criteria for Foods and Food Ingredients (Chapter 11)

Summary responses to 13 specific contract items related to certain aspects of microbiological criteria are given in Appendix A.

INTRODUCTION

Microorganisms are always associated with harvested plants and slaughtered animals, the raw materials of the food industry. Except for foods that are heat processed to the degree that they are sterilized, microorganisms are usually associated with food products. Some of these microorganisms may cause spoilage, others may cause foodborne disease, and still others may bring about desirable changes as a result of growth in foods with which they are associated.

There are two broad categories of foods, i.e., those that are shelf-stable and those that are perishable. The factors responsible for the stability of shelf-stable products must be properly controlled. With perishable foods, processing and storage conditions must be controlled to achieve maximum shelf-life consistent with product safety. Approaches to assurance of control have varied. Among these have been (1) education and training, (2) inspection of facilities and operations, and (3) microbiological testing. The limitations of each are discussed in this report.

The subcommittee concluded that the Hazard Analysis Critical Control Point system (HACCP), first presented at the 1971 National Conference on Food Protection, provides a more specific and critical approach to the control of microbiological hazards in foods than that provided by traditional inspection and quality control approaches (see Chapters 1 and 10). The system consists of (1) identification and assessment of hazards associated with growing, harvesting, processing, marketing, preparation, and use of a given raw material or food product; (2) determination of critical control points to control any identifiable hazard; and (3) establishment of systems to monitor critical control points. Properly applied, the HACCP system separates the essential from the superfluous aspects of microbiological control by focusing attention on those points that directly affect safety and quality and by monitoring to determine whether or not these points are under control.

Monitoring may involve the application of microbiological testing, but more often physical and chemical tests as well as visual observations are used (see Chapter 10).

The HACCP system has been successfully applied to microbiological control of low-acid canned foods, in which case it is mandated by federal law. It is likewise employed by some food processors in the control of products other than low-acid canned foods. But the use of the HACCP system by the food industry is far from universal, despite its merits.

The HACCP system offers the food processor a rational approach to microbiological control. Of equal importance, the application of the HACCP system can lead to more effective and economical utilization of regulatory personnel as the inspector can focus attention on review of monitoring results. If these indicate satisfactory control over critical control points, the inspector has a high degree of assurance that the control of micro-biological hazards has been effective and can expend his efforts elsewhere. Chapter 10 presents the details of the HACCP system and the problems that must be solved if this system is to be embraced by the food industry and regulatory authorities.

BASIC CONSIDERATIONS

Standards, guidelines, and specifications are the terms used to identify the microbiological criteria that are discussed in this report (Chapter 2). A *standard* is part of a law or ordinance and is a mandatory criterion. A *guideline* is a criterion used to assess microbiological conditions during the processing, distribution, and marketing of foods. Guidelines are mandatory in that they signal when there are microbiological problems that require attention. A *specification* is used in purchase agreements between buyers and vendors of a food or ingredient. They may be mandatory or advisory.

The components of a microbiological criterion are described and some of the potential contributions of criteria to food safety and quality are discussed (Chapter 2). The report emphasizes that microbiological criteria should be established and implemented only when there is a need and when the criterion can be shown to be effective and practical. It was concluded that microbiological quality standards such as those recently proposed for seafoods by FDA should be reviewed and evaluated according to the plan proposed in Chapter 11.

There are a number of factors that will determine the foods for which criteria related to safety might be applied (Chapter 3). Of special importance is epidemiological evidence that the food in question is a significant vehicle of disease. Also important are various hazard considerations which include (1) susceptibility of the food to contamination by pathogens, (2) the opportunity for the survival of pathogens, (3) the likelihood of microbial growth during manufacture, storage, distribution, and preparation for serving, (4) whether or not the food is to be cooked prior to serving, and (5) the susceptibility of probable consumers to infectious agents or toxins.

Microorganisms suitable as components of microbiological criteria (standards, guidelines, specifications) have been placed in two categories—pathogens and indicator organisms. *Pathogens* (Chapter 4) suitable for this purpose are those likely to be found in a food or ingredient that thereby becomes a potential vehicle for transmission of the organism or its toxin to consumers. *Indicator organisms* (Chapter 5) are those whose presence in a food indicates (1) that a pathogen or its toxin of concern may be present, (2) that faulty practices occurred that may adversely affect safety or shelf-life of the product, or (3) that the food or ingredient is unsuited for an intended use.

Although the list of foodborne diseases and the microbial agents that cause them is long, only about 20 are known to be transmitted by foods with a consequence and/or frequency serious enough to cause concern. The discussion of each of these organisms[2] includes its relative importance, the status of the method(s) available for its detection and/or enumeration, and conclusions on the suitability of each to be a component of a microbiological criterion; with respect to the latter, specific recommendations have been made.

Indicator organisms and agents were evaluated relative to their use for the assessment of (1) numbers of microorganisms and/or microbial activity,[3] (2) potential human or fecal contamination or potential presence of

---

[2]For emphasis the pathogens have been grouped in three categories according to the severity of the hazard they present:

Severe hazards: *Clostridium botulinum*, *Shigella*, *Vibrio cholerae*, *Salmonella typhi*, *Salmonella paratyphi* A, *Salmonella paratyphi* B, *Salmonella paratyphi* C, *Salmonella sendai*, *Salmonella cholerae-suis*, *Brucella abortus*, *Brucella melitensis*, *Brucella suis*, *Mycobacterium bovis*, hepatitis A virus, fish and shellfish toxins, and certain mycotoxins.

Moderate hazards, potentially extensive spread: *Salmonella* (species other than those given above), pathogenic *Escherichia coli*, and *Streptococcus pyogenes*.

Moderate hazards, limited spread: *Staphylococcus aureus*, *Clostridium perfringens*, *Bacillus cereus*, *Vibrio parahaemolyticus*, *Coxiella burnetii*, *Yersinia enterocolitica*, *Campylobacter fetus* subsp. *jejuni*, *Trichinella spiralis*, and histamine.

[3]Aerobic plate count, thermoduric, psychrotrophic, thermophilic, proteolytic and lipolytic counts, the direct microscopic count, Howard mold count, rot fragment count, "machinery

pathogens,[4] and (3) post-heat processing contamination.[5] Each of these organisms, in addition to agents,[3,6] was discussed relative to its importance, its status and limitation of method of detection or enumeration, and its suitability as a part of a microbiological criterion.

It is recognized that the *sampling plan* and decision criteria are essential components of a microbiological criterion (Chapter 6). They should be based on sound statistical concepts. The International Commission on Microbiological Specifications for Foods (ICMSF) concept of relating the stringency of the sampling plan to the degree of hazard of the food was endorsed by the subcommittee as an effective means in the selection process. Whenever applicable, attributes sampling plans such as the ICMSF 2- and 3-class plans are recommended for microbiological criteria of foods and food ingredients in the United States.

The action taken when the limit of a criterion is exceeded relates to the purpose for which the criterion was established (Chapter 7). Actions that may be taken under the following circumstances are discussed: (1) evidence of existence of a direct health hazard, (2) evidence that a direct health hazard could develop, (3) indications that a product was not produced under conditions assuring safety, (4) indications that a raw material may adversely affect shelf-life, and (5) evidence that a critical control point is not under control.

Microbiological criteria are applied at the *international*, *federal*, and *state* or *local* levels (Chapter 8). The programs of the Joint FAO/WHO Codex Alimentarius Commission, the European Economic Community (EEC) and the ICMSF are described. The Canadian food standards also are discussed.

The role and activities of the Food and Drug Administration (FDA), the U.S. Department of Agriculture (USDA), the U.S. Army Natick Research and Development Center of the Department of Defense, and the National Marine Fisheries Service (NMFS) of the Department of Commerce relative to microbiological criteria for foods are outlined.

---

mold,'' yeast and mold count, heat-resistant molds, and thermophilic spore count. Examination for metabolic products such as by organoleptic examination, dye or indicator reduction time, pH, trimethylamine, total volatile nitrogen, indole, ethanol, diacetyl, histamine, endotoxins (*Limulus* amoebocyte lysate test), extract release volume, and adenosine triphosphate.

[4]Staphylococci, *Escherichia coli*, fecal coliforms, enterococci, and *Pseudomonas aeruginosa*.
[5]Coliform bacteria and *Enterobacteriaceae*.

[6]Thermonuclease and the use of U.V. light are discussed in a section on metabolic products of pathogens that indicate a potential health hazard. Included also is the application of the phosphatase test for milk and milk products.

APPLICATION OF MICROBIOLOGICAL
CRITERIA TO FOODS AND FOOD INGREDIENTS

Detailed information on the application of microbiological criteria to 22 groups of foods and food ingredients is given in Chapter 9.

Dairy Products

Microbiological criteria play an important role as part of overall quality assurance programs applied by both industry and regulatory authorities. Microbiological safety of dairy products can be assured only through (1) pasteurization or more severe heat treatments, (2) prevention of post-heat treatment contamination and, for certain products, (3) end-product testing for appropriate pathogens or toxins. Microbiological criteria for most dairy products are included as an integral part of documents that present in detail the FDA and USDA dairy products control programs. The subcommittee concluded that, with few exceptions, there appears to be no need for imposing more severe or additional criteria.

The *Salmonella* testing of dried milk as provided for in the USDA *Salmonella* Surveillance Program is a case in point. This program has been reviewed in this report, and deficiencies primarily in sampling plans (which directly affect the severity of criteria imposed) have been pointed out. Recommendations for correction of these deficiencies as well as strengthening of the program have been made.

Cheese is the other product for which greater attention to finished-product testing for a pathogen or its toxin is indicated. Of primary concern is *S. aureus*, especially its enterotoxins. The hazard is limited primarily to hard varieties, e.g., Cheddar and similar types and Swiss or Emmenthaler. This hazard has been discussed and suggestions have been made for more rigorous application of microbiological criteria in programs to control this hazard.

The continuous problem of the hazard of consuming raw milk and fresh cheese made from raw milk have been given particular attention. Outbreaks of milkborne disease caused by drinking raw milk purchased legally continue to occur in the United States with regularity. Brucellosis due to consumption of fresh cheese made from raw milk and enterocolitis caused by certain pathogenic strains of *E. coli* are of recent occurrence. A strong position has been taken pointing out that health professionals have a responsibility to encourage efforts to see that the public and policymakers are kept adequately informed so that public policy on raw milk and dairy products made from raw milk is compatible with scientific knowledge and protection of the public's health.

Raw Meats and Poultry

The causes and contributing factors of foodborne illness from meats and poultry have been thoroughly examined. The subcommittee could not establish a need for microbiological standards for pathogens in raw meat and poultry. Efforts to reduce foodborne illness caused by cooked meat and poultry should be directed to improved education, e.g., recognition of the potential presence of pathogens in raw animal foods and proper handling of raw and processed animal foods. In view of this need, renewed efforts to educate all persons that handle raw and processed animal foods of potential risks and proper food-handling practices are of the highest priority.

Factors relating to achieving optimum shelf-life of raw meat and poultry are discussed. These include processing and storage conditions. The application of microbiological guidelines to monitor these operations is indicated.

Present inspection practices of food-processing facilities by regulatory agencies need a more cost-effective approach by application of the HACCP system. Because the vast majority of foodborne disease is the direct result of mishandling of foods in food service operations and homes, the extent of regulatory inspection of food service operations is disproportionate compared with that of food-processing facilities. Therefore, emphasis of inspection should be directed more to those areas where mishandling of animal foods occurs more frequently, namely food service operations.

Fish, Molluscs, and Crustaceans

Measures to promote the safety and shelf-life of fish and shellfish are treated in this report. Although strict adherence to the recommendations of the National Shellfish Sanitation Program (NSSP) generally has resulted in the production of safe shellfish, there is need for more effective measures for monitoring the safety of these products, particularly with reference to the presence of viruses that may cause illness in humans.

Intoxication (ciguatera and scombroid and paralytic shellfish poisoning [PSP]) resulting from consumption of fish and shellfish is a major concern. The regulatory limits for histamine in tuna and PSP toxin in raw shellfish are recognized as useful in the control of these foodborne diseases. Relative to ciguatera there is a need for a simple reliable test to detect toxic fish.

The quality of raw fish can best be assured through application of the HACCP approach by sensory inspection of raw materials, proper temperature control, sanitation of equipment, and proper handling of product by employees.

There are conflicting reports about the botulism hazard of raw fish stored under refrigeration in vacuum packages or in modified atmospheres. Thus, this packaging-storage method is not recommended for raw fish at the present time—there is need for research to examine the safety of this practice.

Except for the NSSP criteria for shellfish, many of the microbiological criteria for fish and seafoods at the state or local level are not based on sound data or experience and are impractical from the standpoint of compliance or enforcement. These criteria need to be reexamined relative to the plans of action proposed in this report. It is recommended that the recently proposed FDA criteria for frozen crab cakes, frozen fish cakes, frozen fish sticks, and raw breaded shrimp be reviewed and evaluated according to the plan proposed in Chapter 11.

Processed Animal Products

Though such products as ground meat, poultry parts, and fish fillets are classified as processed, the safety and spoilage problems involved are the same as discussed above relative to raw animal products.

In the present context, processed animal products are foods that are produced through the application of various physical and/or chemical treatments to raw animal products. Such treatments as pasteurization, curing, salting, and acidulation (including fermentation) tend to destroy or otherwise control the development of the microorganisms that normally spoil the raw products. Likewise, to a greater or lesser extent, these treatments destroy or prevent the growth of foodborne disease agents.

These products vary considerably in their stability. Country cured hams and dry sausages may be stored for long periods at ambient temperatures without spoilage, whereas luncheon meats, cooked poultry, and smoked fish are highly perishable. Similarly, some of these products, if contaminated and subject to temperature abuse, readily support the growth of toxigenic organisms. Ham, for example, has historically been the most important cause of staphylococcal foodborne illness. Others such as dried meats, poultry, and fish will not support the growth of pathogens but may create hazards if abused after reconstitution with water.

The application of the HACCP system to the control of the safety and quality of these products is discussed. In many cases microbiological criteria play a role and where they apply they have been identified; but more often, physical and chemical measurements are the most effective means of monitoring critical control points.

Three products in this category have in recent years caused multiple outbreaks of foodborne illness, namely smoked fish (botulism), dry sausage (staphylococcal intoxication), and cooked roast beef (salmonellosis). Effective control measures are discussed.

Eggs and Egg Products

The regulation of eggs and egg products by the USDA in accordance with the Egg Products Inspection Act of 1970 is probably largely responsible for the dramatic decrease in egg-associated salmonellosis in recent years.

Microbiological criteria play no role in the control of shell egg quality. Defective shell eggs are essentially eliminated from commerce by sorting and candling.

Microbiological guidelines are useful in the monitoring of critical control points in the production of egg products, e.g., equipment sanitation and environmental monitoring. The pasteurizing step is more effectively monitored by observing time/temperature relationships. A microbiological standard is applied to finished egg products and is enforced by the USDA. Deficiencies in the sampling plans embodied in this criterion are discussed and appropriate changes are recommended.

Fruits and Vegetables

Raw fruits and vegetables as marketed may harbor large populations of viable microorganisms, but they have not presented a serious public health problem in the United States and consequently the application of microbiological criteria to these foods is not recommended.

In the processing of fruits and vegetables for canning, drying, and freezing, there are opportunities for microbial buildup on equipment and growth in the food. Guidelines that limit counts of microorganisms or utilize microscopic counts for molds are recommended as a means of monitoring critical control points and promoting good processing conditions.

Fruit Beverages

Because of their high acidity, fruit juice beverages have rarely been vehicles for foodborne pathogens. Guidelines that limit numbers of viable organisms or levels of metabolic products can be useful to monitor critical control points in the processing line. Specifications that restrict spore counts of heat-resistant molds are recommended as a means to minimize spoilage outbreaks of pasteurized fruit beverages.

Canned Foods

The production of low-acid, acid, and water activity-controlled canned foods is regulated by the FDA. Regulations governing this program are contained in the Code of Federal Regulations. These regulations embody the HACCP approach to the control of safety and quality. Canned products were the first foods to which the application of HACCP was mandated by regulation. The success of this program should serve as a model to other segments of the food industry.

Though finished-product microbiological criteria play no role in assuring the acceptability of finished products, guidelines are used in monitoring critical control points including equipment cleaning and sanitizing, microbial buildup during operations, and the microbiological quality of chill water. Further, specifications are applied to critical raw materials to assure that the level of heat-resistant sporeformers does not exceed acceptable limits.

Cereals and Cereal Products

The usefulness of criteria for grains, pasta products, and pastries was considered, as were public health problems associated with these foods. The presence of mycotoxins on grains, contamination of soy and pasta products with salmonellae, and the growth of *Staphylococcus aureus* in certain cream-filled pastries were identified as the major problems. The use of microbiological criteria in support of HACCP programs is recommended for these products.

Fats and Oils

Fats and oils in the presence of moisture and other essential nutrients are subject to degradation by a variety of microorganisms. Such a condition is provided by several processed foods in which fats and oils are major ingredients. Mayonnaise, salad dressings, peanut butter, margarine, and butter are of concern. For each of these products, the application of each or all of the three types of microbiological criteria is useful and in some instances essential to safety. For example, with respect to peanut butter routine testing of raw peanuts for aflatoxin and of the finished product for *Salmonella* is essential.

The characteristics of these products that relate to either microbial growth or inhibition of growth in them are discussed, as are significant sources of contamination with either spoilage organisms or pathogens. Applications of microbiological guidelines for monitoring critical control points of manufacture are described. The need for routine testing of peanut butter for *Salmonella* has been emphasized. The subcommittee recommends amending the standards of identity for mayonnaise and salad dressings to include a specific requirement for a pH of 4.1 or below in the aqueous phase of these products.

Sugar, Cocoa, Chocolate, and Confectioneries

The major microbiological concerns for these foods are the presence of bacterial spores and yeasts in sugar and of salmonellae in cocoa and chocolate. Specifications that limit thermophilic spores in sugar for canning; yeasts, molds, and mesophilic bacteria in sugar for bottled beverages; and osmophilic yeasts for confectionery products are appropriate. The ingredients of confectionery and similar ready-to-eat foods should be free of enteric pathogens, in particular salmonellae.

Spices

Microbiological concerns are governed by end use. Spices to be used as table condiments should be free of salmonellae. Spices containing high numbers of sporeforming bacteria may cause spoilage during the heat processing of certain luncheon meats; those containing thermophilic sporeformers may cause spoilage of canned foods. In these instances, spices as ingredients constitute a critical control point and are generally monitored via specifications. Ethylene oxide and irradiation treatments are appropriate control procedures when necessary.

Yeasts

Salmonellae in yeasts, especially in nutritional yeast that will be eaten without further heating, are a major concern. HACCP programs in the yeast industry must include routine testing for this pathogen. Microbiological guidelines are useful in the yeast industry for monitoring good manufacturing practices. Microbiological testing is also useful for the detection of contaminants that may cause spoilage of products containing yeasts, e.g., rope spores.

Formulated Foods

This broad category of products includes commercially prepared ready-to-cook or ready-to-eat foods containing ingredients from two or more food commodity categories. Beef and chicken potpies, the various packaged meals or "dinners," meat and seafood salads, pizzas, dried infant formulae, dry soup mixes, and cake mixes are only a few examples of the host of such products that are available to the public. It has been emphasized that no useful single microbiological criterion can be developed. Rather, the potential hazards of each product or group of products must be identified. Appropriate programs that embody the HACCP system including microbiological criteria (particularly guidelines as applied at critical control points in manufacture) must be individually designed if microbial growth and resulting hazard to health or of spoilage are to be prevented. Attention has been drawn to regulations of several states that specify a single criterion for all products within diverse groups such as salads. The deficiency of such criteria is presented.

Nuts

With the exception of coconut, the water activity of most nuts is sufficiently low to preclude bacterial growth. Because the growth of molds with the production of mycotoxins is a problem with peanuts and certain tree nuts, testing for these toxins should be part of a HACCP program. Nonsterile coconut should be free of salmonellae.

A standard for *E. coli* on tree nuts has been imposed by the FDA. The presence of this organism is interpreted as an indication of the presence of filth. The subcommittee is not aware of epidemiological evidence that suggests a relationship between the presence of *E. coli* and enteric pathogens in nuts.

Miscellaneous Additives

Gums, enzymes, and food colors are included in this category. There is little published information on their microbiology. Processors using these additives should apply various microbiological criteria, depending on end use, to assure the safety and quality of their products.

Bottled Water, Processing Water, and Ice

Bottled drinking water must be prepared from a safe source and must be processed, bottled, held, and transported under sanitary conditions. There is no epidemiological evidence to indicate that bottled drinking water sold in the United States offers a health hazard to the public. Therefore, there appears to be no need for additions to or modification of current standards. A periodic reassessment of practices in this rapidly expanding industry relative to the microbiological safety of bottled drinking water should be made.

Water and ice come in contact with or become a part of many foods during processing and storage and in food preparation. They have the potential of contributing spoilage bacteria and on occasion pathogens. The microbiological safety and quality of water and ice that come in contact with foods must be ensured.

Pet Foods

A major concern is that intermediate moisture and dry pet foods may harbor viable salmonellae and thus can be a vehicle for infection in the household of the pet owner. Microbiological control procedures by the processor should include (1) specifications that limit salmonellae in ingredients, e.g., rendered products, and (2) guidelines for monitoring critical control points in processing and in the plant environment.

EXPANSION OF THE HACCP SYSTEM IN FOOD PROTECTION PROGRAMS

Despite the successful application of HACCP in the control of the safety and quality of low-acid canned foods, this approach has not been universally adopted by either industry or regulatory agencies in the control of other foods (see Chapter 10).

The successful application of HACCP to low-acid canned foods can be attributed to several important factors: (1) industry and government, working cooperatively, identified critical control points and developed appropriate monitoring systems; (2) FDA required the training of key people involved in processing; (3) FDA inspectors were trained in the elements of HACCP, and plant inspections placed major emphasis upon review of monitoring results; and (4) the use of HACCP was mandated by federal regulation.

If the HACCP system is to be more broadly applied in the food industry, certain requirements must be met, including:

1. Technical expertise must be employed in applying the system to each food. This involves a careful analysis of hazards, the identification of critical control points and the establishment of effective monitoring systems.

2. Those responsible for regulation must be trained in the elements of HACCP and in this approach to inspectional activity.

3. Those responsible for food processing must be trained in the HACCP approach, as was done with key personnel in low-acid canned food plants.

4. The use of the HACCP system by all segments of the food industry relative to microbiological hazards should be mandatory.

Adversary attitudes and lack of cooperation between regulatory agencies and the food industry have presented a serious hindrance to the achievement of common goals of food safety and quality. These problems were largely overcome with the application of HACCP to low-acid canned foods. They continue to be a problem in other segments of the food industry.

A particularly sensitive issue relates to access to industry records. Industry recognizes that records of observations are needed for meaningful food protection, e.g., monitoring results from critical control points. But identification of which records are relevant for regulatory purposes is an issue of major disagreement. Much of the information in question may relate to manufacturing practices that may be proprietary. The regulator should have access to monitoring results at critical control points and the actions taken by the processor when limits are exceeded. The issue of access of records should be reviewed and resolved, as it is a serious impediment to expansion of the HACCP concept. Relative to HACCP, the subcommittee concluded that there should be no need for regulatory access to proprietary information having no relevance to food quality or safety.

PLANS OF ACTION

The subcommittee has proposed two plans of action that should be taken (Chapter 11). The first is a plan of action through which the use of the HACCP system could be applied universally in food protection programs of industry. The second is a plan for the implementation of microbiological criteria.

Recommendations

Specific recommendations developed on the basis of discussions in each of the chapters and sections of this book are summarized below.

INTRODUCTION (CHAPTER 1)

It is recommended that those who are concerned with the use of microbiological criteria take cognizance of the following:

1. With a few exceptions, i.e., canned products receiving a heat process sufficiently severe to render them sterile, microorganisms are associated with foods. Among these are microorganisms capable of causing spoilage, others capable of causing illness if they are not destroyed before the food is consumed, and still others that may produce illness-causing toxins if they multiply in a food before its consumption. In addition, the presence and growth of microorganisms may be associated with the production of some foods, and their presence in the product, sometimes in large numbers, is indicative of desired quality for these foods.

2. Foods may be segregated into two categories with respect to their stability, i.e., those that are shelf-stable and those that are perishable.

a. Shelf-stable foods are not necessarily sterile; in fact most of them are not. Their distinguishing characteristic is that some attribute or combination of attributes prevents the growth of microorganisms, e.g., pH, water activity (a_w), preservatives, etc. The microbiological spoilage of a food purported to be shelf-stable is an unexpected event that generally indicates improper processing (as for example underprocessing of canned foods) or improper handling (as for example the wetting of a dried product).

b. Perishable foods have a limited shelf-life and their microbio-

15

logical spoilage is an expected event. Generally speaking, perishable foods are selective environments. As a consequence the microbial flora that causes spoilage of such foods is characteristic. It follows, as a result, that the manifestations of spoilage of various perishable foods are likewise characteristic, and this constitutes a consumer safeguard.

3. Safety and ''microbiological quality,'' as measured by the numbers of microorganisms present in a food, are not necessarily directly related.

a. Shelf-stable foods may contain low numbers of microorganisms and yet present a health hazard. For example, nonfat dried milk may have a very low aerobic plate count (APC) and be free of coagulase-positive staphylococci, yet contain *Staphylococcus* enterotoxin. Chocolate candy may have a low APC, yet contain salmonellae. Roasted peanuts may be virtually free of microorganisms, yet contain dangerously high levels of mycotoxin.

b. A perishable food may have an exceedingly high APC yet not constitute a health hazard. As a corollary, a perishable food may have a low APC, yet constitute a health hazard.

DEFINITIONS, PURPOSES, AND NEEDS FOR MICROBIOLOGICAL CRITERIA (CHAPTER 2)

1. Microbiological standards should be considered only when:

a. there is evidence to indicate that a problem exists between a food and outbreaks of foodborne disease and that the standard will alleviate the problem;

b. exceeding the limits is evidence that the food contains decomposed ingredients, and/or is evidence of preparation, packaging, or storage of the food under grossly poor conditions; or

c. there is no jurisdiction over processing and distribution practices, such as with certain imported foods, and the standard would eliminate a health hazard and/or reject products produced under questionable conditions.

Wherever a product poses a direct hazard to health, an implied standard exists (see Chapter 1, page 52, note 3).

2. Microbiological guidelines should be used as alerting mechanisms to signal when microbiological conditions during processing, distribution, and marketing of foods are not within the normal range.

3. Purchase specifications should be based on relevant background data and should fill a need.

Microbiological quality standards, such as those recently proposed by the Food and Drug Administration (FDA) for certain frozen seafoods, are not recommended since they are not related to organoleptic quality and since guidelines can serve to monitor good manufacturing and distribution practices.

SELECTION OF FOODS FOR CRITERIA RELATED TO SAFETY (CHAPTER 3)

It is recommended that the following factors provide the primary bases for deciding whether a microbiological criterion for a given food would or would not serve a useful purpose: (1) epidemiological evidence that the food is a significant vehicle for the transmission of foodborne disease, (2) the susceptibility of the food to microbial contaminations, (3) the opportunities for survival of contaminants in the foods, (4) the likelihood that growth of contaminants would occur at some point during manufacture, storage, distribution, and under conditions preparatory to serving, (5) the treatment to which a food may be subjected just prior to its serving, and (6) the susceptibility of probable consumers to infectious or toxic agents.

SELECTION OF PATHOGENS AS COMPONENTS OF MICROBIOLOGICAL CRITERIA (CHAPTER 4)

A pathogen, to be eligible for consideration as a component of a microbiological criterion, must likely be found in a particular food or ingredient with a consequence serious enough to cause concern. Such a food is considered sensitive to the presence of the particular pathogen. Based on current information, the rationale for determining whether a pathogen or toxin of concern should be designated in a microbiological criterion for a food sensitive to it is given in Chapter 4 and provides the bases for the following recommendations:

Pathogens

Clostridium botulinum

1. *C. botulinum* should not be designated in microbiological criteria for application in the routine surveillance of sensitive foods.

2. In the course of epidemiological investigations of botulism outbreaks, suspect foods should be examined for the presence of *C. botulinum* and/or its toxins.

3. For assurance of the safety of low-acid and acidified low-acid canned foods from the botulism hazard, industry and official agencies should rely upon fail-safe mechanisms to be certain that control of heat processing,

pH, and a_w have been adequately accomplished and that container integrity has been maintained.

Shigella

1. Microbiological criteria for *Shigella* should not be established for routine surveillance of foods. Methods of analysis are too complicated and insensitive to be practical for this purpose, but they are useful in the course of epidemiological investigations of outbreaks to examine suspect foods for the presence of *Shigella*.

2. Presence of *Shigella* in foods that are not heated before consumption should cause the food to be rejected.

Vibrio cholerae

1. Microbiological criteria for *V. cholerae* should not be established for routine surveillance of foods.

2. Strict adherence to provisions of the National Shellfish Sanitation Program (NSSP) should be relied upon as the principal means of preventing raw oysters, mussels, and clams from becoming contaminated with *V. cholerae* and serving as vehicles for its transmission to consumers.

3. Adequate heat treatment of crabmeat before eating and use of good sanitary practices in handling crabmeat and other sensitive foods before and after heat treatment should prevail.

Brucella and Mycobacterium bovis

1. Prevention of milkborne brucellosis and tuberculosis is dependent upon pasteurization of milk supplies and adherence to the provisions of the state/federal brucellosis and tuberculosis eradication programs for cattle. As part of these programs serological tests are used to detect *Brucella* and *Mycobacterium bovis* infections in cattle. In this context, microbiological criteria for these organisms are feasible and should continue to be applied.

2. Suspect tuberculosis lesions found during carcass inspection at slaughter are routinely cultured for *Mycobacterium*. In this sense a microbiological criterion is feasible and should continue to be applied.

Viruses

1. Microbiological criteria for viruses in foods should not be established for routine surveillance of foods. At present methods of analysis are impractical for that purpose.

2. Laboratories capable of analyzing foods for viruses should be encouraged to examine suspect foods for them during the course of epidemiological investigations of suspected viral foodborne outbreaks.

Paralytic Shellfish Poison (PSP)

A microbiological standard for PSP is applied regularly to samples of shellfish from growing waters and in accordance with the National Shellfish Sanitation Program. Routine application of the standard to shellfish at wholesale and retail markets would not be an effective control measure and should not be used for this purpose.

Ciguatera Toxin(s)

There are no federal or state surveillance programs for preventing the occurrence of ciguatera fish poisoning other than some educational effort to emphasize the hazard of toxic fish due to the presence of this toxin(s). Until the factors responsible for toxic concentrations of the toxin(s) in fish are clarified and specific and practical assay methods for the toxin(s) become available, microbiological criteria would have no meaning and should not be established.

Mycotoxins

The FDA has set standards (tolerance levels) for aflatoxin B_1 and aflatoxin M_1 for sensitive foods. These criteria have been effective in preventing toxic foods from reaching the public and susceptible animals and should continue to be applied.

Salmonella

1. Microbiological criteria for *Salmonella* are commonly applied by industry and official agencies. They have been effective in preventing contaminated foods from reaching the market and should continue to be applied to sensitive foods and feeds.

2. FDA should be encouraged to abandon the bases currently used for establishing *Salmonella* sampling plans and to return to the system that was used prior to publication of the fourth edition of the Bacteriological Analytical Manual (BAM) (for further discussion refer to Appendix A-I).

Pathogenic Escherichia coli (PEC)

1. Procedures for detection and enumeration of pathogenic *E. coli* are at present not practical for use in routine food surveillance programs.

Microbiological criteria specifically for these *E. coli* biotypes would be impractical and should not be established for this purpose.

2. In the course of investigations of outbreaks, suspect foods should be examined for the presence of PEC. (see also Chapter 5.)

Streptococcus pyogenes

1. Because of the lack of a practical method for detection and enumeration of *S. pyogenes* in foods and the infrequency of foodborne outbreaks caused by this organism, a microbiological criterion would not be useful and should not be established.

2. Pasteurization of milk, adequate heating, and sanitary handling of sensitive foods should be relied upon for prevention of foodborne *S. pyogenes* infections.

Staphylococcus aureus

Microbiological criteria for *S. aureus* are feasible and should be established and applied to appropriate foods to indicate potential presence of enterotoxin or to indicate faulty sanitary and/or production practices.

Clostridium perfringens

1. The presence of low numbers of *C. perfringens* in many foods usually is unrelated to faulty sanitary practices. Only large numbers in a food would be cause for concern. Microbiological criteria for use in routine surveillance programs would not contribute significantly to prevention of outbreaks of *C. perfringens* enteritis and should not be established for that purpose.

2. Suspect foods from outbreaks should be examined for this organism.

3. When temperature abuse of sensitive foods has occurred or is suspected, analysis for presence of alpha toxin (indicator of extensive growth of *C. perfringens*) should be made. In this sense a microbiological criterion for alpha toxin is useful.

Bacillus cereus

1. During investigation of outbreaks in which symptoms observed are similar to those of *C. perfringens* or *S. aureus*, the suspect foods should also be examined for *B. cereus*.

2. Low numbers of *B. cereus* are found in many foods, but only large numbers are cause for concern. It is unlikely that microbiological criteria

for purposes of routine surveillance of foods would be justified. At present, criteria for that purpose should not be established.

Vibrio parahaemolyticus

1. Microbiological criteria for use in routine surveillance of seafoods are not practical at this time and should not be established.
2. Methods for identifying and enumerating pathogenic strains are sufficient for examination of seafoods or seafood products that may be implicated in outbreaks. Examination of such foods for V. parahaemolyticus always should be made.

Coxiella burnetii

Routine use of the agglutination test for the presence of C. burnetii in milk supplies available to the public would not be useful in preventing C. burnetii infections in man and should not be used for this purpose.

Histamine

The practice of much of the fisheries industry to examine routinely susceptible fish for histamine content should be expanded to all of the industry as a means of preventing deteriorated and/or toxic fish from reaching consumers.

Yersinia enterocolitica

Owing to the low incidence of outbreaks caused by Y. enterocolitica and the complexities of quantitative recovery methods for pathogenic strains, microbiological criteria for this organism would be of little value in routine surveillance programs and therefore should not be established until changes in this situation indicate otherwise.

Campylobacter fetus subsp. jejuni

Microbiological criteria for routine application to foods would not be a significant preventive measure for foodborne campylobacteriosis and should not be established at present.

Trichinella spiralis

In view of the procedures specified by USDA for, and the almost universal practice of, cooking raw pork, routine examination of meat for larvae to control trichinellosis is not recommended.

General Actions

Research

Methods should be developed for more rapid detection and quantitative enumeration of those bacterial pathogens and of those viruses, toxic substances, and parasites that are significant causes of foodborne illness. Federal agencies concerned with control of food safety and quality should provide financial support that will foster increased research on microbiological methods for the examination of food.

Morbidity and Mortality Weekly Reports

The benefits derived from the reporting of foodborne disease outbreaks to the Centers for Disease Control (CDC) are many. One of these benefits has been the wide distribution, without cost to the recipient, of reports of these reported outbreaks through CDC's weekly morbidity and mortality reports. By this means personnel of industry, regulatory agencies, universities, and other organizations were kept abreast of the occurrence of outbreaks, the causes of these outbreaks, and often the control measures that were instituted. These reports played a significant role in drawing attention to the ever-present problem of foodborne illness and the need for preventive measures. Accordingly, the CDC should reconsider its decision to curtail free distribution of the *Morbidity and Mortality Weekly Report*.

SELECTION OF INDICATOR ORGANISMS AND AGENTS AS COMPONENTS OF MICROBIOLOGICAL CRITERIA (CHAPTER 5)

Aerobic Plate Count

Because generalizations of the relationship between APCs and sensory quality of foods are not possible and little direct relationship exists between APCs and safety, APCs generally should not be specified in microbiological criteria for these purposes. They can, however, indicate microbial survival of processes or growth at critical control points.

Direct Microscopic Count

Because of the inherent characteristics of the method, microbiological criteria involving direct microscopic count limits should be restricted to those situations where high microbial populations (viable, nonviable, or both) are expected and where information on the microbial history of the food (such as dried milk or eggs) may be useful.

Microscopic Mold Counts

The use of these microscopic mold counts (Howard mold count, rot fragment count) as components of microbiological criteria to detect introduction of decayed tissue of fruits and vegetables into processed product and as an index of manufacturing practices should be continued but re-evaluated in terms of the effect of certain processing practices.

Machinery Mold

Although *Geotrichum candidum* has been used to evaluate sanitation in fruit and vegetable processing plants, additional studies are recommended to relate filament counts to modern processing practices.

Yeast and Mold Counts

Application of yeast and mold counts is often related to special conditions in a food such as low pH and/or low a_w, which are not conducive for bacterial growth but in which many fungi are capable of proliferating. Microbiological criteria for yeasts and molds are useful under such conditions and should be applied to sensitive foods, e.g., sugars, fruit beverages, and soft drinks.

Heat-Resistant Molds

Limits for heat-resistant molds such as *Byssochlamys fulva* and *Aspergillus fisheri* are applicable primarily to thermally processed fruits and fruit juices. Microbiological guidelines for application by industry should be encouraged.

Thermophilic Spore Count

Thermophilic spore counts have been applied extensively in industry for ingredients such as sugars, starches, flour, spices, and cocoa. Their use as components of microbiological criteria for food ingredients to be used in low-acid canned foods should be continued.

Dye or Indicator Reduction Time

Technological advances in the sanitary production of raw milk have outstripped the usefulness of dye reduction tests for grading this product. More sensitive methods are available and use of dye reduction tests should be discouraged. Dye reduction tests have little merit for the evaluation of other foods such as meat, fish, poultry, vegetables and fruits.

pH

Measurements of pH are important to monitor acid production at critical control points in the processing of appropriate foods, particularly dry and semidry fermented sausages, fermented milks, and cheese, and to determine equilibrium pH of acidified canned foods, mayonnaise, and salad dressings.

Trimethylamine and Total Volatile Nitrogen (TMA and TVN)

Although TMA and/or TVN values are often closely related to microbial degradation of certain species of fish, their use for detection of spoilage is subject to severe limitations. At present they should not be used in regulatory criteria for seafoods in the United States. Research should be encouraged to evaluate relationships among these parameters and microbiological deterioration and sensory characteristics of economically important fish species in the United States.

Indole

The indole content is a useful index to detect certain types of microbial decomposition that occurred in imported canned/cooked frozen shrimp prior to heating. The indole level is also a useful index to evaluate the acceptability of imported frozen raw shrimp, provided that it is not used as the sole indicator. In this case it should be of value to assess prior temperature abuse when used in conjunction with other quality tests such as organoleptic examination.

Ethanol

Current information indicates that the ethanol content of salmon may serve as a useful index of microbial decomposition and therefore may have useful application as a component of a criterion to evaluate acceptability. Continued research should be encouraged to further evaluate this relationship.

Diacetyl

The diacetyl content should be applicable as a parameter to monitor the sanitary condition of fruit processing.

Histamine

The histamine content should be applied as part of a microbiological criterion for scombroid fish. The Association of Official Analytical Chemists (AOAC) fluorometric method should be applied where sophisticated laboratory equipment and technicians are available. If collaborative tests indicate that a recently developed rapid screening test has satisfactory sensitivity, it should become a valuable tool to monitor incoming scombroid fish.

LLT and ATP

Although tests such as the *Limulus* amoebocyte lysate test (LLT) and the test for adenosine triphosphate (ATP) are not yet developed where they can be used routinely in the microbiological evaluation of foods, further research on these and other rapid tests is recommended.

Staphylococci

S. aureus counts are applicable as a component of microbiological criteria to indicate the potential presence of enterotoxin and lack of sanitary handling of sensitive foods. The AOAC MPN method should be replaced by the direct plating method because the former is inhibitory to injured cells and offers no advantage with respect to method sensitivity.

Escherichia coli

E. coli is the best indicator of fecal contamination presently available. Microbiological criteria involving *E. coli* should be applied to sensitive foods as indicators of fecal contamination. In the interest of more rapid and sensitive detection and enumeration of *E. coli*, the direct plating method (see *E. coli* section in text) should be further evaluated for application to a broad spectrum of foods.

Fecal Coliforms

A fecal coliform standard is currently used to evaluate the sanitary condition of shellfish growing waters. Its use has been successful and should be continued. However, since the best indicator of fecal contamination is *E. coli*, the direct plating method should be further evaluated for use in this program.

Enterococci

The significance, accuracy, and precision of the methodology is limited and is poorly correlated with safety or sanitary quality characteristics of foods. Therefore microbiological criteria for enterococci should not be applied.

Pseudomonas aeruginosa

The value of *P. aeruginosa* as an index of safety of bottled water should be further evaluated and accurate methods for the detection and enumeration of this organism should be developed.

Coliform Bacteria

Coliform counts are applicable in microbiological criteria for many foods to indicate post-heat processing contamination. However, *E. coli* or a fecal connotation of *E. coli* should not be linked categorically to any food in which coliforms are found.

Enterobacteriaceae

Enterobacteriaceae counts and coliform counts are generally used for the same purpose. The former has not been used to any appreciable extent in the United States, although it is commonly used in Europe. Because the advantages of the *Enterobacteriaceae* count over the coliform count are not substantial, the latter should be the method of choice for use in microbiological criteria in the United States.

Thermonuclease Test (TNase)

The TNase test should be applicable in microbiological criteria for the purpose of screening foods such as certain cheeses and sausages for extensive growth of *S. aureus* and presence of enterotoxin(s).

Aflatoxin Detection by Ultraviolet Light

The use of ultraviolet light as a screening test for detection of aflatoxin in moldy corn and other grains has been successful and should be continued.

Phosphatase Test

Although limited in application, this test is useful in criteria for certain milk and milk products to detect underpasteurization. Its use in the dairy industry should be continued and expanded.

CONSIDERATIONS OF SAMPLING ASSOCIATED WITH A CRITERION (CHAPTER 6)

1. The sampling procedure and decision criteria are essential parts of a microbiological criterion and should be based on sound statistical concepts.

2. The concept of relating the stringency of a sampling plan to the degree of hazard of the food is a meaningful way of making such a selection.

3. Where attributes sampling plans are applicable, the ICMSF 2- and 3-class plans are recommended for microbiological criteria for foods.

4. Further studies are recommended to evaluate the applicability of variables sampling plans to microbiological criteria for foods.

CONSIDERATION OF DECISION (ACTION) TO BE TAKEN WHEN A CRITERION (LIMIT) IS EXCEEDED (CHAPTER 7)

Assuming that microbiological criteria have been established in accordance with the principles set forth in Chapter 2, it is recommended that individuals responsible for the decision-making process take cognizance of the following:

1. When the limit of a criterion (whether it be a standard, a guideline, or a specification) is exceeded, it should trigger action on the part of the responsible authority. The nature of the action depends upon the purpose for which the criterion was established, but if the criterion was established according to the principles set forth in Chapter 2, then failure to meet the established limits set by it should signal decisive action.

2. If analytical results indicate a direct health hazard, it must be decided if the product should be destroyed or if it can be diverted to some use that obviates the hazard.

3. If analytical results indicate the potential for the development of a direct health hazard if the product is mishandled, it must be determined whether or not the product can be diverted into channels where its safe handling can be assured and thus the potential for developing a hazard obviated.

4. If analytical results indicate that the product was not produced under conditions assuring safety, the action taken should vary with the product so as to obviate any potential hazard.

5. If analytical results indicate a raw material may adversely affect the shelf-life of a finished product, the processor must determine whether or not to use the raw material.

6. If an analytical result indicates that a critical control point is not under control, this should trigger immediate action by the food processor.

CURRENT STATUS OF MICROBIOLOGICAL CRITERIA AND LEGISLATIVE BASES (CHAPTER 8)

This chapter is a status report; therefore, recommendations are not appropriate.

APPLICATION OF MICROBIOLOGICAL CRITERIA TO FOODS AND FOOD INGREDIENTS (CHAPTER 9)

Dairy Products

1. The U.S. Department of Agriculture (USDA) should consider amending its recommended bacterial count standard for Grade 2 milk for manufacturing purposes to more adequately reflect use of good sanitary and other handling practices during production, transportation, and storage of raw milk before processing.

2. The current USDA program for *Salmonella* surveillance of domestically produced dried milk products should be strengthened by (a) collecting samples at least monthly rather than quarterly, (b) using sampling plans consistent with recommendations of the NAS/NRC *Salmonella* report, and (c) drawing samples at the time of successive surveys from each dryer located in a plant having more than one dryer rather than from only one as is the current practice.

3. The current practice of most of the dried milk industry to test products for *Salmonella* should be applied by all manufacturers of dried milk, dried cheese, and dried blends composed principally of dairy products. Such

testing should be appropriately monitored through cooperative effort of federal and state regulatory agencies.

4. Programs for *Salmonella* surveillance of dried milk products offered at import should be continued. These programs should be reviewed periodically to ascertain that sampling plans, including methods used, are consistent with the hazards presented and in accord with current developments in methodology and with appropriate statistical concepts.

5. Manufacturers of cheese varieties susceptible to the development of large numbers of *Staphylococcus* should be encouraged to (a) routinely monitor critical control points for presence or indications of staphylococcal growth, and (b) test all such finished cheese for *S. aureus* or thermonuclease or both if abnormal lactic culture activity occurred during manufacture or if other indications of conditions that might lead to extensive staphylococcal growth were encountered.

6. Routine testing of domestically produced cheese by regulatory agencies is not recommended; however, industry testing programs should be monitored by these agencies.

7. FDA should routinely test all susceptible cheese varieties offered at import for presence of thermonuclease. Positive lots should be rejected.

8. FDA should undertake jointly with the French government and industry a comprehensive study of the problems of pathogenic *E. coli* in imported soft cheese with the objective of further reducing the hazard of pathogenic *E. coli* in susceptible varieties. The work should include analytical surveys of cheese offered at import as well as studies at point of production.

9. Regulatory agencies, industry, university extension departments, and other organizations concerned with the public health should (a) more actively emphasize that pasteurization is an essential process in providing milk free of disease-causing microorganisms, (b) cooperatively develop and apply with renewed vigor programs that will discourage consumption of raw milk, and (c) aggressively work toward development of legislation that will declare the sale of raw milk illegal in the United States.

10. The ability of *S. aureus* to grow in whipped butter has been demonstrated. Regulatory agencies should encourage manufacturers of whipped butter to routinely apply in-plant guidelines for the APC and *S. aureus* at critical control points of manufacture.

11. Whey cream as an ingredient in butter manufacture (or any formulated product) should be tested for staphylococcal thermonuclease before use; product showing a positive test should either not be used or be further tested to confirm presence or absence of staphylococcal enterotoxins.

Raw Meats

1. To produce raw red meat with optimum shelf-life, critical control points such as slaughtering-dressing practices, sanitary condition of equipment and utensils, and control of refrigeration temperature should be monitored carefully. Microbiological guidelines are applicable to monitor some of these critical control points.

2. To achieve optimum shelf-life of raw meats, the HACCP concept should be extended to include retail outlets, food service establishments, and homes, particularly as it pertains to handling practices and maintenance of adequate refrigeration.

3. Microbiological standards for raw meats are not recommended since they will prevent neither spoilage nor foodborne illness.

4. Microbiological criteria containing limits for pathogens in raw meats are not recommended.

5. To reduce the health hazards from raw meats the following should prevail:

    a. recognition that small numbers of pathogens may be present on raw meats;

    b. strict adherence to good food preparation practices;

    c. application of new or alternate production and processing practices that reduce the incidence of pathogens;

    d. more effective education on food-handling practices of food plant personnel, food service operators, and homemakers;

    e. increased emphasis on inspection of food service establishments using the HACCP approach.

6. Present inspections of food-processing facilities and operations by regulatory agencies such as the USDA should be made more cost-effective by application of the HACCP concept.

Processed Meats

1. Microbiological guidelines for raw ground beef and for perishable raw salted and salted cured meat should be applied at the processing level to assess the microbiological condition of the raw materials used, the effectiveness of equipment sanitation and the microbiological condition of the freshly processed product. Application of microbiological criteria to these products after they have entered trade channels is of little value.

2. The processor should apply microbiological criteria for *Salmonella* in evaluating cooked roast beef at the processing facility before it is shipped to distribution channels.

3. Microbiological control of shelf-stable raw salted and salted cured meats should be exercised by control of critical control points such as

temperature during curing and humidity during the postcuring drying period.

4. In the processing and handling of cooked cured meats, microbiological guidelines should be applied to evaluate the quality of raw materials, equipment sanitation, and condition of finished product. Microbiological criteria for products that have entered retail channels are inappropriate.

5. Application of criteria involving *S. aureus*, thermonuclease, and/or enterotoxin should be applied to ascertain that proper acid formation during production of fermented sausages has taken place.

6. Microbiological guidelines (APC) should be applied to dried meats as a means of assuring the adequacy of moisture control during the drying process. Criteria for pathogens should be appropriately applied depending upon the ultimate use of the product.

Raw (Eviscerated, Ready-To-Cook) Poultry

Recommendations regarding raw poultry are focused on two objectives, namely to reduce the risk of association of poultry, directly or indirectly, with foodborne disease and to produce a product with optimum quality characteristics and shelf-life.

1. A HACCP system tailored to the specific processing conditions and careful monitoring of critical control points such as sanitary condition of equipment, employee practices, carcass washing, cooling, and storage procedures should be applied to obtain optimum quality characteristics and shelf-life of freshly processed carcasses and to keep the number of pathogens at the lowest possible level.

2. Microbiological guidelines that are part of such HACCP programs should include (a) periodic evaluation of equipment surfaces to check cleaning and sanitation procedures, and (b) evaluation of processing practices by examination (aerobic plate count and coliforms) of freshly processed carcasses.

3. To increase shelf-life of refrigerated poultry, refrigerated storage in vacuum packages or in modified gaseous atmospheres is being considered. Research directed toward determination of the effect of these practices on safety and shelf-life of raw poultry should be intensified.

4. Until infection and contamination of birds on the farm are reduced effectively and/or until a method of decontamination is routinely applied to packaged carcasses, microbiological criteria for raw poultry with limits for pathogens, e.g., *Salmonella*, are considered impractical and should not be applied.

5. Recommendations for the reduction or eradication of *Salmonella* in

raw poultry given in this report (Chapter 9, part D) and in the NRC report on the *Salmonella* problem are considered of the highest priority in efforts to reduce the health hazard from consumption of cooked poultry.

6. Because raw poultry may contain pathogens, food service personnel and homemakers should adhere strictly to good food-handling and preparation practices.

7. Additional studies are recommended to evaluate the role of newly emerging pathogens associated with poultry such as *C. fetus* subsp. *jejuni*, including practical methods for detection, enumeration, and control of these organisms.

Processed Poultry Products

1. To obtain safety and optimum shelf-life of processed poultry, a HACCP system should be developed for each group of products.

2. Shelf-life and quality characteristics of refrigerated tray-pack products should be controlled by monitoring critical control points such as the microbiological condition of carcasses used, sanitary handling of the product during cut-up operations, sanitary condition of equipment, and time-temperature profile of product during processing and storage. Microbiological guidelines involving APC (swab, rinse, or other simple procedures) should be applied at critical control points to evaluate the sanitary condition of poultry carcasses and processing equipment.

3. To obtain safe ready-to-eat poultry, strict adherence to recommended food-handling and preparation practices such as proper cooking, chilling, refrigerated storage, hot-holding, reheating, and avoidance of cross-contamination should be continually emphasized.

4. Safety and shelf-life of perishable cooked further-processed poultry products should be controlled by careful monitoring of critical control points such as microbiological condition of the carcasses, deboning and trimming operations, sanitary condition of equipment, product flow, time-temperature profile during processing, cooking, chilling, slicing, packaging, and storage conditions. Microbiological guidelines should be applied for:

   a. carcasses (APC), particularly if they were from other sources;

   b. checking sanitary condition of equipment (APC by swab, direct contact, or other simple methods) particularly in areas where cooked products are handled;

   c. packaged products (APC, *S. aureus,* coliforms, *Salmonella).*

5. Studies are recommended to improve the design and layout of processing equipment and handling operations to reduce opportunity for post-heat contamination of cooked products.

6. Poultry potpies, particularly heated pies, should not be subjected to temperature abuse; otherwise they may become a health hazard (botulism, *C. perfringens* enteritis). Microbiological criteria, however, should not be used to monitor temperature abuse of potpies.

Eggs and Egg Products

1. It is recommended that the USDA adopt the sampling plans suggested by the National Research Council Committee on *Salmonella* (NRC, *An Evaluation of the* Salmonella *Problem,* 1969). Depending upon the ultimate use of the product, egg products should be classified as Category I or Category II products.

2. The sampling plans utilized by the USDA for confirmation and surveillance are even less stringent than those employed for certification. It is recommended that in connection with these programs Category I or Category II sampling plans be utilized.

3. The USDA provides for retesting of lots found positive for *Salmonella*, though plants with known *Salmonella* problems are not permitted to resample. It is recommended that the practice be reviewed in terms of the "resampling syndrome" discussed in Chapter 6.

4. It is recommended that the sampling frequency, as required by the USDA (see Figure 9-2, Chapter 9, part F), be critically reviewed.

5. The USDA instructions (see Chapter 9, part F) state that no rigid or set sampling pattern is to be followed in connection with surveillance sampling. It is recommended that this "random approach" to sampling be reviewed in terms of its consistency with the principles of statistical quality control.

Fish, Molluscs, and Crustaceans

1. Microbiological standards (National Shellfish Sanitation Program) for shellfish growing waters and for raw shellfish should be updated as new information becomes available on more effective test procedures to monitor contamination of growing waters and shellfish. This is particularly true with respect to the presence of viruses in waters and shellfish that can cause human illness.

2. Since rapid, direct plating methods have recently become available to test water and shellfish directly for *E. coli*, the use of *E. coli* instead of coliforms or fecal coliforms as part of microbiological criteria for shellfish and shellfish growing waters should be evaluated.

3. Regulatory agencies and industry should direct efforts to determine the potential hazards of packaging raw seafoods and holding them under

refrigeration in vacuum or in modified gaseous atmospheres specifically relative to opportunities for growth and toxin production by *C. botulinum*. This packaging/storage method is not recommended for raw seafoods until the safety of this practice is validated.

4. Additional research efforts are recommended to evaluate the significance of *Vibrio* species associated with diseases in humans, specifically to:

a. detect and enumerate more effectively pathogenic strains of *V. parahaemolyticus*;

b. determine the distribution of *V. cholerae* (O1 and non-O1) in seafoods and the effect of processing, storage, and food preparation practices on survival and/or growth of these species;

c. evaluate the potential hazards of *V. mimicus, V. fluvialis, V. fulnificus,* and *V. hollisae* in raw and processed seafoods.

5. Scombroid poisoning, ciguatera, and paralytic shellfish poisoning (PSP) are prominent foodborne diseases associated with the consumption of fish and shellfish. Although knowledge about these diseases has increased greatly in recent years, increased research effort should be directed to the nature of the toxins, toxicity levels to humans and test methods, particularly practical methods, to detect and quantitate toxins in fish and shellfish.

6. Application of HACCP systems is recommended to assure safety and wholesomeness of fish and fishery products. Within this system, microbiological guidelines should be implemented whenever needed to monitor critical control points. For fresh raw products, monitoring of critical control points should consist primarily of inspection of incoming materials for odor and appearance, control of temperature (refrigeration or freezing), equipment sanitation, and employee handling. Additional concerns that should be considered include: for mulluscan shellfish, the fecal coliform count of growing waters and of the wholesale product and the presence and levels of saxitoxin and related toxins; for processed tuna, the level of histamine.

For cooked ready-to-eat products, microbiological guidelines for finished products that include APC, *E. coli*, and *S. aureus* should be implemented.

7. Microbiological criteria for fish set by state and local regulatory agencies are generally not based on sound background data and are impractical from the standpoint of compliance or enforcement. In those instances where there is a need for a microbiological criterion, it should be developed from properly designed and executed studies.

8. Microbiological quality standards recommended by FDA for frozen

crab cakes, frozen fish cakes, and frozen fish sticks should not be accepted by state and local regulatory agencies as standards since these products constitute neither a health hazard nor a serious quality problem.

Fruits and Vegetables

1. Microbiological standards are not recommended for raw and processed fruits and vegetables. In general these foods have had an excellent public health record, and in most instances where they have been the vehicle for foodborne illnesses, standards would not have prevented the problem.

2. It is recommended that guidelines, based on sound data, be used for assessing manufacturing practices in the processing of dried and frozen fruits and vegetables. Where appropriate, aerobic plate counts should be used for evaluating low-acid vegetables while fruits should be cultured for aciduric microorganisms such as yeasts and lactic acid bacteria. There is little evidence that routine tests for coliforms serve any useful purpose. They usually are a part of the normal processing-line microflora. The routine testing for foodborne pathogenic bacteria is not recommended since most samples would be negative for infectious organisms and would yield only low populations of toxigenic species.

3. Microscopic mold counts (Howard, rot fragment, and *G. candidum*) can be useful for assessing the wholesomeness of raw fruits and vegetables and the sanitary status of cannery lines. However, additional research to relate modern processing conditions to the levels of filaments is recommended.

Fruit Beverages

1. Microbiological standards are not recommended for fruit juice beverages since they have rarely been responsible for foodborne illnesses.

2. The use of guidelines is recommended for assessing Good Manufacturing Practices and the quality of the original fruit. The subcommittee recommends culturing for aciduric microorganisms, or testing for microbial metabolic products such as diacetyl in citrus juices and patulin in apple juice, where applicable.

3. Limits for heat-resistant mold spores serve a useful purpose in purchase specifications for ingredients that are to be used in pasteurized fruit drinks. Limits for yeasts, molds, and aciduric bacteria are recommended when the ingredients are to be used in products that depend upon preservatives for their stability.

Canned Foods: Low-Acid, Acid, and Water Activity Controlled

In the United States, thermally processed foods commercially packaged in hermetically sealed containers have an excellent health record. Control of safety and stability of these foods is best accomplished by monitoring a series of critical control points by physical and chemical control tests. These measures, embodied in federal regulations, should be continued and strengthened when necessary.

Cereals and Cereal Products

1. Microbiological standards for cereal grains and most milled products are not recommended because these commodities are not common causes of foodborne illnesses. Cereal products to be used as ingredients in dry-blended or formulated foods that might not receive adequate cooking should be free of infectious pathogens. The current standards for aflatoxins, on the other hand, are appropriate and it is possible that limits for other mycotoxins may be needed as new problems become apparent.

2. Soy products that do not receive a terminal heat process should be examined for salmonellae since these foods are susceptible to contamination by this pathogen.

3. Microbiological guidelines for cereal grains and their milled products generally are not recommended because these foods are raw agricultural products that present little opportunity for microbial growth during their processing.

4. The continued use of specifications that limit the incidence of thermophilic spores in cereal products to be used in canning is recommended.

5. Dried pasta products may be contaminated at times with salmonellae and manufacturers should routinely test for this organism.

6. Although cream- and custard-filled pastries have been implicated in numerous disease outbreaks, usually due to staphylococci, standards are not recommended for these foods. Prevention is better achieved by observing Good Manufacturing Practices and proper refrigeration during marketing.

Fats and Oils

Peanut Butter

1. Peanut butter manufacturers should be encouraged to provide for complete separation between raw peanuts and the peanut butter processing areas.

2. Use of water for cleaning and sanitizing should be avoided if possible.

3. A microbiological standard for *Salmonella* in peanut butter is appropriate.

Salad Dressings and Mayonnaise

The microbiological safety of these products relates directly to the pH (4.1 or below) and the acetic acid content of the moisture phase. The federal standards of identity for mayonnaise and for salad dressing do not specify a pH level for either of these products. Also, no specific concentration of acetic acid is specified for salad dressing.

The FDA should consider amending the standard of identity for mayonnaise to include a specified pH level of 4.1 or below and amending the standard of identity for salad dressings to include both a specified pH level of 4.1 or below and an acidity of not less than 2.5% calculated as acetic acid.

Sugar, Cocoa, Chocolate, and Confectioneries

1. Microbiological specifications now applied to sugar used as an ingredient in low-acid canned foods (thermophilic spores), beverages (mesophilic bacteria, yeasts, and molds), and confectioneries (osmophilic yeasts) should be continued.

2. Microbiological specifications for thermophilic spores should be applied for cocoa to be used in retorted products.

3. The *Salmonella* hazard in cocoa and chocolate manufacture should be controlled by testing raw materials, finished products, and environmental samples for *Salmonella*, preferably as part of a HACCP program.

4. In the manufacture of confectionery products, microbiological criteria should be applicable to sensitive ingredients. Guidelines and specifications for osmophilic yeasts should be applicable for sweeteners. Ingredients such as cocoa, coconut, dried milk, and eggs should be examined for *Salmonella*. Nuts should be tested for aflatoxins.

Spices

1. Microbiological criteria for spices should be closely related to their end use. For spices to be used in foods that receive no further heat treatment the criterion should be focused on absence of infectious pathogens such as *Salmonella*. For spices to be used in low-acid canned food, limits on thermophilic spores should be included. When used as an ingredient in

cooked cured meats, the emphasis should be on control of aerobic spore-formers.

2. Where appropriate, reduction of the intrinsic microflora of spices by treatment such as approved gaseous "sterilants" and by irradiation is recommended.

Yeasts

1. The continued routine testing for salmonellae in yeast products is recommended since they are at times prone to contamination by this pathogen.

2. The establishment of guidelines for nonpathogenic bacteria, wild yeasts, and molds is encouraged to assess Good Manufacturing Practices.

Formulated Foods

1. Because of the diversity and different characteristics of the various formulated foods, no single microbiological criterion is appropriate for these foods.

2. Potential hazards of each type of formulated food should be identified. Appropriate programs that embody the HACCP system including microbiological criteria (particularly guidelines as applied at critical control points) should be individually designed for each type of formulated food.

Nuts

1. Coconut should be tested routinely for salmonellae.

2. Aflatoxin standards should be continued for peanuts and for those tree nuts that are susceptible to contamination by *Aspergillus flavus* and *Aspergillus parasiticus*.

3. Purchase specifications that limit molds and other spoilage organisms may be useful when the nuts are to be used as ingredients of foods such as bakery items.

Miscellaneous Additives

Since little is published about the microbiology of these additives with the exception of carmine color, specific regulatory criteria other than judgments based on the provisions of Section 402(a) 1,3,4, of the Food,

Drug and Cosmetic Act (See Chapter 1) cannot be recommended at this time. Manufacturers should routinely test these products to assure their safety and quality.

Bottled Water, Processing Water, and Ice

1. There appears to be little evidence of need at the present time for additions to or modifications of existing criteria in FDA regulations for bottled water; however, in view of recent proliferation of vendors of bottled waters including imports, and the variety of water sources used, FDA should reassess periodically the practices of this industry relative to the microbiological and chemical safety of bottled water offered to the public and the adequacy of the present microbiological standards for this product.

2. Water or ice that comes in contact with or becomes part of a food should be from a potable supply and the microbiological criteria for them should at a minimum meet the U.S. Public Health Service's Drinking Water Standards.

3. Increased research efforts should be made toward development of more effective indicators to assure the microbiological safety of drinking water and to develop more rapid, simple, and less costly methods to detect viruses that cause human illness and are transmitted through drinking water or water and ice used in the food industry.

Pet Foods

1. Microbiological criteria should be utilized to assure that pet foods are free of Salmonella.

2. Specifications to limit the level of salmonellae in dry and intermediate moisture pet food ingredients are recommended as a means of reducing opportunities for contamination of the finished product.

3. Processors of dry and intermediate moisture pet foods should use microbiological guidelines to aid in assessing the sanitation of processing lines and the efficacy of the critical control points.

IMPLEMENTATION OF THE HACCP SYSTEM IN FOOD PROTECTION SYSTEMS (CHAPTER 10)

For HACCP use to be broadly realized, it is likely that the utilization of this system relative to microbiological hazards of foods will have to be required by regulation.

1. The regulation should include:

   a. a statement to identify the basic elements of the HACCP system;

   b. a provision requiring ready availability of monitoring records relating to critical control points and other appropriate information for review by regulatory inspection personnel.

2. Details of the mechanism of applying the HACCP system should be the prerogative of industry.

3. Regulatory authorities should have the option to assess the appropriateness of selected critical control points, the adequacy of the monitoring procedures and the actions taken when monitoring results indicate the need for corrective action.

4. Regulatory inspection personnel should be trained in the elements of the HACCP system so that their activities focus on the review of monitoring records as the primary basis for assessing the adequacy of food processor's control programs.

5. The HACCP system should likewise be applied at points in the food chain other than the processing level, i.e., in production, storage, transport, retail sales, and at food service establishments.

PLANS OF ACTION FOR IMPLEMENTATION
OF THE HACCP SYSTEM AND OF MICROBIOLOGICAL CRITERIA
(CHAPTER 11)

Implementation of the HACCP system and development and implementation of microbiological criteria for foods and food ingredients should be in accordance with the plans of action proposed in Chapter 11 of this report.

1

Introduction

SOURCES OF MICROORGANISMS IN FOODS

Man's food supply consists primarily of plants and animals and products derived from them. Microorganisms are naturally present in the soil, water, and air, and therefore exterior surfaces of plants and animals are contaminated with a variety of microorganisms. There is little specificity to this microflora since it reflects that of the environment in which the plants were grown and the animals were raised. Interior tissues of plants and animals usually contain few, if any, microorganisms. The gastrointestinal tracts of animals, however, contain large numbers of organisms. But if proper slaughtering-dressing procedures are used, contamination of interior muscle tissue can be avoided.

From the time of slaughter, catch, or harvest, the surface and interior tissues of animals and plants are subject to contamination. This is due in part to the breakdown of normal defense mechanisms, particularly in animals. Each processing step subjects the raw material to additional opportunities for contamination. Sources of contamination include surfaces of the harvested plant or slaughtered animal, water, equipment, utensils, workers, and the processing environment.

MICROBIAL ACTIVITIES IN FOODS

Historical Aspects

During their existence, human beings have been confronted with the problem of limited shelf-life of animal and plant foods in part due to

41

microbial activities. During the last 5,000 to 10,000 years a variety of techniques (such as drying, salting, heating, fermentation, refrigeration, or freezing) evolved empirically and contributed to the increased shelf-life of plant and animal foods. These techniques, which controlled microbial activity to a greater or lesser extent, were applied before the mechanism of their effect was understood. In the early 1800s Francois Nicholas Appert was awarded a patent for a practical method of food preservation, namely, "canning." Since that time, and particularly during the last 40 years, new processes have been developed to extend shelf-life of foods. Although some others may have suggested microbial involvement in food spoilage at earlier dates, it was Louis Pasteur who in the mid-1800s first established a scientific basis for the direct relationship between food spoilage and microbial activity. Microorganisms responsible for foodborne diseases were first recognized around 1880. Since that time, the number of microbial agents recognized as involved in foodborne illness has increased steadily.

Spoilage, Pathogenic, and Useful Microorganisms

Microorganisms associated with foods can be categorized as "spoilage," "pathogenic," or "useful." Spoilage microorganisms are those that can grow in a food and cause undesirable changes in flavor, consistency (body and texture), color, or appearance. Also bacterial enzymes may effect slow deterioration of frozen or dried foods during long-time storage. These changes diminish the quality characteristics of foods and may render them ultimately unfit for human consumption. For example, refrigerated perishable foods such as milk, fresh meat, poultry, fish, fruits, and vegetables lose some quality characteristics during normal storage and ultimately spoil, due in part to the activity of microorganisms capable of growth at refrigeration temperatures. Usually, extensive microbial growth (millions of organisms per g or cm^2) occurs before quality losses are perceptible. These changes, when perceived by the consumer, serve as an alert that extensive microbial activity has taken place.

Pathogenic microorganisms can render foods harmful to humans in a variety of ways. Foods may serve as the vehicle for the introduction of infectious microorganisms into the gastrointestinal tract, e.g., *Salmonella* and *Shigella*. Multiplication of certain microorganisms in foods prior to consumption may result in production of toxins, e.g., *Clostridium botulinum*, *Staphylococcus aureus*, and *Bacillus cereus*. Foods may also be the vehicle for microorganisms that form toxins *in vivo*, e.g., *Clostridium perfringens* and certain pathogenic *Escherichia coli*.

With some foods, conditions are chosen to favor the development of useful microorganisms such as lactic acid bacteria and yeasts, which are either naturally present or added intentionally. Such foods as cheeses, yogurt, breads, pickles, and fermented sausages offer desirable organoleptic properties and shelf-life.

Food as a Selective Environment

Microbial activities in foods can be viewed from the perspective of the food as a "selective environment," despite the diversity of microorganisms that contaminate the surfaces of the raw materials. The selectivity is imposed by the physical-chemical characteristics of the food, the additives it contains, the processing techniques, the packaging material, and the storage conditions. It is necessary to distinguish between the shelf-life of two broad categories of foods, namely those that are shelf-stable and those that are perishable. For this discussion, shelf-life will be treated as it relates to microbial activity only.

Microbiological shelf-stability of many foods is related to storage conditions. For example, dried and frozen foods are microbiologically shelf-stable as long as they remain dry or frozen. Shelf-stable foods are not necessarily sterile; indeed, many do contain microorganisms. Some shelf-stable canned foods may undergo microbiological spoilage if they are exposed to elevated temperatures permitting the growth of surviving thermophilic sporeforming bacteria, whereas these organisms are inactive at ambient temperatures and indeed tend to die during normal storage. Shelf-stable food is distinguished from perishable food in that an attribute or attributes of the shelf-stable food prevent(s) the growth of contaminating microorganisms. For example, certain canned products are heat processed to the degree that they are sterile; the attribute assuring stability of such products is elimination of all living forms. With many shelf-stable foods, other attributes prevent microbial growth. Dried beans are shelf-stable because they contain insufficient moisture to permit microbial growth. Mayonnaise is shelf-stable because it contains sufficient quantities of acetic acid in the moisture phase of the product to prevent growth of contaminating organisms. Certain canned cured meats are shelf-stable, not because they are sterile, but because sublethal heat treatment so injures surviving spores that they are incapable of outgrowth in the presence of salt and nitrite. The distinguishing characteristic of shelf-stable foods, then, is their resistance to microbiological spoilage. Microbial growth in such products is an abnormal and unexpected event.

Perishable foods, on the other hand, have a finite shelf-life and if not consumed, will spoil at some time during storage. The exact time of spoilage depends upon a great number of variables. Though various processing procedures, additives, packaging methods, and storage conditions may be applied to increase shelf-life, microorganisms capable of growth survive and ultimately grow. When such growth proceeds to the extent that undesirable changes are perceptible to the processor, preparer, or consumer, the food is deemed of inferior quality or spoiled and is rejected. The distinguishing feature of perishable foods, in contrast to shelf-stable foods, is that microbiological spoilage is an expected event. It will ultimately occur even if the food has been prepared from wholesome raw materials and has been properly processed, packaged, and stored.

Microflora of Processed Foods

Although the microflora of raw materials is usually heterogeneous, processing of foods (except those that are sterile) often imposes a characteristic and highly specific microbiological flora. The normal flora of severely heat processed, but not sterilized, low-acid canned foods is comprised of thermophilic sporeforming bacteria, the most heat-resistant microbial components of the raw materials. The predominating flora of shelf-stable canned cured meats consists of mesophilic aerobic and anaerobic sporeforming bacteria, the predominant organisms resistant to the heat process applied to these products. The normal flora of mayonnaise and salad dressing is comprised of small numbers of sporeforming bacteria, yeasts, and lactic acid bacteria. Aerobic sporeforming bacteria predominate in dry spices and in a number of dry vegetable products. Molds and yeasts predominate in dried fruits. The normal flora in carbonated beverages is comprised of yeasts. In each of the foregoing, the surviving and predominating microflora reflects the nature of the raw materials, processing conditions, packaging, and storage of the shelf-stable product. However, spoilage is still possible. If the severely heat-processed canned foods were exposed to high temperatures during storage, spoilage due to the germination and outgrowth of thermophilic sporeforming bacteria might occur. If shelf-stable canned cured meat were to contain excessive numbers of aerobic sporeforming bacteria, growth of these organisms might result in spoilage, despite an adequate heat process and normal levels of salt and nitrite. Excessive levels of yeasts or lactic acid bacteria might result in their growth and subsequent spoilage of the mayonnaise, despite levels of acetic acid that would assure the stability of a product containing "normal" levels of the same organisms. Time/temperature abuse of an ingredient of a carbonated beverage (for example, a flavor) may lead to the development of large numbers of yeasts that could overcome the effect of carbonic acid, which would normally render the same beverage stable. The normal flora in microbiologically shelf-stable products is, therefore, rather specific. If the stabilizing nature of the system should be overcome, this microflora may multiply and cause spoilage—an unexpected event.

With perishable products, the microflora that survives processing may be heterogeneous, but that portion of it developing during storage and causing spoilage is usually quite specific. For example, a heterogeneous flora exists on raw red meats, poultry, and fish as a result of contamination from the animal and/or the processing environment. Yet, during refrigerated storage of such products, spoilage is caused predominantly by a highly specific group of microorganisms, namely *Pseudomonas* and closely related aerobic, psychrotrophic gram-negative bacteria. If the same products are vacuum-packed in oxygen-impermeable films, a different microflora becomes predominant, namely, lactic acid bacteria that grow under both aerobic and anaerobic conditions. In both examples, despite the heterogeneous flora of the finished product, a rather restricted group of microorganisms may develop and ultimately cause sensory changes in the product. Similar relationships exist for many other perishable foods.

It follows that since most classes of perishable foods constitute selective environments for rather restricted groups of microorganisms, the spoilage caused by the growth of these microorganisms manifests itself in a characteristic manner, i.e., normal spoilage pattern. For example, when pseudomonads and other closely related gram-negative psychrotrophic aerobic bacteria grow to large numbers on the surface of refrigerated fresh meat, poultry, and fish, sensory changes occur. The first manifestation of spoilage is development of off-odor. As growth proceeds, slime may develop and the off-odor may intensify. The normal spoilage pattern of a perishable food can be a safeguard, since under certain situations it warns the processor, preparer, or consumer that the food is no longer edible.

Changes in processing of perishable foods must take into account the effect these changes may have on the spoilage flora, and thus on the normal spoilage pattern of the food involved. If such changes tend to alter the normal patterns of spoilage the public health aspects must be taken into account. A classic example of this relates to the merchandising of smoked whitefish. For generations this product was merchandised under conditions where the fish was exposed to air. Spoilage was evidenced by the development of bacteria which produced off-odors and slime that were readily recognized by the consumer and caused rejection of the product. Then it was discovered that the shelf-life of smoked fish could be significantly increased if the product was packed in an oxygen-impermeable film. With extended storage of the product under these conditions, *C. botulinum* type E was able to grow and produce toxin, just as it would have been able to do in the conventionally packaged product. However, under these storage conditions the aerobic bacteria producing off-odor and slime could not develop and the normal spoilage flora was now comprised of lactic acid bacteria that did not produce off-odors. This change in the normal spoilage pattern of the product reduced the probability that the consumer would reject a product that had been held in storage out of refrigeration for an extended period of time. This led to a multistate outbreak of type E botulism (Kautter, 1964). Thus, it is essential that if changes are made in the processing or merchandising of a perishable product, the influence of these changes on the normal spoilage patterns of the product be taken into account.

CONTROL OF MICROORGANISMS IN FOODS

Control must be exercised over three different categories of microorganisms that may be present in foods: (1) those that have the potential for producing foodborne disease, (2) those that cause food spoilage, and (3) those that grow in food and produce desirable changes.

Effective food control programs eliminate the potential for foodborne illness in a variety of ways. Processing techniques that cause destruction of pathogens may be employed, e.g., the pasteurization of milk to destroy *Coxiella burnetii* and *Mycobacterium tuberculosis* and less heat resistant pathogens such as the diphtheria bacillus, salmonellae, and pyogenic streptococci, and the 12-D process[1] for the destruction of *C. botulinum* in low-acid canned foods. In other cases, toxigenic and infectious microorganisms are controlled by product formulation (acetic acid in mayonnaise) or storage conditions (the refrigeration of perishable pasteurized canned cured meats to control the growth of *C. botulinum*). In yet other situations, the ultimate control is exercised by the person who prepares the food (adequate cooking of poultry to eliminate salmonellae and of pork to eliminate trichinellae). Despite such efforts, food control programs have fallen short of their goals for controlling foodborne pathogens (see in particular Chapter 4 where foodborne illness of microbiological origin is treated in detail).

Control measures directed toward prevention of spoilage have also fallen short of the ideal. Although precise figures are difficult to obtain, it is estimated that one-fourth of the world's food supply is lost through microbial activity alone. The control of food spoilage is a prime economic objective of control programs. For products designed to be shelf-stable,

---

[1]The 12-D process is the minimum heat treatment applied to low-acid canned foods; it provides for the reduction of 10^{12} heat-resistant spores of *C. botulinum* to one. This requires approximately 2.5 minutes exposure at 121.1°C (250°F) or its equivalent.

control is accomplished through processing and/or formulation procedures that result in the inhibition of spoilage organisms. With perishable foods, the object is to achieve the longest possible shelf-life consistent with product safety. In general, this is attempted by instituting measures that will result in products with low microbial loads, since shelf-life and initial level of contamination are usually directly related in perishable foods. Control of remaining microorganisms is most often achieved by proper refrigerated storage.

The desirable organoleptic properties (taste, odor, body, and texture) of such foods as cheeses, yogurt, cultured buttermilk, sour cream, pickles, and fermented sausages result in part from the activities of a specific microbial flora. Extensive microbiological control procedures are needed to produce "cultured products" of high quality and to ensure that the microbial activities are guided in such a manner that the end products have the desirable sensory properties. For example, in cultured dairy products this is achieved by (1) proper selection and handling of starter cultures, (2) control of the presence of antibiotics and bacteriophages, and (3) checking by chemical and organoleptic means the progress of microbial activity in raw and finished products. These measures can influence both the quality and the safety of the food. For example, the lack of acidity caused by culture failure can allow the development of *S. aureus,* which could result in cheese containing staphylococcal enterotoxin.

Another objective of food control programs is to keep filth and other foreign substances out of food. In some cases, extraneous matter is of public health concern, e.g., rodent pellets and hairs; in other instances, the foreign material is of aesthetic rather than health significance, e.g., certain cereal insects.

Finally, another objective of food control programs is to ensure that packaging, storage, handling, transportation, display, and sale of foods are all properly carried out. Processors and regulatory officials can exert control over a product while it is packaged, stored, and readied for distribution from the plant of origin. But beyond that point, the intensity of control rapidly diminishes.

The bulk of the problems with foodborne disease and food spoilage results from events that occur after food has left the processing plant— during transport, during retail sales, and ultimately in the food service establishment or home (CDC, 1981). In these locations, control on occasion either does not exist or is executed ineffectively, thus producing the weakest link in the food chain. Many improvements in food control that are made at the processing level will be nullified if handling procedures beyond the plant are not effectively controlled.

APPROACHES TO MICROBIOLOGICAL CONTROL IN FOODS

Traditionally, three principal means have been used by regulatory agencies and food processors to control microorganisms in foods. These are (1) education and training, (2) inspection of facilities and operations, and (3) microbiological testing.

Although food handlers have the potential for contaminating foods with disease-producing microorganisms, i.e., staphylococci, salmonellae, and hepatitus virus, health examination of food handlers is a nonproductive approach to the control of foodborne illness. Specimens from food handlers have traditionally been examined only for a few microorganisms, and such tests do not always detect carriers. Screening tests cannot be made with sufficient frequency to be effective in detecting the carrier status in persons who are continually exposed to the risk of acquiring foodborne pathogens. Negative tests convey to food handlers, managers, and public health personnel the erroneous concept that the workers are free of infections and therefore incapable of transmitting foodborne pathogens to the foods they handle. Although direct transfer of pathogens from food handlers to food is a hazard, far more frequently improper food-handling practices create a hazard that is not circumvented by health examinations.

Education and Training Programs

These programs are directed primarily toward developing an understanding of the causes and consequences of microbial contamination and of measures to prevent contamination and subsequent growth. The extent of training required of personnel within processing plants and food service establishments depends upon the technical complexity of the food operation and the level of responsibility of the individuals being trained. In-depth training may be necessary for supervisory personnel, while for others training may relate only to specific aspects of a food operation. Although education and training are necessary parts of any food control program, standing alone they have certain limitations and shortcomings. Personnel turnover in the food industry is both constant and rapid, and thus education of workers must be a continuing rather than a sporadic exercise. It is essential that supervisory personnel be properly trained with respect to the hazards associated with the operations for which they have responsibility.

Inspection of Facilities and Operations

Inspections of facilities and operations are commonly used to evaluate adherence to good handling practices. The U.S. Department of Agriculture

(USDA) relies almost entirely upon this approach in the regulation of meat and poultry operations. Resident inspectors observe all phases of processing from the live animal to the finished product. Little reliance is placed upon microbiological testing in the meat and poultry control programs. In its activities with respect to dried milk and egg processing, the USDA relies not only on inspections but also on microbiological testing of the finished products.

The Food and Drug Administration (FDA) also relies heavily on inspection of facilities and operations. In addition, both in-process and finished product samples are collected and analyzed. Results of such analyses are used to corroborate observations made during inspections; they are not intended to perform the processors' responsibility of microbiological control on a day-to-day basis. The FDA inspection program is designed to determine whether or not processors are operating in compliance with the Federal Food, Drug and Cosmetic Act. Thus, this activity is in sharp contrast to that of the USDA meat and poultry inspection, wherein resident inspectors are charged to assure that plants are in compliance with the Federal Meat Inspection Act and Poultry Products Inspection Act on a day-to-day basis.

Procedures vary widely at the state, county, and municipal levels, but the approach to regulatory control is primarily through periodic inspection of facilities and operations.

Just as with the education and training approach to food control, inspection of facilities and operations alone is not sufficient. Generally, the inspector relies upon advisory or mandatory documents such as Good Manufacturing Practice (GMP) guidelines and Codes of Hygienic Practice or local food control laws, ordinances, or regulations. Unfortunately, such documents often refer to stated requirements without specifying what is considered to be in compliance with the requirements.[2] This lack of specificity, or failure to indicate the relative importance of the requirements, leaves interpretation of compliance solely at the discretion of the inspector. Lack of discrimination between important and relatively unimportant requirements may result in overemphasis upon unnecessary or relatively minor requirements, and thus increase costs without significantly reducing hazards. Requirements that are critical to the safety of the product may be overlooked or underestimated.

---

[2] A notable exception is the USPHS/FDA Grade A Pasteurized Milk Ordinance wherein for each requirement a statement is given that specifies what constitutes compliance with the requirement.

Microbiological Testing

Samples of ingredients, materials obtained from selected points during the course of processing or handling, and finished products may be examined microbiologically to determine adherence to Good Manufacturing Practices. In some instances, foods are examined for a specific pathogen or its toxins, but more often examinations are made to detect organisms that are indicative of the possible presence of pathogens or spoilage or to detect presence of the specific spoilage organisms or their products. Microbiological testing is absolutely essential to the control of certain products, e.g., to assure that dried milk and eggs and confectionery products are free of a *Salmonella* hazard. Testing is essential to assure that critical raw materials are satisfactory for their intended use, e.g., to assure that the sugar used in canning meets established standards and to assure that critical products used in dried blends are free of *Salmonella*.

Microbiological testing has severe limitations as a control option. The most serious shortcoming is the constraint of time. Most microbiological test results are not available until several days after testing. Therefore, if finished product acceptability must be measured by microbiological testing, the product is held pending results. With perishable foods, this is generally not possible; with shelf-stable foods, the warehousing of finished product increases costs. If in-line samples are collected and analyzed, the results are of retrospective value since the finished product has already been produced. Other difficulties are related to sampling (see Chapter 6), analytical methods (see Chapters 4 and 5), and the use of indicator organisms for pathogens (see Chapter 5).

Composite Programs

Sophisticated microbiological control programs encompass the three approaches, namely education and training, inspection of facilities and operations, and microbiological testing. The emphasis varies from plant to plant, product to product, and establishment to establishment, as does the success of the various microbiological control programs.

The Hazard Analysis Critical Control Point (HACCP) System

The HACCP system, first presented at the 1971 National Conference on Food Protection (APHA, 1971), provides a more specific and critical approach to the control of microbiological hazards than that achievable by traditional inspection and quality control procedures. The system consists of: (1) identification and assessment of hazards associated with growing, harvesting, processing-manufacturing, marketing, preparation, and/ or use of a given raw material or food product; (2) determination of critical control points to control any identifiable hazard(s); and (3) establishment of procedures to monitor critical control points. Analysis of factors to be considered in hazard analyses, detailed in Chapter 3, leads to establishment of the control points to be monitored. Depending upon the situation, the monitoring may involve inspections, physical or chemical measurements, and/or microbiological testing.

The HACCP system is a structured approach to microbiological quality control. The key lies in the meaning of "critical control point," which is a location or a process that, if not correctly controlled, could lead to contamination of the product with foodborne pathogens or spoilage microorganisms or their survival or unacceptable growth. A careful hazard analysis leads to the identification of critical control points. Once the critical control points have been identified, the final problem involves finding the most effective and practical means for monitoring these points. Properly applied, the HACCP system separates the essential from the superfluous aspects of microbiological control. As discussed in Chapter 10, use of the HACCP system by industry not only offers the food processor a rational approach to microbiological control, but also leads to more effective and economical utilization of regulatory manpower. The inspector focuses initial attention on monitoring records and, if the results indicate satisfactory control over critical control points, logically concludes that efforts could be more effectively expended on other food-processing operations either with the same or with other food-processing plants.

The HACCP system has been successfully applied to the microbiological control of low-acid canned foods. Indeed, in the United States monitoring of critical control points in the production of these products is subject to federal regulations. Many industrial organizations have adopted the HACCP system as a means of microbiological control over products other than low-acid canned foods. The system has also been applied to microbiological control over food service establishments and has even been used in the home. Unfortunately, only limited use has been made of the HACCP system by regulatory authorities. Impediments to its more widespread use are discussed in detail in Chapter 10.

THE CURRENT ROLE OF CRITERIA
IN MICROBIOLOGICAL CONTROL IN FOODS

Microbiological criteria in one form or another have been in existence in the United States since the early part of this century. The more prominent microbiological standards formulated and enforced by federal regulatory agencies are those for milk, water, shellfish, and egg products. Other standards exist for aflatoxins, scombroid toxin, paralytic shellfish toxin in specific foods, and defect action levels for specific foods. The enforcement of these standards has contributed to significant improvements in the microbiological safety and quality of these products. At the federal level no formal microbiological standards exist for other foods. Despite this lack, existing laws provide sufficient authority for the removal from the marketplace of products with microbiological conditions that pose a threat to health. Therefore, "implied" microbiological standards do exist.[3] Even in the absence of a threat to health, existing federal laws provide sufficient authority for seizure of products if there is direct or indirect evidence that a product is contaminated with filth, e.g., seizure of tree nuts contaminated with *E. coli* and seizure of raw shrimp contaminated with salmonellae. In the latter case, seizure is based not on a health hazard, but on the premise that the presence of salmonellae is indicative of insanitation in the processing of the shrimp. Federal laws also give sufficient authority for seizure of products for aesthetic reasons. If GMPs were held to have the force of law, they could provide authority to the FDA to use microbiological criteria therein in the assessment of good manufacturing practices. However, with few exceptions, umbrella GMPs are inadequate for such purposes as they lack precise, achievable standards (*U.S. v. An Article of Food*, 1972).

Thus, at the federal level, though limited use has been made of formal standards, the law has nevertheless provided adequate authority for seizure of foods known to present health hazards. A detailed discussion of the current status of microbiological criteria and their legislative bases is

---

[3]Section 402(a)(1) of the Food, Drug and Cosmetic Act (U.S. Congress, 1980) specifies that a food that bears or contains any poisonous or deleterious substance that may render it injurious to health is deemed to be adulterated. Pathogens or their toxins may be considered as deleterious or poisonous substances, respectively. However, the presence of certain pathogens in any number in a food available to consumers must not be tolerated (e.g., *Shigella dysenteriae, Vibrio cholerae* O-1); the mere presence of certain others is not hazardous although high populations of them would be (e.g., *C. perfringens, B. cereus*). Section 402 (a)(1) does not make this distinction. Accordingly, microbiological criteria become useful in interpreting this section of the act as they specify the pathogen or toxin of concern, the analytical method by which they may be detected, the sampling plan for obtaining the food to be analyzed, and the level of population of a pathogen or concentration of toxin that must not be exceeded. Nevertheless, in the absence of such criteria "implied" standards for pathogens do exist by the very nature of the wording of Section 402(a)(1), and have been enforced by the FDA when in its judgment a direct health hazard exists, i.e., a food contains a deleterious agent that may render it injurious to health. Thus, microbiological criteria provide a means for interpreting the provisions of 402(a)(1) as it pertains to pathogens.

presented in Chapter 8. Microbiological criteria adopted by state, county, and local health agencies are also included in this review. Twenty-five states have microbiological criteria, usually guidelines, for one or more foods (Wehr, 1982).

Microbiological quality standards have recently been proposed by the FDA. These standards do not purport to have any relationship to safety. As yet, none has been adopted. For further discussion of microbiological quality standards, see Chapter 2.

Microbiological criteria have long been used by industry to assess the microbiological safety and quality of its products, for in-process monitoring, and for microbiological inspection of raw ingredients. Generally, these criteria are internally generated and proprietary, though some companies publish the microbiological criteria relating to their finished products for sales promotion purposes. Microbiological criteria are also used by industry in connection with purchase specifications. These criteria are included in purchase contracts between vendors and purchasers of products. Industry "standards" exist for certain raw materials, the best examples being the National Food Processors Association standards for sporeforming bacteria in sugar and starches and the National Soft Drink Association standard for the presence of yeasts, molds, and bacteria in sugar.

CONSIDERATIONS IN ESTABLISHING CRITERIA

The establishment of a meaningful microbiological criterion is not a simple process. In 1964, the Food Protection Committee of the National Research Council proposed three basic principles for setting a microbiological criterion (NRC, 1964). These principles were that microbiological criteria for foods should: (1) accomplish what they purport to do, i.e., reduce public health hazards; (2) be technically feasible, i.e., attainable under conditions of good commercial practice; and (3) be adminstratively feasible.

Difficult questions must be answered before a useful microbiological criterion can be established. For example, what foods should be subject to microbiological criteria and on what basis? What contaminants should be specified (pathogens, indicator organisms, toxins, etc.)? What limits should be placed on the presence of each contaminant? How large a sample of each food should be examined and by what method? The most comprehensive discussion of these questions on the international level is provided by the International Commission on Microbiological Specifications for Foods (ICMSF, 1985) and the Codex General Principles for the Establishment and Application of Microbiological Criteria for Foods (see Appendix B).

THE CURRENT REPORT

This book is the result of the Subcommittee on Microbiological Criteria's examination of the value of microbiological criteria in the control of food quality and safety. The subcommittee tried to bring the uses of microbiological criteria into perspective with respect to their place in a total program for microbiological control of foods in the United States. The book contains chapters on the purpose of microbiological criteria and definitions of terms used in relation to them, on factors that influence the selection of foods to be considered for criteria, on the selection of microorganisms as components for criteria, on the selection of sampling plans, and on the action to be taken when a criterion is exceeded. Foods of several major commodity groups are identified as appropriate candidates for microbiological criteria on the basis of recognized problems related to safety and quality. Finally, plans of action are presented for implementation of the HACCP system and development of meaningful microbiological criteria. The subcommittee's responses to specific questions raised by the sponsoring agencies and the general recommendations of the subcommittee are presented in sections devoted to those purposes.

REFERENCES

APHA (American Public Health Association)
  1971   Proceedings of the 1971 National Conference on Food Protection. Washington, D.C.: U.S. Department of Health, Education and Welfare, Public Health Service, Food and Drug Administration.
CDC (Centers for Disease Control)
  1981   Foodborne Disease Outbreaks. Annual Summary 1979. Issued April 1981. Atlanta: U.S. Department of Health and Human Services, Public Health Service, Centers for Disease Control.
ICMSF (International Commission on Microbiological Specifications for Foods)
  1985   Microorganisms in Foods. 2. Sampling for microbiological analysis: Principles and specific applications. 2nd Ed. In preparation.
Kautter, D. A.
  1964   *Clostridium botulinum* type E in smoked fish. J. Food Sci. 29:843-849.
NRC (National Research Council)
  1964   An Evaluation of Public Health Hazards from Microbiological Contamination of Foods. Food Protection Committee. Washington D.C.: National Academy of Sciences-National Research Council.
U.S. Congress
  1980   Federal Food, Drug and Cosmetic Act, as amended. Washington, D.C.: U.S. Government Printing Office.
U.S. v. *An Article of Food*
  1972   Pasteurized whole eggs, 339 F. Supp. 131 (N.D. Ga., 1972).
Wehr, H. M.
  1982   Attitudes and policies of governmental agencies on microbial criteria for foods—an update. Food Technol. 36(9):45-54, 92.

2

Definitions, Purposes, and Needs for Microbiological Criteria

A meaningful discussion on the use of microbiological criteria for foods and food ingredients requires a precise description of terms used when applying microbiological limits to foods. In this chapter, definitions are given for the various types of microbiological criteria. In addition, the purposes and needs for microbiological criteria for foods and food ingredients in the United States are examined. Because controversy exists about the application of microbiological criteria as quality standards of foods, attributes of quality amenable to measurement by microbiological criteria also are examined.

DEFINITIONS

A criterion is a yardstick on which a judgment or decision can be made. For this report, a microbiological criterion will stipulate that a type of microorganism, group of microorganisms, or toxin produced by a microorganism must either not be present at all, be present in only a limited number of samples, or be present as less than a specified number or amount in a given quantity of a food or food ingredient.

Components of a Microbiological Criterion

A microbiological criterion should include the following:

1. a statement describing the identity of the food or food ingredient,
2. a statement of the contaminant of concern, i.e., the microorganism or group of microorganisms and/or its toxin or other agent,

55

3. the analytical method to be used for the detection, enumeration, or quantification of the contaminant of concern,
4. the sampling plan (see Chapter 6), and
5. the microbiological limits considered appropriate to the food and commensurate with the sampling plan used.

Mandatory and Advisory Criteria

A mandatory limit is one that the food cannot exceed. Food that does not meet the criterion must be subjected to some action (see Chapter 7). For example, it may be rejected by the purchaser, destroyed, reprocessed, sold as an inferior grade, or diverted to a use where the contaminant is not of concern. Certain mandatory criteria also may result in the loss of license to process food when limits are consistently exceeded.

Advisory criteria often serve as an alert to deficiencies in processing, distribution, storage, or marketing. They are not mandatory but permit judgments to be made when limits are not met.

Types of Microbiological Criteria

The terms standard, guideline, and specification are widely used in the United States and other nations to describe microbiological criteria for foods. There appears to be no need for additional terms. The following definitions of these terms are recommended by the subcommittee for application by the food industry and governmental agencies in the United States and will be used throughout this report.

Standard

A microbiological standard is a microbiological criterion that is a part of a law, ordinance, or administrative regulation. A standard is a mandatory criterion. Failure to comply with it constitutes violation of the law, ordinance, or regulation and will be subject to the enforcement policy of the regulatory agency having jurisdiction.

Guideline

A microbiological guideline is a criterion that often is used by the food industry or a regulatory agency to monitor a manufacturing process. Guidelines function as alert mechanisms to signal whether microbiological conditions prevailing at critical control points or in the finished product are within the normal range. Hence, they are used to assess processing efficiency at critical control points and conformity with Good Manufacturing Practices. A microbiological guideline is an advisory criterion in that a given lot of food exceeding the limit for a nonpathogenic organism would not be taken off the market or even downgraded. Guidelines may be mandatory, however, in the sense that food company management and regulatory agencies may demand that the conditions responsible for persistent microbiological deficiencies be corrected without delay (see Chapter 7).

Specification

A microbiological specification is a microbiological criterion that is used as a purchase requirement whereby conformance with it becomes a condition of purchase between buyer and vendor of a food or ingredient. A microbiological specification can be either mandatory or advisory.

PURPOSES

Microbiological criteria as described above may be used to assess:

1. the safety of a food,
2. adherence to good manufacturing practices,
3. the utility (suitability) of a food or ingredient for a particular purpose, and
4. the keeping quality (shelf-life) of certain perishable foods.

Evaluation of the safety of a food may involve tests for the pathogens or toxins of concern. Alternatively, it may involve tests for indicator organisms, where a relationship has been shown between the occurrence of the indicator organism and the safety of the food. For some pathogens and toxins, the numbers or concentrations present in a food are significant in that lower figures do not pose a health hazard whereas higher ones do (see Chapter 4). Examples of criteria broadly meeting the definition of microbiological standards are those applied to milk and shellfish (US-DHEW, 1965; USPHS/FDA, 1978). The purpose of these criteria is to protect the consumer's health.

The Howard mold count limits as applied to tomato and certain fruit products are standards that were designed to minimize the amount of decayed raw produce that might be introduced into such foods. Although there is now an awareness that certain molds produce mycotoxins, the mold count standards (Defect Action Levels) were not established to reduce a health hazard.

Criteria often are used for making decisions related to the acceptability of products since they may measure adherence to Good Manufacturing Practices. They can also be used to assess the utility of a food or food ingredient for a specific purpose; for example, canners of fruit products must limit the number of heat-resistant ascospores of *Byssochlamys fulva* in ingredients such as fruit juice concentrates and tapioca starch.

Industry quality control/assurance departments may use microbiological criteria to monitor the potential shelf-life of perishable foods. Products with small numbers of spoilage microorganisms are more likely to have a longer shelf-life than are those with larger numbers. Such results are of retrospective value: while they do not extend the shelf-life of the lot that was analyzed, they do alert the processor to problems that must be corrected in order to achieve satisfactory preservation of future production.

NEED FOR ESTABLISHMENT

A microbiological criterion for a food or food ingredient should be established and implemented in the United States only when there is a need for it and when it can be shown to be effective and practical. The criterion must accomplish its objective, i.e., adequately measure the contaminants of concern, be technically attainable under commercial conditions by Good Manufacturing Practices, and be administratively feasible. There are additional factors that should be considered before the need for a specific microbiological criterion can be established. These should include (see Chapters 1 and 3):

1. evidence of a hazard to health based on epidemiological data or a hazard analysis (see also Chapter 4);

2. the nature of the natural and commonly acquired microflora of the food and the ability of the food to support microbial growth;

3. the effect of processing on the microflora of the food;

4. the potential for microbial contamination and/or growth during processing, handling, storage, and distribution;

5. the category of consumers at risk;

6. the state in which food is distributed, e.g., frozen, refrigerated, heat processed, etc.;

7. potential for abuse at the consumer level;

8. spoilage potential, utility, and GMPs;

9. the manner in which the food is prepared for ultimate consumption, i.e., heated or not;

10. reliability of methods available to detect and/or quantify the microorganism(s) and toxins of concern (see Chapter 4); and

11. the costs/benefits associated with the application of the criterion.

APPLICATIONS OF CRITERIA

Standards

Microbiological standards may be useful when epidemiological evidence indicates that a food is frequently a vehicle of disease. Several factors should be considered before a microbiological standard is established. Most important, the standard must attain its stated objective, namely the elimination or reduction of foodborne disease. (Although potpies have been involved in outbreaks of botulism, standards related to the presence of *Clostridium botulinum* spores in the frozen product would be highly impractical since in each outbreak, illness was caused by extreme abuse of the food by the consumer.) Currently existing "implied" microbiological standards for foods should also be considered (see Chapter 1, page 52 note 3).

A criticism of standards based on fixed numbers of nonpathogenic microorganisms is that they can result in the recall or downgrading of significant quantities of what otherwise may be wholesome food. One means of minimizing this would be the approach used in the Grade A Pasteurized Milk Ordinance (USPHS/FDA, 1978). Here a given lot is not automatically rejected when standard plate counts or numbers of coliforms exceed the prescribed limit, but penalty provisions, which can include suspension of the permit to process milk, may be instituted on repeated violations, e.g., when three out of five of the last analyses within a specified period of time exceed the standard. This system affords the correction of undesirable conditions with minimal loss of food, and thus with minimal cost to the consumer.

Guidelines

Microbiological guidelines are used by food processors to monitor the microbiological condition of raw products, of a food at critical control points during processing, of process equipment surfaces, and of the finished product. Industry quality control/assurance departments commonly establish microbiological limits, often based on many years of experience, that should be achievable in foods at critical control points or in the finished product if good manufacturing practices are observed. Results that exceed these limits serve to signal some divergence from accepted good manufacturing practices and may suggest remedial measures. Industry guidelines often are of a proprietary nature and may vary from company to company, even for the same product.

Microbiological guidelines can aid regulatory agencies in the assessment of good manufacturing practices when analyses are conducted in conjunction with plant inspection. Before this can be done, a relationship between the microbiology of the food and the factory conditions would have to be established, usually for each product and process under consideration.

There is a use for published guidelines such as those offered for finished products at ports of entry by the International Commission on Microbiological Specifications for Foods (ICMSF, 1985) and in certain Codex Codes of Hygienic Practice (see below). When based on good manufacturing practices, statistically valid data, or appropriate experience, such guidelines permit the processor and others to assess the conditions under which certain foods have been processed and stored.

Specifications

Microbiological specifications are used in the United States to determine the acceptability of a raw material or finished product in a contractual agreement between two parties (buyer and vendor). Specifications are used by governmental agencies to assess microbiological acceptability of foods purchased for use in government programs. As with other microbiological criteria, specifications should be based on relevant background data and should fill a need.

RELATIONSHIP TO CODEX

With some exceptions, the definitions, components, types, and purposes of microbiological criteria described in this report are similar to those published by the Codex Alimentarius Commission (1980, 1981). Codex microbiological criteria, however, are tied closely to Codex codes of hygienic practice and Codex concerns are with international commerce, while the mission of this subcommittee is to address the needs of governmental agencies and the food industry within the United States. The differences noted below stem from this fact.

A Codex microbiological criterion is mandatory when contained in a Codex Alimentarius Standard. When introduced, it shall not be *de novo* but shall be derived from microbiological end-product specifications that have accompanied Codes of Practice through the Codex Procedure and have been extensively applied to the food. In addition, a Codex microbiological standard "should, whenever possible, contain limits only for pathogenic microorganisms of public health significance in the food concerned, although limits for nonpathogenic microorganisms may be necessary" (Codex Alimentarius Commission, 1980).

The term "specification" in the Codex "General Principles" document

(Codex Alimentarius Commission, 1980; see also Appendix B) refers only to a microbiological end-product specification and is intended to increase assurance that the provisions of hygienic significance in the code have been met. This Codex document does not contain a definition of a microbiological specification as a limit to determine the acceptability of raw materials, ingredients, or foods in contractual agreement between two parties.

ATTRIBUTES OF QUALITY AMENABLE TO MEASUREMENT BY MICROBIOLOGICAL CRITERIA

The term quality usually refers to the property, inherent nature, characteristic or attribute, or degree or grade of excellence of something. The term quality as commonly applied to food summarizes in one word its desirable characteristics. Quality of a food as perceived by the consumer can be described as a value related to flavor, color, and texture. It also includes imperceptible traits such as nutritional and aesthetic values and safety. Exclusive of discussions of safety, for the purpose of this report, microbiological aspects of quality include:

1. shelf-life, as perceived by attributes such as flavor and appearance;
2. adherence to good manufacturing practices;
3. utility of a food.

Each of these attributes is measurable to some extent microbiologically; the decisive question, however, is to what extent. Although subsequent sections of this report will deal with this question in more detail, some discussion of the subject is presented below.

The ultimate shelf-life of a perishable product can be estimated to some degree through the application of microbiological criteria. Assuming identical storage conditions, a perishable food with a low number of spoilage microorganisms will have a longer shelf-life than the same product with larger numbers of such organisms. In practice, products with unacceptable shelf-life will soon be recognized and rejected by customers in the market place. Regulatory agency or industry use of microbiological criteria to grade foods for shelf-life often is an impractical task because of variable conditions during storage. Furthermore, relationships among common microbiological parameters such as total counts and coliform counts, and the shelf-life of a food are inexact. Some types of microorganisms, because of enzyme systems acting upon the constituents of the food, cause marked changes in perceptible quality characteristics of a food while others are relatively inert biochemically and thus produce little change. In addition, the effect of certain levels and/or types of microorganisms on perceptible quality characteristics often differs from food to food and is also subject to changes in environmental conditions such as temperature and gaseous atmosphere.

Lack of adherence to good manufacturing practices can often be related to levels and types of microorganisms in excess of those present in a product produced and held under good conditions. The use of poor quality materials, careless handling, or insanitation may result in a higher bacterial count in the finished product. However, a heat treatment or other lethal process can reduce the higher bacterial counts that result from malpractice; furthermore organisms may die off during storage of frozen, dried, or fermented foods. Low counts, therefore, do not necessarily indicate good commercial practices or even food safety. The absence of viable staphylococci in cheese, for example, does not guarantee the absence of staphylococcal enterotoxin. High aerobic plate counts (APC), on the other hand, do not necessarily mean careless handling or lack of wholesomeness. For example, ground beef is likely to yield a high APC, but this may merely reflect the growth of harmless psychrotrophic bacteria during refrigerated storage.

The relationship between the microbiology of a food and adherence to good manufacturing practices must be established by conducting repeated surveys of processing lines to obtain statistically valid data. The critical control points in the HACCP approach (see Chapter 10) must be identified and the microbiology of the food at different stages of processing must be determined. Through these studies, numbers and types of organisms that characterize the flora of a food produced under a given set of conditions can be identified and thus provide a basis for the establishment of a microbiological criterion. Even then, an allowance has to be made for variations due to differences in processing procedures and equipment.

Finished foods with microbial counts that exceed the criterion might reasonably be expected to have been mishandled in some manner during production and/or storage. As pointed out earlier, however, low counts do not always reflect good manufacturing practices because a lethal step in the process or significant die-off of microorganisms during storage may have occurred.

The relationship between good commercial practices and quality often is a question of aesthetics. A frozen food, for example, might be processed under conditions of sanitation that a discriminating person would find objectionable. While these conditions would be reflected in the microbiology of the food, the usual quality attributes of nutritional value, flavor, texture, color, safety, and shelf-life might not be altered.

Microbiological criteria can be useful to determine the utility of a food or ingredient. The limits for thermophilic spores in sugar and starches to be used in canning are an example of this application (National Canners Association, 1968).

In recent years microbiological quality standards have been proposed for various foods under Section 401 of the Food, Drug and Cosmetic Act (U.S. Congress, 1938), which authorizes the establishment of standards of indentity and quality (see Chapter 8). Limits for APC and numbers of coliforms were based on extensive market surveys. No data were published that showed a correlation between organoleptic quality of the foods and the levels of microorganisms, and since the samples were collected from retail markets, the microbiological findings could not be related to the quality of the raw product or processing conditions. As a result of such surveys, FDA has recommended that state and local agencies consider the adoption of microbiological quality standards for frozen fish sticks, fish cakes, and crab cakes (FDA, 1980, 1981).

Although microbiological quality standards are not purported to be related to safety and a consumer might not perceive any effect on quality due to the high counts, these standards have been justified on the basis that microbial levels are indicative of (1) the excellence of raw materials and ingredients used, (2) the degree of control during processing, and (3) the conditions of distribution and storage (FDA, 1972). Additional justifications (FDA, 1976, 1980) were that minimal standards would be maintained for foods prone to microbial growth or other quality defects, and that the microbial quality standards would promote honesty and fair dealing in the interest of the consumer.

A difficulty with microbiological quality standards is that they are predicated on the basic assumption that quality varies inversely with numbers of microorganisms. This appears to be true only with some foods processed under certain conditions. Good-quality frozen peas were found to yield APC figures approximately 20-fold higher than the poor quality, overmature product (Pederson, 1947). The former were more tender and thus more subject to bruising with the release of microbial growth-promoting juices. With frozen foods, best quality usually is achieved by very rapid freezing followed by storage of the food at the lowest possible temperature (USDA, 1960). These also are the conditions that permit the highest survival of microorganisms. A common means for reducing the number of viable microorganisms on a food is to expose it to sprays or flumes containing relatively high concentrations of chlorine. While such treatments improve microbiological quality, other quality attributes may be affected adversely since chlorine reacts with numerous food constituents such as amino acids, lipids, and chlorophyll. At present it is not known whether these different chloro-organic compounds are completely innocuous.

REFERENCES

Codex Alimentarius Commission
  1980   General principles for the establishment and application of microbiological criteria for foods. Appendix II in Report of the 17th Session of the Committee on Food Hygiene. Rome: Food and Agriculture Organization.
  1981   Report of the 14th session of the Codex Alimentarius Commission. Rome: Food and Agriculture Organization.

FDA (Food and Drug Administration)
  1972   Proposed microbiological quality standards. Federal Register 37(186):20038–20040.
  1976   Standards of quality for foods for which there are no standards of identity. Amendment and confirmation of effective date. Federal Register 41(154):33249–33253.
  1980   Frozen fish sticks, frozen fish cakes, and frozen crab cakes; Recommended microbiological quality standards. Docket No. 79N-081. Federal Register 45(108):37524–37526.
  1981   Frozen fish sticks, frozen fish cakes, and frozen crab cakes; Recommended microbiological quality standards. Docket No. 79N-0081. Federal Register 46(113):31067–31068.

ICMSF (International Commission on Microbiological Specifications for Foods)
  1985   Microorganisms in Foods. 2. Sampling for microbiological analysis: Principles and specific applications. 2nd Ed. In preparation.

National Canners Association
  1968   Laboratory Manual for Food Canners and Processors. Vol. 1. Westport, Conn.: AVI Publishing.

Pederson, C. S.
  1947   Significance of bacteria in frozen vegetables. Food Research 12:1–10.

U.S. Congress
  1938   Federal Food, Drug and Cosmetic Act of 1938. Pub. L. 717 (June 25) 52 Stat. 1040. Washington D.C.: U.S. Government Printing Office.

USDA (U.S. Department of Agriculture)
  1960   Conference on frozen food quality, Western Regional Research Laboratory. Publication ARS-74-21. Washington D.C.: USDA.

USDHEW (U.S. Department of Health, Education and Welfare)
  1965   National Shellfish Sanitation Program, Manual of Operations. Part 1. Sanitation of Shellfish Growing Areas. Washington D.C.: U.S. Government Printing Office.

USPHS/FDA (U.S. Public Health Service/Food and Drug Administration)
  1978   Grade A Pasteurized Milk Ordinance. 1978 Recommendations. USPHS/FDA Publication No. 229. Washington, D.C.: U.S. Government Printing Office.

3

Selection of Foods
for Criteria Related to Safety

As discussed in Chapter 2, microbiological criteria can serve several purposes. They may give an indication of safety of a product; they may reveal breaches in good manufacturing and handling practices; they may tell something of the keeping quality or shelf-life of a product; and they may reflect suitability for special uses such as canning, infant feeding, or long-term refrigerated storage.

Every microbiological criterion specifies some kind of test. A criterion may require the absence of certain pathogenic organisms or their toxins from a specific quantity of the product. Such a criterion is routine for *Salmonella* spp. in milk chocolate, milk powder, dried eggs, and other ready-to-eat products that have a history of *Salmonella* contamination. Normally foods are tested for pathogenic or toxigenic microorganisms only if there is reason to believe they may be present. For example, cheese that is suspected in a staphylococcal food poisoning outbreak may be tested directly for enterotoxins. Similarly, a low-acid canned food that is suspected of being underprocessed may be tested for *Clostridium botulinum* or its toxin.

However, microbiological criteria that are aimed at assuring safety often rely on tests for organisms that indicate a possibility of hazard, not the hazard itself. Coliforms in drinking water, for example, often indicate a failure of the purification process with the possibility that sewage and therefore salmonellae or other intestinal microorganisms might be present. Excessive numbers of fecal coliforms in raw shellfish also may indicate sewage contamination and the presence of pathogens. Large numbers of coagulase-positive staphylococci in cheese, fermented sausage, or frozen

65

food suggest that enterotoxin may be present or that mistreatment may lead rapidly to its formation.

It should be emphasized that direct tests for pathogenic microorganisms and their toxins, excepting *Salmonella* spp. and *Staphylococcus aureus*, are not routinely applied to foods for quality control purposes. Most criteria aimed at assuring safety are based on tests for indicator organisms whose presence suggests the possibility of hazard; the tests do not reveal the hazard itself.

It is impractical and unnecessary to develop microbiological criteria for every food. Instead, criteria should be developed only for those foods with potential danger that can be reduced or eliminated by the imposition of microbiological criteria. The following sections describe some of the factors that go into the selection of candidate foods. These factors form the basis of the ICMSF "case plan" (ICMSF, 1985), which reflects varying degrees of health hazard (see Table 6-1). Exactly the same considerations go into the Hazard Analysis Critical Control Point system, which is discussed further in Chapters 1 and 10.

EPIDEMIOLOGICAL EXPERIENCE

Around the turn of the century many countries, including the United States, suffered devastating outbreaks of milkborne disease. Thousands of people contracted typhoid fever, brucellosis, tuberculosis, scarlet fever, diarrheal disease, and diphtheria from commercial dairy products. Even as late as the mid-1920s, 50 to 60 people died every year in the United States from milkborne disease (Bryan, 1983; Foster, 1973). Public health authorities and the dairy industry then imposed controls on milk production, developed safe and effective pasteurization procedures, and set sensible microbiological limits that ensured a better quality of commercial milk supplies. The net effect of these measures was to change milk from one of the United States' most dangerous foods to one of its safest. How much of this can be attributed to microbiological criteria is not clear, but surely they helped.

A similar story can be told for drinking-water. A combination of water purification, waste treatment, and microbiological criteria has led to the production of safe municipal water supplies throughout the nation. Likewise, the problem of *Salmonella* in processed egg products, first revealed by epidemiological observations during World War II, has been solved by mandatory pasteurization and the application of microbiological criteria to the finished products. Thus the recognition of foodborne disease outbreaks is an important first step in the consideration of the application of microbiological criteria aimed at assuring a safe food supply. On the other hand, while raw meat and poultry are notorious as vehicles in foodborne salmonellosis outbreaks, the application of microbiological criteria for these products would be impractical as a control means as they would not lessen the problem (see Chapter 9, parts B and D).

OPPORTUNITIES FOR CONTAMINATION

Some raw foods are commonly contaminated with potentially dangerous pathogenic and toxigenic microorganisms. *Salmonella* spp. and *Campylobacter* spp. are frequently found on raw meat and poultry. Recent surveys have shown that 37% of the broiler chickens on the market carried viable salmonellae. The incidence of these organisms in fresh pork is somewhat lower than that in poultry, and in beef it is lower still (Bryan et al., 1979; Tompkin, 1978). Salmonellae cannot be assumed to be absent from any raw animal product and have been ruled by the courts as an inherent defect in red meats and poultry (*APHA* v. *Butz*, 1974).

Vegetables may carry spores of *C. botulinum, Clostridium perfringens,* and *Bacillus cereus* from the soil. Also, up to 50% of food handlers shed staphylococci from their upper respiratory tracts. While small numbers of these organisms can be expected in foods, they present no hazard. Microbiological criteria, therefore, are not indicated unless opportunities for growth occur. Shellfish from polluted waters may be contaminated with various intestinal pathogens, including salmonellae and viruses (e.g., hepatitis A, ECHO, and Norwalk-like agent). Use of microbiological criteria as part of the National Shellfish Sanitation Program assists in providing protection from these agents.

On the other hand, marine fish and crustaceans, particularly those from warm waters, often carry *Vibrio parahaemolyticus*. In this instance, microbiological criteria for this bacterium would be unwise (see Chapter 4). It would be unrealistic to exclude these and similar raw products from the food supply simply because they contain a potentially dangerous microorganism; they can be rendered safe by appropriate processing and cooking.

OPPORTUNITIES FOR GROWTH

Growth of pathogenic microorganisms in a food increases the likelihood of disease. Multiplication of hazardous microorganisms in a food is determined by the usual conditions that affect growth, i.e., available nutrients, pH, water activity, concentration of inhibitory chemicals (e.g., sulfur dioxide, nitrite, phosphate, salt, sugar), temperature of storage, gaseous atmosphere within the container, and the presence of competing microorganisms. In fermented foods, for example, harmless and desirable organisms are often added to the raw product as starter cultures, and conditions are provided for their rapid growth and fermentation. The resulting acid or alcohol normally serves as an effective preservative against organisms that can cause disease.

Under normal circumstances, one or more of the above conditions is deliberately manipulated to prevent growth of undesirable microbes and thereby effect preservation. Safety exists when the appropriate preservative factors are under control. However, danger can result when events do not follow the expected course. *S. aureus* may grow during the manufacture of cheese and fermented sausage if the lactic starter culture does not produce acid fast enough. Botulinal toxin has developed in homemade dill pickles that did not contain enough salt. There have been instances of botulism from home-canned tomatoes that had mold growth on the surface—apparently the mold metabolized the acid, the pH rose, and conditions became suitable for growth of *C. botulinum*.

New technological procedures and marketing methods may introduce hazards that did not exist before. For example, the application of vacuum packing to Great Lakes smoked fish (see Chapter 1) greatly extended the keeping time, but it also provided time for *C. botulinum* to grow when the fish was not properly refrigerated. This happened in 1960 and again in 1963 when two outbreaks of Type E botulism led to 19 cases and 7 deaths (CDC, 1979; Osheroff et al., 1964).

Canned mushrooms present another example of hazard resulting from technological change. When mushroom canners switched to vibrating fillers, they consequently packed more product into each can. This changed the heat penetration characteristics with the result that the heat processes previously used were no longer adequate. Underprocessing resulted and a serious botulism hazard was created. During 1973 five mushroom processors recalled products because of survival of *C. botulinum;* no deaths, however, were reported from these products (FDA, 1973).

Pressures to reduce the concentration of inhibitory chemicals in foods can be expected to increase the incidence of disease. Some nations severely limit the concentration of sulfur dioxide. The United States has already reduced the amount of nitrite in cured meats, and individuals are being urged to restrict the intake of salt. Phosphate, a rather effective antibotulinal agent in cheese spreads, faces mounting opposition to its use at current levels. Foods affected by these actions will have reduced stability and safety and may thereby become candidates for microbiological criteria.

OPPORTUNITIES FOR SURVIVAL

As a general rule, foodborne pathogens will survive for long periods in dry or frozen foods. Salmonellae will die off slowly in milk chocolate or dried eggs, but there is never certainty that all are dead. Spores, of course, will survive indefinitely. These facts argue for the usefulness of microbiological criteria in judging the safety of a processed product.

Special situations that require careful interpretations do exist. For example, enterotoxigenic strains of *S. aureus* sometimes grow in cheese during manufacture. Population levels of one to five million cells per gram of food produce detectable amounts of enterotoxin. During ripening the numbers of staphylococci may decline substantially, but the active enterotoxin level remains unchanged and the product continues to be hazardous. A viable count of 10,000 *S. aureus* per gram of aged cheese has been proposed as a suitable basis for suspecting that enterotoxin may be present (NRC, 1975; see also Chapter 4 and Chapter 9, part A). A positive test for thermonuclease (TNase) strengthens this suspicion and justifies testing for enterotoxin itself.

On the other hand, commercial mayonnaise provides an extremely hostile environment to enteric pathogens. Both salmonellae and staphylococci die within a few days when exposed to the acidity of mayonnaise (Smittle, 1977) and therefore no microbiological criteria for these organisms are needed. However, microbiological criteria to control spoilage organisms are usefully applied during the manufacture of mayonnaise and salad dressing (see Chapter 9, part N).

PROCESSING CONDITIONS

Many processes include a bactericidal treatment that will eliminate some or all organisms of public health significance. Such treatments range in severity from the pasteurization of eggs, which will eliminate salmonellae, through the pasteurization of milk, which will destroy all nonsporeforming pathogens, to the commercial sterilization of low-acid canned foods, which will inactivate the spores of *C. botulinum*. Acidification of certain canned foods such as palm hearts and pimientos reduces the heat treatment necessary for preservation. Another bactericidal agent of limited use is ethylene oxide, which can be applied to spices and a few other items. The effectiveness of all these treatments is known; the need is to ensure that they are carried out properly.

Direct measurements are often simpler and more effective for assuring safety than are microbiological criteria. Examples include temperature in processing of pork products to destroy trichinellae, pH in monitoring fermentation in dry and semidry sausages, residual chlorine in cannery cooling water, and phosphatase to detect faulty pasteurization. These measurements provide information at the time of processing when it is most needed.

While certain processing steps can reduce the incidence of foodborne pathogens in a product, other steps can do the reverse. Staphylococci may be added to crab meat during hand picking. Exposure of cooked food to work surfaces and utensils previously used for raw animal products can result in transfer of salmonellae to the finished food. Even canned foods can become recontaminated from cooling water through minute defects in the containers.

SUSCEPTIBILITY OF PROBABLE CONSUMERS

Infants, the aged, the malnourished, and the infirm are more susceptible to salmonellae and other infectious agents than are healthy adults. Therefore, foods intended primarily for these susceptible groups are expected to meet more rigid microbiological requirements than are foods for the general population (NRC, 1969).

ULTIMATE TREATMENT

Although regulatory agencies make no special point of the ultimate treatment before consumption, the fact remains that food to be cooked shortly before eating is less likely to carry viable pathogenic organisms than is food prepared and last handled some time previously. That is to say, a *Salmonella* organism in a dry turkey soup mix that will be cooked before eating is less hazardous than another *Salmonella* in a bar of milk chocolate. Thus, microbiological criteria have less importance with food that must be cooked than they have for ready-to-use products.

REFERENCES

APHA v. *Butz*
  1974   *American Public Health Association, et al., Appellants* v. *Earl Butz, Secretary of Agriculture, et al.* D.C. Civil Court. Suit to enjoin Secretary of Agriculture against alleged violations of the Wholesome Meat Act. Pp. 331–338. 511 F. 2d. 331 (D.C. Civ. 1974).
Bryan, F. L.
  1983   Epidemiology of milk-borne diseases. J. Food Prot. 46:637–649.
Bryan, F. L., M. S. Fanelli, and H. Riemann
  1979   *Salmonella* infections. In Food-borne Infections and Intoxications, H. Riemann and F. L. Bryan, eds. New York: Academic Press.

CDC (Center for Disease Control)
  1979   Botulism in the United States, 1899–1977. Handbook for Epidemiologists, Clinicians, and Laboratory Workers. Atlanta: CDC.
FDA (Food and Drug Administration)
  1973   FDA orders examination of all canned mushrooms. FDA Consumer, October, p. 28.
Foster, E. M.
  1973   Preservation of foodstuffs and beverages. Pasteur Sesquicentenniel Commemorative Symposium. ASM News 39(1): 32–35.
ICMSF (International Commission on Microbiological Specifications for Foods)
  1985   Microorganisms in Foods. 2. Sampling for microbiological analysis: Principles and specific applications. 2nd Ed. In preparation.
NRC (National Research Council)
  1969   An Evaluation of the *Salmonella* Problem. Committee on *Salmonella*. Washington, D.C.: National Academy of Sciences.
  1975   Prevention of Microbial and Parasitic Hazards Associated with Processed Foods. A Guide for the Food Processor. Committee on Food Protection. Washington, D.C.: National Academy of Sciences, pp. 82–83.
Osheroff, B. J., G. G. Slocum, and W. M. Decker
  1964   Status of botulism in the United States. Pub. Health Reports: 79(10):871.
Smittle, R. B.
  1977   Microbiology of mayonnaise and salad dressing: A review. J. Food Prot. 40:415–422.
Tompkin, R. B.
  1978   The red meat processor's role in salmonellosis prevention. In Proceedings, National Salmonellosis Seminar, W. B. Bixler, ed. Washington, D.C.

4

Selection of Pathogens as Components of Microbiological Criteria

INTRODUCTION

Microorganisms as components of microbiological criteria for foods may be grouped into two categories: pathogens, including their harmful toxins, and indicator organisms. Pathogens suitable as components of a criterion are those likely to be found in the food or ingredient which thereby becomes a potential vehicle for its transmission to consumers. Suitable indicator organisms or agents are those whose presence in the food or ingredient indicates: (1) the likelihood that a pathogen(s) or harmful toxin(s) of concern also may be present; (2) the likelihood that faulty practices occurred during production, processing, or distribution that may adversely affect the safety and/or the shelf-life of the product; or (3) that the food or ingredient is unsuited for an intended use. Furthermore, adequate and practical methods must be available for detection and/or enumeration of selected pathogens or indicator organisms. Other ancillary factors that relate to the selection of contaminants, as well as other components of microbiological criteria, are presented elsewhere (see Chapters 2, 3, and 6). Indicator organisms that may be useful for the purposes indicated above are treated in Chapter 5.

This chapter deals with the various foodborne pathogens that are of particular concern. Each pathogen is grouped in one of three categories according to the severity of the hazard it may present. The discussion of each organism or group of organisms includes its relative importance, the status of the method(s) available for its detection and/or enumeration, and conclusions on suitability of the organism as a component of a microbiological criterion.

PATHOGENS

An extensive listing of foodborne diseases and the agents that cause them has been prepared by Bryan (1982). Included in this manual are brief but pertinent summaries of the nature of the organism, incubation period and symptoms of the disease, likely sources and reservoirs of the organisms, the foods most likely involved, and the most useful specimens for laboratory examination. Similar listings with emphasis on only the more commonly occurring and important foodborne diseases also are available (Bryan, 1980a; Sanders et al., 1984).

Although the list of foodborne diseases of microbial etiology is long, only about 20 are known to be transmitted by foods with a consequence serious and frequent enough to cause concern relative to microbiological criteria (see listing below). As for the others, either proof of their transmission by foods is inconclusive or suspect or they are so infrequently foodborne that their involvement is remote. Table 4-1 presents a summary of reported foodborne disease outbreaks in the United States during the years 1977-1981 (CDC, 1983). Similar data are available for Japan (Okabe, 1974), the United Kingdom (Vernon, 1977), and Canada (Health and Welfare Canada, 1981).

The number of foodborne disease organisms required to produce disease has been investigated to some extent, largely through feeding studies using healthy adult volunteers. A summary of a series of such studies is given in Table 4-2. Except for *Shigella dysenteriae*, the results indicate that large numbers were necessary to cause illness in the volunteers. However, it would be imprudent to conclude that small dosages are relatively harmless. Host parasite susceptibility varies, the more susceptible being infants, the aged, and debilitated persons. Studies in connection with investigations of certain *Salmonella* foodborne outbreaks indicate that relatively few cells of several serotypes caused illness. A summary of these studies in which the number of cells found in the causative vehicles were quantitated is shown in Table 4-3. Compared to those given in Table 4-2, the numbers are surprisingly low. Assuming that a reasonable serving was consumed, e.g., approximately 3 ounces of chocolate, the number causing illness would approximate 0.6-6 cells of *Salmonella eastbourne*. A 3-ounce serving of cereal would have contained approximately 600-1,200 cells of *Salmonella muenchen*.

It must be recognized that investigation and reporting of foodborne disease outbreaks are grossly incomplete. For example, about 400-500 outbreaks and 10,000-20,000 cases are reported annually in the United States. The actual incidence, however, may be 100 times or more the reported figures (CDC, 1981a; Hauschild and Bryan, 1980). Although

TABLE 4-1 Confirmed Foodborne Disease Outbreaks, by Etiology, United States, 1977–1981

Etiology	1977 No. (%)	1978 No. (%)	1979 No. (%)	1980 No. (%)	1981 No. (%)
BACTERIAL					
A. hinshawii	1 (0.6)	—	—	—	—
B. cereus	—	6 (3.9)	2 (1.3)	9 (4.1)	8 (3.2)
C. jejuni	—	—	—	5 (2.3)	10 (4.0)
C. botulinum	20 (12.7)	12 (7.8)	7 (4.0)	14 (6.3)	11 (4.4)
C. perfringens	6 (3.8)	9 (5.9)	20 (11.6)	25 (11.3)	28 (11.2)
E. cloacae	—	—	1 (0.6)	—	—
E. coli	—	1 (0.7)	—	1 (0.5)	—
Salmonella	41 (26.1)	45 (29.3)	44 (25.5)	39 (17.7)	66 (26.4)
Shigella	5 (3.2)	4 (2.6)	7 (4.0)	11 (5.0)	9 (3.6)
S. aureus	25 (15.9)	23 (14.9)	34 (19.7)	27 (12.2)	44 (17.6)
Streptococcus Group A	—	—	—	—	2 (0.8)
Streptococcus Group D	—	1 (0.7)	—	—	1 (0.4)
Streptococcus Group G	—	—	1 (0.6)	—	—
V. cholerae O1	—	1 (0.7)	—	—	—
V. cholerae non-O1	1 (0.6)	—	1 (0.6)	—	1 (0.4)
V. parahaemolyticus	2 (1.3)	2 (1.3)	2 (1.3)	4 (1.8)	2 (0.8)
Y. enterocolitica	—	—	—	—	2 (0.8)
Other	—	1 (0.7)	—	1 (0.5)	1 (0.4)
TOTAL	101 (64.2)	105 (68.5)	119 (69.2)	136 (61.7)	185 (74.0)

CHEMICAL					
Ciguatoxin	3 (1.9)	19 (12.3)	18 (10.4)	15 (6.8)	15 (6.0)
Heavy metals	8 (5.1)	1 (0.7)	1 (0.6)	1 (0.5)	2 (0.8)
Monosodium glutamate	2 (1.3)	—	—	—	2 (0.8)
Mushroom poisoning	5 (3.2)	1 (0.6)	1 (0.6)	—	11 (4.4)
Paralytic shellfish	—	4 (2.6)	—	5 (2.2)	—
Scombrotoxin	13 (8.3)	7 (4.5)	12 (7.0)	29 (13.0)	7 (2.8)
Other	6 (3.8)	5 (3.2)	4 (2.3)	16 (7.2)	14 (5.6)
TOTAL	37 (23.6)	37 (23.9)	36 (20.9)	66 (29.7)	51 (20.4)
PARASITIC					
Anisakidae	1 (0.6)	—	—	—	—
Trichinella spiralis	14 (8.9)	7 (4.5)	11 (6.4)	5 (2.3)	7 (2.8)
Other	—	—	—	2 (0.9)	1 (0.4)
TOTAL	15 (9.5)	7 (4.5)	11 (6.4)	7 (3.2)	8 (3.2)
VIRAL					
Hepatitis A	4 (2.5)	5 (3.2)	5 (2.9)	10 (4.5)	6 (2.4)
Other	—	—	1 (0.6)	2 (0.9)	—
TOTAL	4 (2.5)	5 (3.2)	6 (3.5)	12 (5.4)	6 (2.4)
CONFIRMED TOTAL	157 (100.0)	154 (100.0)	172 (100.0)	221 (100.0)	250 (100.0)

SOURCE: Centers for Disease Control, 1983.

TABLE 4-2   Summary of Various Organisms Found to Induce Illness in Volunteer Feeding Studies[a]

Organism	Number Causing Illness[b]	Reference
Campylobacter jejuni	10^6	Steele and McDermott, 1978
	5×10^2	Robinson, 1981
Clostridium perfringens		
type A, heat resistant	10^8-10^9	Dische and Elek, 1957
type A, heat sensitive	10^9	Hauschild and Thatcher, 1967
Escherichia coli	10^6-10^{10}	DuPont et al., 1971; Ferguson and June, 1952; June et al., 1953; Kirby et al., 1950
Salmonella anatum	10^5-10^8	McCullough and Eisele, 1951a,b
Salmonella derby	10^7	McCullough and Eisele, 1951c
Salmonella bareilly	10^5-10^6	McCullough and Eisele, 1951c
Salmonella meleagridis	10^6-10^7	McCullough and Eisele, 1951a,b
Salmonella newport	10^6	McCullough and Eisele, 1951c
Salmonella pullorum	10^9-10^{10}	McCullough and Eisele, 1951d
Salmonella typhi	10^4-10^9	Hornick et al., 1970a,b; DuPont et al., 1970
Shigella flexneri	10^2-10^9	Shaughnessy et al., 1946; DuPont et al., 1969, 1972
Shigella dysenteriae	10^1-10^4	Levine et al., 1973
Streptococcus faecalis subsp. *liquefaciens*	10^9-10^{10}	Sedova, 1970
Vibrio cholerae		
(unbuffered)	10^8-10^{11}	Hornick et al., 1971
(buffered)	10^3-10^4	Hornick et al., 1971
Vibrio parahaemolyticus		
(buffered)	10^{5-7}	Sanyal and Sen, 1974
Yersinia enterocolitica	10^9	Szita et al., 1973

[a]Adapted from Bryan (1977).
[b]In some studies no attempt was made to determine lowest levels. In others, such attempts were made for *C. perfringens*, *V. cholerae.*, *S. typhi*, *S. anatum*, *S. meleagridis*, *S. derby*, *E. coli*, *S. faecalis* subsp. *liquefaciens*, *Y. enterocolitica*. Adults were subjects for all studies except for *E. coli* studies in which some nonadults were included.

incomplete, the reporting at current levels through the efforts of the Centers for Disease Control (CDC) and other federal and state agencies does help to provide a continuing assessment of trends in etiologic agents and food vehicles. Furthermore, such efforts contribute to (1) identification and removal of contaminated products from the market, (2) correction of faulty food-handling practices, (3) identification and treatment of human carriers, and (4) detection of newly emerging agents of foodborne disease. Items (1) and (2) are of particular significance with respect to microbiological criteria.

Many sources of information, those referred to above and others (Bryan, 1972; Riemann and Bryan, 1979; Sours and Smith, 1980), amply justify

TABLE 4-3 Number of Various Organisms Found in Foods Involved as Vehicles in Foodborne Outbreaks

Vehicle	Strain/Serotype	Number	Reference
Ham	S. infantis	23,000/g	Angelotti et al., 1961
Frozen egg yolk	S. typhimurium	0.6/g	CDC, 1967
Carmine dye	S. cubana	30,000/0.3 g	Lang et al., 1967
Protein dietary supplement			
Spice flavored	S. minnesota	11/100 g	Andrews and Wilson, 1976
Apricot flavored	S. minnesota	13/100 g	
Chocolate	S. eastbourne	1.7/100 g	Deibel[a]
		0.6/100 g	
		6/100 g	
		2/100 g	
		2.5/g	Craven et al., 1975
		0.2–0.9/g	D'Aoust et al., 1975
Cereal	S. muenchen	7–14/g	Silverstolpe et al., 1962
Frozen dessert (Chiffonade)	S. typhimurium and S. braenderup	113/75 g	Armstrong et al., 1970
Raw hamburger	S. newport	60-2300/100 g	Fontaine et al., 1978

[a]R. H. Deibel, Department of Bacteriology, University of Wisconsin, Madison, personal communication, 1974.

the listing of the organisms and/or toxins given below as being of concern as causative agents of foodborne disease in the United States. The agents are grouped according to the seriousness of the hazard they present when found in food. The grouping parallels that of the International Commission on Microbiological Specifications for Foods (see Chapter 4 and Table 7 of ICMSF, 1974). Some rearrangement within categories was necessary as the scope of the current report is confined to the United States.

Severe Hazards: *Clostridium botulinum, Shigella, Vibrio cholerae, Salmonella typhi, Salmonella paratyphi A, Salmonella paratyphi B, Salmonella paratyphi C, Salmonella sendai, Salmonella cholerae-suis, Brucella abortus, Brucella melitensis* and *Brucella suis, Mycobacterium bovis,* hepatitis A virus, fish and shellfish toxins, and certain mycotoxins.

C. botulinum causes botulism, which frequently results in death. Shiga dysentery, caused by *S. dysenteriae,* is an example of a disease that, without specific treatment, may result in high mortalities (ICMSF, 1978). While the illness caused by the other three species of *Shigella (S. flexneri, S. boydii, S. sonnei)* is usually less severe, considerable variation in severity occurs; hence, these species are included. Cholera may be severe and result in death if untreated; however, mild to asymptomatic infections are common. Salmonellae more or less strictly adapted to humans are

S. typhi, S. paratyphi A, S. paratyphi B, S. paratyphi C, and *S. sendai.* These species and *S. cholerae-suis* (primary host, swine) generally produce a systemic syndrome as opposed to the gastroenteritis caused by other *Salmonella* (NRC, 1969). Brucellosis and tuberculosis, although now rarely foodborne in the United States, result in serious consequences for those affected. The effects of hepatitis A virus infection may range from asymptomatic to acute liver disease resulting in severe debilitation and even death. Paralytic shellfish poisoning is a severe intoxication that may result in respiratory failure and death. Ciguatera fish poisoning results in gastrointestinal and neurological symptoms with disability lasting several days, several months, or longer. The disease implications of mycotoxins for man are still not clear; however, aflatoxin is a known carcinogen.

Moderate Hazards with potentially extensive spread: *Salmonella,* pathogenic *Escherichia coli* (PEC), and *Streptococcus pyogenes.*

Moderate Hazards with limited spread: *Staphylococcus aureus, Clostridium perfringens, Bacillus cereus, Vibrio parahaemolyticus, Coxiella burnetii, Yersinia enterocolitica, Campylobacter fetus* subsp. *jejuni, Trichinella spiralis,* and histamine.

The agents listed as "moderate" hazards generally cause illnesses milder than those caused by the agents listed as "severe" hazards. Agents with potential for extensive spread are often initially spread by specific foods; however, secondary spread to other foods commonly occurs from environmental contamination and cross-contamination within processing plants and food preparation areas including homes. The illness dose for these agents may be low.

Agents in the lowest risk group (moderate hazards, limited spread) are found in many foods, usually in small numbers. Generally, illness is caused only when ingested foods contain large numbers of the pathogens, e.g., *C. perfringens,* or have at some time contained large enough numbers to produce sufficient toxin to cause illness, e.g., *S. aureus.* Outbreaks are usually restricted to consumers of a particular meal or a particular kind of food, e.g., milk in the instance of *C. burnetii. Y. enterocolitica* and *C. fetus* subsp. *jejuni* are included as moderate hazards although the full importance of these species is not clear, nor are the factors governing secondary spread to other foods.

Severe Hazards

Clostridium botulinum

The importance of the botulism hazard in foods is well known and needs no further elaboration here. Food containing botulinal toxin in any amount is unacceptable. Excellent methods are available for detection of *C. botulinum* and its toxins (AOAC, 1980). They are invaluable for the examination of foods implicated in botulism outbreaks and for other investigational purposes. However, the expertise required in application of the methods and in the interpretation of results precludes their use in most laboratories that routinely analyze food. Sampling and testing for purposes of routine surveillance of the botulism hazard in foods is ill advised. The probability that the examination of any reasonable size sample of a low-acid canned food contaminated with *C. botulinum* would result in. detection of the organism is too low to assure the level of safety necessary. Safety of low-acid canned foods must depend primarily on instrumentation and other process assurance mechanisms to be certain that processing has been adequately accomplished and that container integrity has been maintained (FDA, 1979). Control of the botulism hazard in perishable foods must be based on adherence to food-handling practices that will prevent growth of *C. botulinum*.

Shigella

The importance and epidemiology of shigellosis as a foodborne disease has been reviewed by Morris (1984) and Bryan (1979). Briefly, *Shigella* is host-adapted to humans and higher primates. Shigellosis is an infectious disease transmitted most commonly by close person-to-person contact via the fecal-oral route. Poor personal hygiene, inadequate sanitation, and crowded living conditions are important factors in the spread of this disease. Migrant workers often are victims and outbreaks among younger children and others confined in hospital wards are not uncommon. Processed foods are rarely involved as vehicles of transmission; however, food may be easily contaminated during preparation by infected food handlers, particularly by convalescent carriers. The infectious dose can be as low as 10 organisms. The mere presence of *Shigella* in a food that will not be subsequently cooked presents a serious hazard.

Detection of *Shigella* in foods is usually done by an enrichment procedure followed by subculturing to a variety of selective/differential media (Morris, 1984). The procedures are useful for the examination of suspect foods in the investigation of outbreaks and should be applied when indicated. The method for their detection in foods is not sensitive and quantitation is rarely done.

Because processed foods are rarely involved and analytical procedures are relatively insensitive and complicated, routine sampling and testing for *Shigella* would not be practical in routine surveillance programs. Sanitary handling of food prior to serving, strict adherence to good personal hygiene practices, and proper temperature control should be relied upon as effective preventive measures.

Vibrio cholerae

Cholera is an acute diarrheal disease caused by *V. cholerae*. This species includes the strains that cause cholera epidemics (*V. cholerae* O group 1) and others that are similar to the epidemic strains but have not been associated with epidemic disease; these organisms, now referred to as non-O1 *V. cholerae*, were formerly referred to as nonagglutinating vibrios (NAGs) or noncholera vibrios (NCVs) (CDC, 1979a). The number of *V. cholerae* O1 and non-O1 infections found in the United States has increased in recent years. Recent outbreaks have been reported from several states (Blake et al., 1980; CDC, 1979a,b, 1980). Raw oysters and steamed crabs were often epidemiologically associated with infections.

V. cholerae O1 produces an enterotoxin that causes excretion and severe loss of fluid and electrolytes from the body. The mortality rate for severe cases where rapid replacement of fluid and electrolytes is not provided may reach 30-40% (WHO, 1976). Non-O1 *V. cholerae* infections are characterized by diarrhea, nausea and vomiting, abdominal cramps and fever (Morris et al., 1981), and the symptoms may range from mild to severe. Certain of the non-O1 strains produce a toxin similar to that of O1 strains. The pathogenic mechanism for the nontoxigenic strains, however, is not well defined.

Detection of *V. cholerae* in foods (Twedt et al., 1984) requires primary enrichment. Subsequently, subculturing usually is done in selective media. Suspect colonies are confirmed by biochemical and serological procedures and other tests, including a mouse adrenal cell assay for cholera toxin. The method has proven useful in the examination of Moore swabs and gauze filters used in investigations of suspect water areas for presence of *V. cholerae* (CDC, 1979b). However, it is too insensitive and time-consuming for routine application to oysters, crabs, and other seafoods in surveillance programs. Further, experience has shown that testing crabs from suspect waters was not an effective and beneficial means of monitoring such areas (CDC 1979b). Over 2,000 crabs were examined in one such program and *V. cholerae* was found in none. Thus, microbiological criteria with *V. cholerae* as the designated contaminant are not indicated. Strict adherence to measures specified under the National Shellfish Sanitation Program should be relied upon as the principal means of minimizing the risk of raw oysters, clams, and mussels contaminated with *V. cholerae* from reaching the consumer. Furthermore, adequate heat treatment of crabmeat before eating and use of good sanitary practices during the handling of crabmeat before and after heat treatment (especially avoidance of cross-contamination between raw and heated product) should prevail.

Salmonella

With respect to the establishment and application of microbiological criteria for *Salmonella* in foods, there is little if any present justification to consider the human-adapted species and *S. cholerae-suis* mentioned above (see "Pathogens, severe hazards") differently from the other *Salmonella*. All are considered pathogenic for human beings and methods for their detection and enumeration are equally applicable; therefore, see the discussion of *Salmonella* below under "Moderate Hazards."

Brucella abortus, Brucella melitensis, Brucella suis, and Mycobacterium bovis

Brucellosis and tuberculosis in man are serious diseases often resulting in long-term illness and serious complications. Brucellosis is primarily an occupational disease of workers in the meat-processing and livestock industries. However, since the organisms may be shed in milk from infected animals, the disease may be acquired by drinking raw milk, usually from infected cattle and goats, or by eating fresh cheese made from such raw milk. Similarily *M. bovis* may be shed in milk from infected cattle and goats and be transmitted to human beings through the milk. The organisms, however, do not survive commercial milk pasteurization processes.

The methods for detection of *Brucella* and *Mycobacterium* in foods are insensitive and lengthy and are unsuited for routine application to milk or other foods.

The likelihood of brucellosis in man being acquired from milk is remote for several reasons. First, availability of pasteurized milk in the United States is virtually universal. Second, the National Cooperative State/Federal Brucellosis Eradication Program in cattle (USDA, 1982), which has been operative over a period of many years, has reduced the incidence of this disease in cattle to an extremely low level. For example, 11 states are now certified as brucellosis-free and all but 4 of the remaining states are nearly brucellosis-free. Finally, the public has been repeatedly warned of the risk of acquiring milkborne diseases by consuming raw milk. Nevertheless a few, some perhaps in ignorance, persist in ignoring the hazards involved. Others, overly impressed by often unwarranted emphasis on attributes of so-called "natural foods", continue to seek out raw milk for their fluid milk needs. Consequently, occasional outbreaks of diseases, including brucellosis and tuberculosis, do occur through the consumption of raw milk and products such as unripened cheese prepared from raw milk.

As part of the brucellosis eradication program, serological techniques are used in testing the milk of dairy cattle to detect *Brucella* infections. In this circumstance, a microbiological criterion is applicable, effective, and widely applied.

Milkborne tuberculosis in the United States is rare, largely due to the reasons stated above for brucellosis. The State/Federal Tuberculosis Eradication Program for cattle (USDA, 1981a) has practically eliminated the disease from milking animals. Milk pasteurization has been an effective measure. At one time, the mandatory time-temperature requirements for milk pasteurization were based on those necessary for the destruction of *M. tuberculosis;* present requirements are even more stringent. Also, educational programs warning of the hazards of raw milk consumption have contributed to reducing the exposure to infection.

While serological methods are used in testing cattle for tuberculosis infection, neither these tests nor cultural methods are applied routinely to milk available for purchase by the public. However, suspect tuberculosis lesions found at time of carcass inspection at slaughter are routinely cultured for *Mycobacterium*. This is an important part of the state/federal eradication program. In this circumstance, a microbiological criterion is appropriate, effective, and routinely applied.

Viruses

Viruses as agents of foodborne disease have been reviewed extensively by Cliver (1979) and Cliver et al. (1984). Hepatitis A, the cause of infectious hepatitis, is a virus frequently transmitted to humans by food. The consequences of infection range from asymptomatic (inapparent infection) to severe liver involvement and damage, and even death. Infected persons shed large numbers of the virus in the feces several days before onset of symptoms and during the acute stage of infection. Raw or inadequately cooked shellfish that have been harvested from sewage-polluted waters have been the most frequent food vehicles for transmission. Contamination of foods may occur during handling and processing by infected persons during the incubation period of the disease.

Viral diarrhea may be transmitted through foods. The agents most commonly involved resemble the "Norwalk" virus. The severity of the disease however is less than for hepatitis A. Poliomyelitis also may be foodborne.

Viruses are detected on the basis of their infectivity; therefore, a susceptible living host must be available for testing. Cell cultures are most frequently used. However, some viruses are difficult to isolate and others have not been successfully grown in the laboratory. Only recently has hepatitis A been grown in cell culture. Poliomyelitis virus can be readily isolated and cultured.

Microbiological criteria for viruses in foods are not practical at present because of the lack of readily applied analytical methods. Control measures for hepatitis A must depend primarily upon surveillance of shellfish growing waters (see Chapter 5 on fecal coliforms). Prevention of contamination of other foods, including shellfish, with hepatitis A and the diarrheal viruses must depend upon the application of personal hygiene and sanitary handling practices in processing plants and food preparation and serving areas. Poliomyelitis is effectively controlled by universal vaccination.

Fish and Shellfish Toxins

Poisonings through eating toxic fish and shellfish are significant causes of human illness. Outbreaks are due primarily to two types of poisoning: ciguatera poisoning and paralytic shellfish poisoning.

Ciguatera.   This is a type of human poisoning caused by eating fish containing ciguatoxin and perhaps other closely related toxins. The toxin(s) is(are) synthesized by the dinoflagellate *Gambierdiscus toxicus* and possibly by certain other dinoflagellate species (Bagnis et al., 1980). Numerous species of fish may feed on these organisms and thereby accumulate the toxin(s) in their tissues. Toxicity may be magnified by transfer through the fish food chain, e.g., large carnivores tend to be more toxic than herbivores and small carnivores. Between 1977 and 1981 ciguatera fish poisoning was the most common foodborne disease in the United States associated with eating fish (Bryan, 1980b; CDC, 1983).

Much confusion has been associated with ciguatoxin poisoning. Withers (1982) has presented a comprehensive review of this problem. Until recently, it was thought that eating fish containing the toxin(s) produced by the dinoflagellate *Ptychodicus breve* (formerly named *Gymnodinium breve*) was the cause of ciguatoxin poisoning of humans. Extensive fish kills in Gulf coastal waters are due to ingestion of this organism by fish. The organism is often present in massive numbers in the "red tides" that occur sporadically in Gulf coastal waters. It has recently become apparent that the toxin(s) of *Ptychodicus breve* is(are) not the cause of ciguatoxin poisoning in humans. Rather it is the toxin(s) of *G. toxicus* that now appear to be the principal cause of the fish poisoning in humans.

The factors that trigger the buildup of toxic concentrations of the toxin(s) of *G. toxicus* and possibly those of other dinoflagellate species are not clear. Further, the toxins, other than ciguatoxin, are not well defined and assay methods for them are neither precise nor specific. Because of the lack of sufficient knowledge in these areas there are no federal or state surveillance programs for preventing the occurrence of ciguatoxin poisoning. At present, there is no basis for establishment and application of a microbiological criterion. However, research is under way to determine the conditions that lead to the occurrence of toxic fish and the nature of the toxin(s) involved, and to develop methods for quantitation of the toxins. For further details see the reviews by Withers (1982) and DeSilva and Poli (1982).

Paralytic Shellfish Poisoning.   Paralytic shellfish poisoning (PSP) is one of the most toxic forms of food poisoning. Certain species of dinoflagellates, most notably *Gonyaulax catenella* and *Gonyaulax tamarensis,* produce saxitoxin, which is known to cause PSP. However, recent studies (Oshima et al., 1977; Shimizu, 1979) have shown that toxic shellfish may contain multiple toxins and that saxitoxin represents only a part of the total toxicity. These newly discovered toxins are related to saxitoxin and their pharmacological action seems to be similar to that of saxitoxin. Shellfish ingest the dinoflagellates and concentrate the toxins in their tissues. Ingestion of toxic shellfish of sufficient toxicity causes acute toxicity in humans. Quantitation of saxitoxin and related toxins is done by mouse bioassay (APHA, 1970).

There are medical records of over 1,650 cases of PSP worldwide that have resulted in at least 300 fatalities (Dale and Yentsch, 1978). Outbreaks, although infrequent, occur sporadically along the Atlantic and Pacific coasts of the United States (CDC, 1983). Shellfish involved most frequently are mussels, clams, soft-shelled clams, butter clams, and occasionally, scallops.

Routine sampling and testing for saxitoxins in shellfish obtained at wholesale or retail markets is not practiced, nor is it necessary. However, a microbiological criterion for PSP is applied, as state authorities regularly assay representative samples of shellfish from growing areas. If toxin content reaches 80 μg per 100 g of edible portion of raw shellfish meat, the area is closed to harvesting of the species involved. These actions and other preventive measures are undertaken in accordance with the National Shellfish Sanitation Program (NSSP), a federal/state/ industry cooperative program described in an operations manual (USDHEW, 1965). Although cases of PSP continue to occur, undoubtedly the incidence would be much higher in the absence of this program.

Mycotoxins

A brief and pertinent review of the problem of foodborne mycotoxicosis was prepared by Stoloff (1984). There is serious concern about the possibility that cancer or delayed organ damage can result from repeated ingestion of subacute levels of mycotoxins. The most intensive effort to determine toxicologic significance has been concentrated on the aflatoxins because of their known widespread natural occurrence in foods and feeds. Yet after two decades of intensive research, the implication of aflatoxins for man is still not clear. Accordingly, control efforts are based more on prudence than on demonstrated danger.

Other mycotoxins found in foods or feeds that have prompted toxicological studies are ochratoxin, patulin, penicillic acid, and zearalenone. Results of such studies provide no cause for concern about the incidence and levels of these toxins that have been encountered in foods in the United States.

Mold contamination of raw farm commodities is not completely preventable. Nevertheless, measures to reduce contamination and subsequent growth are effective in reducing the levels of mycotoxins likely to be found in such commodities and subsequently in processed products.

Chemical methods are used for the detection and quantitation of mycotoxins. The development and validation of methods is achieved through a Joint Mycotoxin Committee representing the Association of Official Analytical Chemists (AOAC), the American Association of Cereal Chemists, the American Oil Chemists Society, and the International Union of Pure and Applied Chemistry. All methods validated to date under the aegis of the Joint Mycotoxin Committee have been adopted by AOAC (AOAC, 1980).

At present, FDA has set tolerance levels only for aflatoxins (20 ppb, aflatoxin B_1 wherever encountered; and 0.05 ppb, aflatoxin M_1 in milk). Susceptible foods and feeds are monitored regularly. Thus, in this instance, a microbiological criterion is applicable and widely applied.

Moderate Hazards, Potentially Extensive Spread

Salmonella

Salmonella continues to rank among the three most frequent causative agents of foodborne disease in the United States. As shown in Table 4-1, *Salmonella* was the most frequently reported etiologic agent in the 5-year period 1977-1981.

The problem of foodborne salmonellosis in the United States was extensively evaluated by the *Salmonella* Committee of the National Research Council (NRC, 1969). The committee was primarily concerned with human health; thus, the review was organized around two viewpoints: (1) the disease: its importance, causal organism, and means by which humans become infected; and (2) how humans can be protected. Means of protection included minimizing exposure by reducing the incidence of animal salmonellosis, avoiding contamination of raw and processed foods, and bactericidal treatment and prevention of growth; surveillance, investigation, and control by industry and regulatory agencies; education; and research. Fifty-five recommendations and suggestions for implementation were made by the committee. Because *Salmonella* may be found in many foods (some more sensitive to contamination than others), two of the recommendations are of particular significance relative to the establishment and application of microbiological criteria. They are: (1) development of a realistic assessment of the degree of hazards imposed by various foods and drugs; and (2) development of sampling plans commensurate with the likely degree of hazard inherent in the food and based on the probability that *Salmonella* are present at less than a statistically defined level. The committee proposed such a classification and sampling system. Sampling plans for raw meat, poultry, and fish were not included. The plans suggested by the committee were not designed to replace testing or other routine surveillance operations of food manufacturers or government agencies. They were intended for use in arriving at a final decision on whether to accept or reject a particular lot in question. In an interesting departure from this principle, FDA has taken the position that the sampling plan, including the acceptance criterion, is applicable to any lot of product tested in connection with any of FDA's surveillance or compliance programs and is not restricted to use with questionable lots.

The current state of analytical methods is no barrier to the designation of *Salmonella* in microbiological criteria. An AOAC official method exists and it is used successfully by many. Also, because of coordination of the efforts of AOAC, the International Standards Organization (ISO), and the International Dairy Federation (IDF), the methods issued by each for the detection of *Salmonella* are essentially the same.

In spite of implementation of some of the National Research Council committee's recommendations and other ancillary control programs, there has been little evidence of change in the magnitude of the *Salmonella* problem over the last 10-15 years (Gangarosa, 1978; Silliker, 1980). Nevertheless, containment of the problem within its present dimension has been a significant accomplishment; for it to remain so or be improved will continue to require major effort.

From the above, it is evident that microbiological criteria in which *Salmonella* is the designated contaminant are appropriate for inclusion with other control measures to reduce the hazard of *Salmonella* in foods, provided that sampling plans are based on a realistic assessment of the hazard the candidate food may present. The *Salmonella* committee provided principles and guidance for such assessment that currently are fully applicable (NRC, 1969).

Pathogenic Escherichia coli (PEC)

Certain biotypes of *E. coli* cause gastrointestinal illness in man and in several other animals. The biotypes include toxigenic and invasive biotypes and others that appear, on the basis of tests for these attributes, to be neither toxigenic nor invasive.

While the importance of *E. coli* in diarrheal disease is well established, outbreaks of *E. coli* foodborne illness in the United States are rare, only three outbreaks having been reported to CDC. One, due to imported soft cheese, occurred in several incidents during late 1971 and early 1972 (Marier et al., 1973). The second, in which the vehicle was beef, occurred in 1978 (CDC, 1981b). Recently, sporadic cases of hemorrhagic colitis due to *E. coli* 0157:H7 were reported in the United States (CDC, 1982b; Riley et al., 1983; Wells et al., 1983) and two outbreaks were reported in Canada (Health and Welfare Canada, 1983a,b). Inadequately cooked hamburger was the vehicle in certain of these cases. It is quite possible that the incidence of PEC outbreaks is underestimated for several reasons, primarily because of the complexities involved in recovery and recognition of PEC from foods.

Methods for recovery of *E. coli* and pathogenic biotypes of *E. coli* are available (Mehlman, 1984). Briefly, the standard enrichment and plating procedures for enumeration of *E. coli* that are so routinely applied in food laboratories neither quantitatively recover pathogenic biotypes nor differentiate them from other *E. coli*. Recognition of pathogenic *E. coli* requires a regimen of serological, pathological (requiring laboratory animals), and biochemical-physiological tests that are costly and require expertise not common to most laboratories that routinely examine foods. Furthermore, these tests, in lieu of controlled primate feeding studies, while highly indicative of human pathogenicity, are not unequivocal. However, the current interest in this foodborne illness might well result in more rapid and specific techniques for recovery and identification of PEC types.

Microbiological criteria for *E. coli* are widely applied (see Chapter 5). However, in view of the lack of procedures that can be routinely applied for detection and enumeration of pathogenic biotypes and the likely low incidence of foodborne PEC illness, establishment of microbiological criteria specifically for these organisms in foods is presently impractical.

Streptococcus pyogenes (Lancefield Group A, beta hemolytic)

Prior to widespread acceptance and availability of pasteurized milk, raw milk was responsible for most of the many outbreaks of scarlet fever and septic sore throat caused by *S. pyogenes*. Cross-infection of cows via milking personnel often resulted in mastitis and subsequent shedding of *S. pyogenes* in the milk from infected udders. Infected food handlers, including carriers, may contaminate foods when preparing them for serving. However, *S. pyogenes* infection is currently infrequently foodborne, and only a few outbreaks were reported during the 5-year period 1977-1981 (see Table 4-1).

Methods that are sufficiently selective and quantitative for routine examination of foods are not available. Accordingly, lack of an adequate method and the infrequency of *S. pyogenes* foodborne outbreaks preclude establishment and application of microbiological criteria as a control measure. Pasteurization of milk, adequate heating of other sensitive foods and sanitary food handling practices are effective measures of preventing foodborne *S. pyogenes* infections.

Moderate Hazards, Limited Spread

Staphylococcus aureus

Staphylococcal food poisoning outbreaks usually are the second most frequently reported causes of foodborne illness in the United States (see Table 4-1). Illness is caused by one or more of several heat-stable enterotoxins produced by certain strains of this species. Bergdoll (1979) provided a comprehensive review of the organism, its nature, the disease it causes, its epidemiology, applicable methodology, and preventive measures for control of the disease.

The number of *S. aureus* required to produce detectable amounts of enterotoxin exceeds one million per gram. The presence of enterotoxin in food, rather than the organism per se, is the principal concern. Large numbers of organisms without associated toxin may be tolerated via ingestion.

Methods for detection and enumeration of *S. aureus* are adequate and practical for purposes of microbiological criteria (Tatini et al., 1984). Certain of these methods provide for resuscitation of injured cells that otherwise would not be detected.

Application of microbiological criteria with *S. aureus* as the designated contaminant is feasible either (1) to indicate the possible presence of detectable enterotoxin in a susceptible food, or (2) to indicate faulty sanitary or production practices in the preparation of food. Small numbers of *S. aureus* are to be expected in foods that have been exposed to or handled by food handlers. Small numbers do not, however, assure safety because the organism can grow and produce enterotoxin and then die off during storage or be killed during subsequent processing (usually heat) of the food; preformed toxin, however, usually will remain in the food. For application of the thermonuclease test to detect possible presence of staphylococcal enterotoxin in food, see Chapter 5 and Chapter 9, Part A.

Clostridium perfringens

C. perfringens enteritis is consistently among the three most frequently reported causes of foodborne illnesses that occur in the United States. Although the presence of small numbers of *C. perfringens* in many foods is unavoidable, large numbers may be indicative of mishandling, including temperature abuse. Several hundred thousand or more per gram of food are usually found in foods involved in outbreaks. An enterotoxin released in the intestine by sporulating cells causes the illness. Hobbs (1979) has provided a comprehensive review of this organism as a foodborne agent.

An adequate and official AOAC method is available for detection and enumeration of *C. perfringens* in foods (Harmon and Duncan, 1984). However, several factors limit its application in routine surveillance of foods. One of these is that vegetative cells of *C. perfringens* lose viability in foods that are frozen or held under refrigeration such as may occur during shipment of samples to laboratories.

The presence of *C. perfringens* in low numbers in many foods usually is unrelated to faulty sanitary practices, and only relatively large numbers in a food are cause for concern. Therefore, the use of *C. perfringens* microbiological criteria in routine surveillance programs would not contribute significantly to prevention of outbreaks of this foodborne illness. Prompt and proper refrigeration and adequate reheating of "leftovers" of sensitive foods should be relied upon as control measures. It is emphasized, however, that foods that are suspect vehicles in gastroenteritis outbreaks and in which *C. perfringens* is likely to be found should be examined quantitatively for this organism. Analysis of foods for this purpose is well within the capabilities of most microbiological laboratories. Also, such foods, especially when their temperature history is unknown, should be tested for the presence of the alpha toxin of *C. perfringens* (Harmon and Duncan, 1984). A detectable quantity of alpha toxin is produced when cell numbers reach about 10^6 *C. perfringens* cells per gram, and the titer or amount of alpha toxin increases as the numbers increase. Since the alpha toxin is little affected by freezing or refrigerated storage of foods, its presence in any detectable amount indicates that the *C. perfringens* population probably was sufficient to cause illness.

Bacillus cereus

Only a few confirmed outbreaks and cases of *B. cereus* foodborne illness have been reported in the United States in recent years (Table 4-1). The lack of greater incidence of reported outbreaks may be due to several factors. The organism is so widely distributed in many environments and foods that it is commonly viewed as relatively harmless under most circumstances. Until recently, methods for its detection and enumeration were somewhat lacking in specificity. As a consequence, the organism was not sought regularly in analysis of foods involved in foodborne outbreaks. In addition, two syndromes of *B. cereus* illness have been recognized; one closely resembles that caused by *S. aureus* and the other resembles that caused by *C. perfringens*. Thus, failure to look for *B. cereus* in suspect foods and the similarity of its disease syndromes to those of *S. aureus* and *C. perfringens* may in large measure account for the infrequent recognition of *B. cereus* foodborne disease. For a detailed discussion of the nature and epidemiology of *B. cereus* gastroenteritis, and in particular its occurrence in the United Kingdom, reference is made to the review by Gilbert (1979).

Currently, the greatest need for sampling and testing for *B. cereus* is in application to suspect foods associated with disease outbreaks. If such analyses are routinely done, a more accurate estimate of the incidence of *B. cereus* in foodborne diseases soon would be obtained, and the more common food vehicles for its transmission would be identified.

At present, *B. cereus* can be enumerated in foods by a plating procedure (Harmon and Goepfert, 1984). However, considerable difficulty may be encountered in obtaining quantitative counts of *B. cereus* in foods containing large numbers of competitive organisms. Colonies of such organisms may overgrow the plates, making *B. cereus* colonies difficult to discern or masking them completely. This overgrowth and other factors largely restrict use of the method to foods that do not contain a large competitive flora. A presumptive plate count can be obtained in 24 hours. If necessary, uncomplicated confirmatory tests can be applied to selected colonies. Generally, presumptive counts would be sufficient for use in surveys to determine population levels likely to be encountered in foods. Similarly, presumptive counts in foods suspect as causes of outbreaks are useful to determine whether or not *B. cereus* was the likely causative agent.

As *B. cereus* is found in low numbers in many foods, it is questionable that application of *B. cereus* microbiological criteria for purposes of routine surveillance of foods would be worthwhile; however, for those foods such as cooked rice products that become more clearly identified as frequent vehicles in *B. cereus* food poisoning outbreaks, a microbiological criterion may be useful.

Vibrio parahaemolyticus

The first reported outbreak outside Japan of foodborne disease caused by this species occurred in Maryland in 1971. Since then 11 confirmed and 8 suspected outbreaks have occurred through 1978 (Bryan, 1980b). In Japan raw fish is the principle vehicle for transmission; in contrast, cooked seafoods (crustaceans) were vehicles in the United States, except for one outbreak in which raw oysters were suspect.

It appears that foodborne disease outbreaks caused by *V. parahaemolyticus* do not occur frequently in the United States. Also, the method for enumeration of *V. parahaemolyticus* is time-consuming and the method for identifying pathogenic strains (Twedt et al., 1984) is complicated. Therefore, microbiological criteria would not be justified in the United States. However, various methods have been helpful in investigations of outbreaks and surveys of susceptible foods. All confirmed outbreaks in the United States resulted from gross cross-contamination of cooked product from contaminated raw product or seawater coupled with subsequent temperature abuse. Therefore, sanitary handling, especially of the cooked product, and refrigerated storage are the most productive preventive measures.

Other *Vibrio* species such as *V. alginolyticus, V. vulnificus, V. fluvialis, V. mimicus, V. metschnikovii,* and *V. hollisae* are associated with human disease (Hickman et al., 1982). More needs to be learned about their ecology, epidemiology, and role in human disease before they can be firmly associated with causes of foodborne illness.

Coxiella burnetii

C. burnetii causes the rickettsial disease Q-fever in man. In infected cattle, sheep, and goats, the organism may be found in large numbers in placental tissues and fluids and feces and also may be shed in the milk.

Q-fever infection in man is usually acquired via the respiratory route as a result of casual or occupational exposure to infected animals and contaminated premises, and can also be acquired through consumption of raw milk. Outbreaks of Q-fever acquired through milk are rare, primarily due to the widespread use of pasteurized milk. No cases were reported to CDC during 1977-1981 (Table 4-1). Present pasteurization time-temperature requirements (USPHS/FDA, 1978) are based on those necessary for the destruction of *C. burnetii* (Enright, 1961; Enright et al., 1956).

C. burnetii is usually detected in milk by either guinea pig inoculation or agglutination tests (Ormsbee, 1980). The former test requires several weeks before results are obtained; the latter is a simple and rapid procedure that is useful in surveys to determine the infection status of dairy animals.

Routine application of microbiological criteria for *C. burnetii* in milk (via serological tests) would not be a practical measure for preventing Q-fever in man in view of the effectiveness, ready availability, and widespread use of pasteurized milk.

Histamine Poisoning

This is the second most frequently reported fishborne illness in the United States (CDC, 1981a). Illness results from eating fish, usually of the *Scombridae* family, which have become toxic after having undergone some microbial decomposition, although overt signs of spoilage may not be evident. Symptoms of scombroid poisoning include flushing, rapid pulse, headache, dizziness, nausea, and diarrhea. With the exception of cheese (see below), foods other than fish are rarely involved.

The occurrence, mechanism of formation, and catabolism of biologically active amines in foods were reviewed by Rice et al. (1976), Voigt and Eitenmiller (1978), and Voigt et al. (1974). Histamine, formed by decarboxylation of histidine, is the apparent principal toxic agent. Scombroid fish normally have a high concentration of the amino acid histidine in their tissues. Many species of bacteria have been associated with histamine formation in various scombroid fish. These include *Proteus morganii, Klebsiella pneumoniae, C. perfringens,* certain coliforms, and others.

Toxic concentrations of histamine and tyramine occasionally occur in certain cheeses (Edwards and Sandine, 1981). Tyramine is the decarboxylation product of tyrosine, which is common in aged cheese including Cheddar, Swiss (Emmenthaler), Gruyere, Roquefort, and certain others. Tyramine can cause critical increases in blood pressure, especially in persons receiving monoamine oxidase inhibiting (MAOI) drugs. Bacterial isolates from cheese that produce amines include certain coliforms, enterococci, and lactobacilli.

An assay method for histamine is available (AOAC, 1980) and is applicable for routine use in a well-equipped and -staffed laboratory. It is common commercial practice within the fisheries industry to organoleptically inspect scombroid-type fish at point of receipt and in-plant at time of evisceration for off-odors and other evidence of mishandling that could result in histamine formation; also, routine examination for histamine is common even though decomposition is not evident. Scombroid fish, usually tuna, offered at import frequently are inspected for evidence of deterioration and are analyzed for histamine content by FDA. Canned albacore, skipjack, and yellow fin tuna with histamine levels of 20 mg or more per 100 g are subject to regulatory action by FDA as being suspect of deterioration. The agency will consider regulatory action against any tuna found to contain between 10 and 20 mg of histamine per 100 g when a second indication of decomposition is present (FDA, 1982a). Furthermore, FDA has established on an interim basis a level of 50 mg of histamine per 100 g of tuna as the level of histamine in tuna that it considers a health hazard. This value may be changed after evaluation of additional data (FDA, 1982b). Accordingly, a microbiological criterion with histamine as the designated contaminant is useful when applied as indicated above to prevent deteriorated fish as well as toxic fish from reaching the processor or consumer. The histamine problem in cheese is not of sufficient incidence to justify routine testing for histamine or tyramine.

Yersinia enterocolitica

The most common symptoms of *Y. enterocolitica* infections are gastroenteritis and terminal ileitis. This organism has been isolated from a wide variety of foods and animals and therefore is of concern as a cause of foodborne illness. Reviews by Lee (1977), Stern and Pierson (1979), and Swaminathan et al. (1982) provide details on *Y. enterocolitica* as a foodborne pathogen. Current methods for its recovery from food and tests for pathogenicity are provided by Feeley and Schiemann (1984).

Currently, members of the species *Y. enterocolitica* include biochemically and serologically diverse strains. In addition to the typical strains of *Y. enterocolitica*, there are closely related species often referred to as *Y. enterocolitica*-like bacteria. The species also includes nonpathogenic strains. Recently, it has been proposed to separate the group into four species, i.e., *Y. enterocolitica, Y. intermedia, Y. frederiksenii,* and *Y. kristensenii* (Bercovier et al., 1980; Brenner, 1980).

Although frequently found in swine and other food animals and often reported as causing illness in humans in many countries, only three documented outbreaks of foodborne illness due to *Y. enterocolitica* have been reported in the United States. One was due to recontaminated chocolate milk (Black et al., 1978), another to tofu (soybean curd packed in water) (Aulisio et al., 1983), and the third to recontaminated pasteurized milk (CDC, 1982a).

Methods for recovery of *Y. enterocolitica* from foods have been improved in recent years; however, no single method is suitable for recovery of all types of this species from various foods. Since not all strains are pathogenic, isolates must be tested for pathogenicity. Primary and secondary or selective enrichment procedures, followed by determination of biochemical and serological characteristics of cultural isolates, are required. Recently, however, a simple method based on reaction of *Y. enterocolitica* with Congo red has been proposed to differentiate pathogenic from nonpathogenic strains (Prpic et al., 1983, 1984). If confirmed, this finding will fulfill an important need.

In view of the limited occurrence of known foodborne outbreaks of *Y. enterocolitica* infections and the complexities of recovery methods, the application of microbiological criteria would currently be of little value. Methods, however, are adequate and their use should be encouraged for investigational purposes whenever foodborne outbreaks occur and in surveys to determine the incidence of potential pathogenic strains in suspect foods.

Campylobacter

The nature and significance of *Campylobacter* as a cause of illness in man were presented in reviews by Doyle (1981) and Bokkenheuser and Mosenthal (1981). The two species pathogenic for humans are *C. fetus* subsp. *jejuni*[1] and *C. fetus* subsp. *intestinalis*. Infections with the subspecies *intestinalis* rarely are foodborne and have been almost entirely limited to compromised patients such as those afflicted with cirrhosis, diabetes, or cancer. On the other hand, *C. fetus* subsp. *jejuni* is recognized as a common cause of gastroenteritis in humans. It is commonly found as a commensal or pathogen in cattle, sheep, fowl, swine, and rodents. In spite of the widespread animal reservoir, few foodborne outbreaks of *Campylobacter* enterocolitis have been reported in the United States. In those few, raw milk and perhaps undercooked poultry were the principal vehicles of transmission (Bryan, 1983; Park et al., 1984).

C. fetus subsp. *jejuni* has been inappropriately termed thermophilic, as it is neither thermophilic nor heat resistant. However, an outstanding characteristic of *C. fetus* subsp. *jejuni* is its growth at 42-43°C (107.6-109.4°F) with poorer growth at 37°C (98.6°F) and no growth at 25°C (77°F). Also, the organism is microaerophilic and requires an atmosphere of reduced oxygen for growth. Because of its sensitivity to air and the relatively high temperature required for growth, growth of *C. fetus* subsp. *jejuni* in foods would be unlikely under ordinary conditions of food han-

---

[1]Taxonomic uncertainty existed over the nomenclature for members of this species. In the eighth edition of "Bergey's Manual" (Buchanan and Gibbons, 1974), they are classified as a single species, *C. fetus* subsp. *jejuni*. In the classification by Veron and Chatelain (1973) and in the Approved Lists of Bacterial Names of the International Committee on Systematic Bacteriology, they are divided into the two species *C. jejuni* and *C. coli*.

dling. Until recently, *C. fetus* subsp. *jejuni* was not usually sought in foods suspect in gastroenteritis outbreaks. Also, while the animal reservoirs are well known, little is known of the incidence of this organism in food supplies in general.

Methods for detecting *C. fetus* subsp. *jejuni* in foods are available (Park et al., 1984). The following conditions are required for accurate analysis: (1) large sample size, (2) suitable microaerophilic condition, (3) selective broth enrichment, (4) filtration to separate the small filterable campylobacters from other nonfilterable organisms in the enrichment cultures, and (5) selective plating agar.

Routine analysis of foods for the presence of *C. fetus* subsp. *jejuni* at the present is not practical because procedures for its recovery from foods are in a state of rapid development. While published data on the incidence of foodborne *Campylobacter* enteritis in the United States are limited, unofficial information appears to indicate that campylobacteriosis is more widespread. Sanitary handling, proper cooking, and prevention of temperature abuse of sensitive foods and avoidance of consumption of raw milk would be far more effective control measures. While microbiological criteria would not be applicable, surveys to ascertain the incidence of this organism in the general food supply should be encouraged and investigations of foodborne gastroenteritis outbreaks should include examination of suspect food for the presence of *C. fetus* subsp. *jejuni*.

Trichinella spiralis

This nematode, which infects many species of animals, causes a frequently severe parasitic disease, trichinellosis, in humans. The most important source of human infection is inadequately cooked pork. Human infection occurs only when the meat of host animals is eaten raw or in an undercooked state. Several outbreaks of trichinellosis are reported annually in the United States. Forty-four outbreaks were reported from 1977 through 1981 (see Table 4-1). For a brief summary of the sources of the parasite and the nature and consequences of infection see Healy and Juranek (1979).

Symptoms of trichinellosis in humans that occur at time of initial invasion include vomiting, diarrhea, and fever. Later, during the phase of parasite distribution to various tissues, joint manifestations, edema, and even myocarditis, encephalitis, and neuritis may occur.

The larvae of *T. spiralis* (trichinellae) in meat can be detected by several methods, including microscopic examination of fresh or digested meat and by enzyme-linked immunosorbent assay (ELISA). While larvae detection methods are routinely used in many countries for examination of swine after slaughter, they are not used in the United States as a means of preventing infected meat from reaching the consumer. Rather, the processing procedures specified in USDA regulations for destroying tri-chinellae in infected meat are emphasized by regulatory agencies and others. These procedures—thorough cooking of pork (to at least 58°C [137°F]), proper meat curing conditions, and specified freezing conditions (USDA, 1973, 1981b)—are considered more effective in preventing human infection as well as less expensive than is routine examination of meat by larvae detection methods.

REFERENCES

Andrews, W. H., and C. R. Wilson
  1976   Salmonella contamination in a protein dietary supplement. Pp. 219–220 in FDA Byliner No. 5. Washington, D.C.: Food and Drug Administration.
Angelotti, R., G. C. Bailey, M. J. Foter, and K. H. Lewis
  1961   Salmonella infantis isolated from ham in food poisoning incident. Public Health Reports 76:771–776.
AOAC (Association of Offical Analytical Chemists)
  1980   Official Methods of Analysis. 13th Ed. Washington, D.C.: AOAC.
APHA (American Public Health Association)
  1970   Recommended Procedures for the Examination of Sea Water and Shellfish. 4th Ed. Washington, D.C.: APHA.
Armstrong, R. W., T. Fodor, G. T. Curlin, A. B. Cohen, G. K. Morris, W. T. Martin, and J. Feldman
  1970   Epidemic Salmonella gastroenteritis due to contaminated imitation ice cream. Am. J. Epidemiol. 91:300–307.
Aulisio, C.C.G., J. T. Stanfield, S. W. Weagant, and W. E. Hill
  1983   Yersiniosis associated with tofu consumption. Serological, biochemical and patho-genicity studies of Yersinia enterocolitica isolates. J. Food Prot. 46:226–230, 234.
Bagnis, R., S. Chanteau, E. Chungue, J. M. Hurtel, T. Yasumoto, and A. Inoue
  1980   Origins of ciguatera fish poisoning: a new dinoflagellate, Gambierdiscus toxicus Adachi and Fukuyo, definitely involved as a causal agent. Toxicon 18:199–208.
Bercovier, H., D. J. Brenner, J. Ursing, A. G. Steigerwalt, G. R. Fanning, J. M. Alonzo, G. P. Carter, and H. H. Mollaret
  1980   Characterization of Yersinia enterocolitica sensu stricto. Curr. Microbiol. 4:201–206.
Bergdoll, M. S.
  1979   Staphylococcal intoxications. Pp. 443–494 in Food-borne Infections and Intoxica-tions. 2nd Ed. H. Riemann and F. L. Bryan, eds. New York: Academic Press.
Black, R. E., R. J. Jackson, T. Tsai, M. Medevesky, M. Shayegani, J. C. Feeley, K.J.E. McLeod, and A. W. Wakelee
  1978   Epidemic Yersinia enterocolitica infection due to contaminated chocolate milk. N. Engl. J. Med. 298(2):76–79.
Blake, P. A., D. T. Allegra, J. D. Snyder, T. J. Barrett, L. McFarland, C. T. Caraway, J. C. Feeley, J. P. Craig, J. V. Lee, N. D. Puhr, and R. A. Feldman
  1980   Cholera—a possible endemic focus in the United States. N. Engl. J. Med. 302:305–309.
Bokkenheuser, V. D., and A. C. Mosenthal
  1981   Campylobacteriosis: A foodborne disease. J. Food Safety 3:127–143.

Brenner, D. J.
  1980   Classification of *Yersinia enterocolitica*. In *Yersinia enterocolitica*. E. J. Bottone,
          ed. Boca Raton, Fla.: CRC Press.
Bryan, F. L.
  1972   Emerging foodborne diseases. I. Their surveillance and epidemiology. J. Milk Food
          Technol. 35:618–625.
  1977   Diseases transmitted by foods contaminated by wastewater. J. Food Prot. 40:45–56.
  1979   Infections and intoxications caused by other bacteria. Pp. 211–297 in Food-borne
          Infections and Intoxications. 2nd Ed. H. Riemann and F. L. Bryan, eds. New York:
          Academic Press.
  1980a   Procedures to use during outbreaks of foodborne disease. Pp. 40–51 in Manual of
          Clinical Microbiology. 3rd Ed. E. H. Lennette, A. Balows, W. J. Hausler, Jr., and
          J. P. Truant, eds. Washington, D.C.: American Society for Microbiology.
  1980b   Epidemiology of foodborne diseases transmitted by fish, shellfish and marine crus-
          taceans in the United States, 1970-1978. J. Food Prot. 43:859–876.
  1982   Diseases transmitted by foods—A classification and summary. 2nd Ed. Atlanta:
          Centers for Disease Control.
  1983   Epidemiology of milk-borne diseases. J. Food Prot. 46:637–649.
Buchanan, R. E., and N. E. Gibbons
  1974   Bergey's Manual of Determinative Bacteriology. 8th Ed. Baltimore, Md.: Williams
          and Wilkins.
CDC (Center for Disease Control)
  1967   *Salmonella* Surveillance Report No. 61 (and supplement dated Oct. 23, 1967). Atlanta:
          Center for Disease Control.
  1979a   Non-O1 *Vibrio cholerae* infections—Florida. Morb. Mort. Weekly Rpt. 28:571–572,
          577.
  1979b   *Vibrio cholerae* O-group 1 infections in Louisiana, 1978. EPI-78-102-2. Atlanta:
          Center for Disease Control.
CDC (Centers for Disease Control)
  1980   Cholera—Florida. Morb. Mort. Weekly Rpt. 29:601.
  1981a   Foodborne disease outbreaks. Annual Summary 1979. Atlanta: Centers for Disease
          Control.
  1981b   Foodborne disease surveillance. Annual Summary 1978 (revised). Reissued February
          1981. Atlanta: Centers for Disease Control.
  1982a   Multi-state outbreak of yersiniosis. Morb. Mort. Weekly Rpt. 31:505–506.
  1982b   Isolation of *E. coli* 0157:H7 from sporadic cases of hemorrhagic colitis—United
          States. Morb. Mort. Weekly Rpt. 31:580, 585.
  1983   Foodborne disease outbreaks. Annual Summary 1981. Atlanta: Centers for Disease
          Control.
Cliver, D. O
  1979   Viral Infections. Pp. 299–342 in Food-Borne Infections and Intoxications, 2nd Ed.,
          H. Riemann and F. L. Bryan, eds. New York: Academic Press.
Cliver, D. O., R. D. Ellender, and M. D. Sobsey
  1984   Foodborne Viruses. In Compendium of Methods for the Microbiological Examination
          of Foods. 2nd Ed. M. L. Speck, ed. Washington, D.C.: American Public Health
          Association.
Craven, P. C., W. B. Baine, D. C. Mackel, W. H. Barker, E. J. Gangarosa, M. Goldfield,
H. Rosenfeld, R. Altman, G. Lachapelle, J. W. Davies, and R. C. Swanson
  1975   International outbreak of *Salmonella eastbourne* infection traced to contaminated
          chocolate. Lancet 1:788–793, April 5.
Dale, B., and C. M. Yentsch
  1978   Red tide and paralytic shellfish poisoning. Oceans 21:41–49.

D'Aoust, J. Y., B. J. Aris, P. Thisdale, A. Durante, N. Brisson, D. Dragon, G. Lachapelle, M. Johnston, and R. Laidley
> 1975   *Salmonella eastbourne* outbreak associated with chocolate. Can. Inst. Food Sci. Technol. J. 8:181–184.

DeSilva, D. P., and M. Poli
> 1982   Ciguatera-tropical fish poisoning. Annual Yearbook. International Game Fish Association.

Dische, F. E., and S. D. Elek
> 1957   Experimental food poisoning by *Clostridium welchii*. Lancet 2:71–74.

Doyle, M. P.
> 1981   *Campylobacter fetus* subsp. *jejuni:* An old pathogen of new concern. J. Food Prot. 44:480–488.

DuPont, H. L., R. B. Hornick, A. T. Dawkins, M. J. Snyder, and S. B. Formal
> 1969   The response of man to virulent *Shigella flexneri* 2a. J. Infect. Dis. 119:296–299.

DuPont, H. L., R. B. Hornick, M. J. Snyder, J. P. Libonati, and T. E. Woodward
> 1970   Immunity in typhoid fever: evaluation of live streptomycin-dependent vaccine. Pp. 236–239 in Proceedings of 10th Interscience Conference on Antimicrobial Agents and Chemotherapy. G. L. Hobby, ed. Oct. 18–21.

DuPont, H. L., S. B. Formal, R. B. Hornick, M. J. Snyder, J. P. Libonati, D. G. Sheahan, E. H. LaBrec, and J. P. Kalas
> 1971   Pathogenesis of *Escherichia coli* diarrhea. N. Engl. J. Med. 285:1–9.

DuPont, H. L., R. B. Hornick, M. J. Snyder, J. P. Libonati, S. B. Formal, and E. J. Gangarosa
> 1972   Immunity in shigellosis. II. Protection induced by oral live vaccine or primary infection. J. Infect. Dis. 125:12–16.

Edwards, S. T., and W. E. Sandine
> 1981   Public health significance of amines in cheese. J. Dairy Sci. 64:2431–2438.

Enright, J. B.
> 1961   The pasteurization of cream, chocolate milk and ice cream mixes containing the organism of Q-fever. J. Milk Food Technol. 24:351–355.

Enright, J. B., W. W. Sadler, and R. C. Thomas
> 1956   Observations on the thermal inactivation of the organism of Q-fever in milk. J. Milk Food Technol. 19:313–318.

FDA (Food and Drug Administration)
> 1979   Thermally processed foods packaged in hermetically sealed containers. Code of Federal Regulations 21 CFR 113.
> 1982a   Defect action levels for histamine. Supplementary information. Federal Register 47(178):40487–40488.
> 1982b   FDA Compliance Policy Guide 7108-24. Dockets Management Branch. Rockville, Md.: Food and Drug Administration.

Feeley, J. C., and D. A. Schiemann
> 1984   *Yersinia*. In Compendium of Methods for the Microbiological Examination of Foods. 2nd Ed. American Public Health Association. M. L. Speck, ed. Washington, D.C.: American Public Health Association.

Ferguson, W. W., and R. C. June
> 1952   Experiments on feeding adult volunteers with *Escherichia coli* 111, B_4, a coliform organism associated with infant diarrhea. Am. J. Hyg. 55:155–169.

Fontaine, R. E., S. Arnon, W. T. Martin, T. M. Vernon, E. J. Gangarosa, J. J. Farmer, A. B. Moran, J. H. Silliker, and D. L. Decker
> 1978   Raw hamburger: An interstate common source of human salmonellosis. Am. J. Epidemiol. 107:36–45.

Gangaroso, E. J.
   1978   What have we learned from 15 years of *Salmonella* surveillance? In Proceedings,
          National Salmonellosis Seminar, Jan. 10–11. Washington, D.C.: U.S. Department
          of Agriculture.

Gilbert, R. S.
   1979   *Bacillus cereus* gastroenteritis. Pp. 495–518 in Food-borne Infections and Intoxi-
          cations. 2nd Ed. H. Riemann and F. L. Bryan, eds. New York: Academic Press.

Harmon, S. M., and C. L. Duncan
   1984   *Clostridium perfringens*. In Compendium of Methods for the Microbiological Ex-
          amination of Foods. 2nd Ed. M. L. Speck, ed. Washington, D.C.: American Public
          Health Association.

Harmon, S. M., and J. M. Goepfert
   1984   *Bacillus cereus*. In Compendium of Methods for the Microbiological Examination of
          Foods. 2nd Ed. M. L. Speck, ed. Washington, D.C.: American Public Health As-
          sociation.

Hauschild, A.H.W., and F. S. Thatcher
   1967   Experimental food poisoning with heat-susceptible *Clostridium perfringens* type A.
          J. Food Sci. 32:467–469.

Hauschild, A. H. W., and F. L. Bryan
   1980   Estimate of cases of food- and waterborne illness in Canada and the United States.
          J. Food Prot. 43:435–440.

Health and Welfare Canada
   1981   Foodborne and Waterborne Disease in Canada. Annual Summary 1977. Ottawa:
          Health Protection Branch, Health and Welfare Canada.
   1983a Hemorrhagic colitis in a home for the aged—Ontario. Canada Diseases Weekly
          Report: 9(8):29–32.
   1983b Hemorrhagic colitis following the consumption of hamburger—Quebec. Canada Dis-
          eases Weekly Report 9(13):50–51.

Healy, G. R., and D. D. Juranek
   1979   Parasitic infections. Pp. 343–385 in Food-borne Infections and Intoxications. H.
          Riemann and F. L. Bryan, eds. New York: Academic Press.

Hickman, F. W., J. J. Farmer III, D. G. Hollis, G. R. Fanning, A. G. Steigerwalt, R. E.
Weaver, and D. J. Brenner
   1982   Identification of *Vibrio hollisae* sp. nov. from patients with diarrhea. J. Clin. Mi-
          crobiol. 15:395–401.

Hobbs, B. C.
   1979   *Clostridum perfringens* gastroenteritis. Pp. 131-171 in Food-borne Infections and
          Intoxications. 2nd Ed. H. Riemann and F. L. Bryan, eds. New York: Academic
          Press.

Hornick, R. B., S. E. Greisman, T. E. Woodward, H. L. DuPont, A. T. Dawkins, and M. J.
Snyder
   1970a Typhoid fever: pathogenesis and immunologic control (I). N. Engl. J. Med. 283:686–
          691.
   1970b Typhoid fever: pathogenesis and immunologic control (II). N. Engl. J. Med. 283:739–
          746.

Hornick, R. B., S. I. Music, R. Wenzel, R. Cash, J. P. Libonati, M. J. Snyder, and T. E.
Woodward
   1971   The broad street pump revisited: Response of volunteers to ingested cholera vibrios.
          Bull. N.Y. Acad. Med. 47: 1181–1191.

ICMSF (International Commission on Microbiological Specifications for Foods)
    1974   Microorganisms in Foods. 2.Sampling for microbiological analysis: Principles and
            specific applications. Toronto: University of Toronto Press.
    1978   Microorganisms in Foods. 1.Their significance and methods of enumeration. Toronto:
            University of Toronto Press.
June, R. C., W. W. Ferguson, and M. T. Worfel
    1953   Experiments in feeding adult volunteers with *Escherichia coli* 55, B$_5$, a coliform
            organism associated with infant diarrhea. Am. J. Hyg. 57:222–236.
Kirby, A. C., E. G. Hall, and W. Coackley
    1950   Neonatal diarrhoea and vomiting. Outbreaks in the same maternity unit. Lancet 2:201–
            207.
Lang, D. J., L. J. Kunz, A. R. Martin, S. A. Schroeder, and L. A. Thomson
    1967   Carmine as a source of nosocomial salmonellosis. N. Engl. J. Med. 276:829–832.
Lee, W. H.
    1977   An assessment of *Yersinia enterocolitica* and its presence in foods. J. Food Prot.
            40:486–489.
Levine, M. M., H. L. DuPont, S. B. Formal, R. B. Hornick, A. Takeuchi, E. J. Gangarosa,
M. J. Snyder, and J. P. Libonati
    1973   Pathogenesis of *Shigella dysenteriae* I (Shiga) dysentery. J. Infect. Dis. 127:261–
            270.
Marier, R., J. G. Wells, R. C. Swanson, W. Callahan, and I. J. Mehlman
    1973   An outbreak of enteropathogenic *Escherichia coli* foodborne disease traced to imported
            French cheese. Lancet 2:1376–1378.
McCullough, N. B., and C. W. Eisele
    1951a   Experimental human salmonellosis. I. Pathogenicity of strains of *Salmonella melea-
            gridis* and *Salmonella anatum* obtained from spray-dried whole egg. J. Infect. Dis.
            88:278–289.
    1951b   Experimental human salmonellosis. II. Immunity studies following experimental ill-
            ness with *Salmonella meleagridis* and *Salmonella anatum*. J. Immunol. 66:595–608.
    1951c   Experimental human salmonellosis. III. Pathogenicity of strains of *Salmonella new-
            port, Salmonella derby* and *Salmonella bareilly* obtained from spray-dried whole egg.
            J. Infect. Dis. 89:209–213.
    1951d   Experimental human salmonellosis. IV. Pathogenicity of strains of *Salmonella pul-
            lorum* obtained from spray-dried whole egg. J. Infect. Dis. 89:259–265.
Mehlman, I. J.
    1984   Coliforms, fecal coliforms, *Escherichia coli* and enteropathogenic *E. coli*. In Com-
            pendium of Methods for the Microbiological Examination of Foods. 2nd Ed. M. L.
            Speck, ed. Washington, D.C.: American Public Health Association.
Morris, G. K.
    1984   Shigella. In Compendium of Methods for the Microbiological Examination of Foods.
            2nd Ed. M. L. Speck, ed. Washington, D.C.: American Public Health Association.
Morris, J. G., R. Wilson, B. R. Davis, I. K. Wachsmuth, C. F. Riddle, H. G. Wathen, R. A.
Pollard, and P. A. Blake
    1981   Non-O Group 1 *Vibrio cholerae* gastroenteritis in the United States. Clinical, epi-
            demiologic and laboratory characteristics of sporadic cases. Ann. Intern. Med. 94:656–
            658.
NRC (National Research Council)
    1969   An Evaluation of the Salmonella Problem. Committee on Salmonella. Washington,
            DC.: National Academy of Sciences.

Okabe, S.
1974 Statistical review of food poisoning in Japan —Especially that by *Vibrio parahae-molyticus*. In Proceedings, International Symposium on *Vibrio parahaemolyticus*. T. Fujino, G. Sakaguchi, R. Sakazaki, and Y. Takeda, eds. Tokyo: Saikon Publishing.

Ormsbee, R. A.
1980 Rickettsiae. Pp. 922–933 in Manual of Clinical Microbiology. 3rd Ed. E. H. Lennette, A. Balows, W. J. Hausler, Jr., and J. P. Truant, eds. Washington, D.C.: American Society for Microbiology.

Oshima, Y., L. J. Buckley, M. Alam, and Y. Shimizu
1977 Heterogeneity of paralytic shellfish poisons. Three new toxins from cultured *Gonyaulax tamarensis* cells, *Mya arenaria* and *Saxidomas gigantens*. Comp. Biochem. Physiol. 57:31–34.

Park, C. E., R. M. Smibert, M. J. Blaser, C. Vanderzant, and N. J. Stern
1984 Campylobacter. In Compendium of Methods for the Microbiological Examination of Foods. 2nd Ed. M. L. Speck, ed. Washington, D.C.: American Public Health Association.

Prpic, J. K., R. M. Robins-Browne, and R. B. Davey
1983 Differentiation between virulent and nonvirulent *Yersinia enterocolitica* isolates by using Congo red agar. J. Clin. Microbiol. 18:486–490.

1984 Differentiation between virulent and nonvirulent *Yersinia enterocolitica* isolates by using Congo red agar. Erratum. J. Clin. Microbiol. 19:446.

Rice, S. L., R. R. Eitenmiller, and P. E. Koehler
1976 Biologically active amines in food. A review. J. Milk Food Technol. 39:353–358.

Riemann, H., and F. L. Bryan, eds.
1979 Food-borne Infections and Intoxications. 2nd Ed. New York: Academic Press. 748 pp.

Riley, L. W., R. S. Remis, S. D. Helgerson, H. B. McGee, J. G. Wells, B. R. Davis, R. J. Hebert, E. S. Olcott, L. M. Johnson, N. T. Hargrett, P. A. Blake, and M. L. Cohen
1983 Hemorrhagic colitis associated with a rare *Escherichia coli* serotype. New. Engl. J. Med. 308:681–685.

Robinson, D. A.
1981 Infective dose of *Campylobacter jejuni* in milk. Br. Med. J. 282:1584.

Sanders, A. C., F. L. Bryan, J. C. Olson, Jr., and J. M. Madden
1984 Foodborne illness—Suggested approaches for the analysis of foods and specimens obtained in outbreaks. In Compendium of Methods for the Microbiological Examination of Foods. 2nd Ed. M. L. Speck, ed. Washington, D.C.: American Public Health Association.

Sanyal, S. C., and P. C. Sen
1974 Human volunteer study on the pathogenicity of *Vibrio parahaemolyticus*. In Proceedings, International Symposium on *Vibrio parahaemolyticus*. F. Fujino, G. Sakaguchi, R. Sakazaki, and Y. Takeda, eds. Tokyo: Saikon Publishing.

Sedova, N. N.
1970 Study of the role of enterococci in the etiology of bacterial food poisoning. Vopr. Pitan. 29:82–87.

Shaughnessy, H. J., R. C. Olsson, K. Bass, F. Friewer, and S. O. Levinson
1946 Experimental human bacillary dysentery. J. Am. Med. Assoc. 132:362–368.

Shimizu, Y.
1979 Developments in the study of paralytic shellfish toxins. In Proceedings of the Second International Conference on Toxic Dinoflagellate Blooms. D. K. Taylor and H. H. Seliger, eds. New York: Elsevier/North Holland.

Silliker, J. H.
  1980   Status of *Salmonella*—Ten years later. J. Food Prot. 43:307–313.
Silverstolpe, L., U. Plazikowski, J. Kjellander, and G. Vahlne
  1962   An epidemic among infants caused by *Salmonella muenchen*. J. Appl. Bacteriol.
          24:134–142.
Sours, H. E., and D. G. Smith
  1980   Outbreaks of foodborne disease in the United States. 1972–1978. J. Infect. Dis.
          142:122–125.
Steele, T. W., and S. McDermott
  1978   *Campylobacter enteritis* in South Austrialia. Med. J. Austr. 2:404–406.
Stern, N. J., and M. D. Pierson
  1979   *Yersinia enterocolitica:* A review of the psychrotrophic water and foodborne pathogen.
          J. Food. Sci. 44:1736–1742.
Stoloff, L.
  1984   Toxigenic Fungi. In Compendium of Methods for the Microbiological Examination
          of Foods. 2nd Ed. M. L. Speck, ed. Washington, D.C.: American Public Health
          Association.
Swaminathan, B., M. C. Harmon, and I. J. Mehlman
  1982   A review: *Yersinia enterocolitica*. J. Appl. Bacteriol. 52:151–183.
Szita, J., M. Kali, and B. Redey
  1973   Incidence of *Yersinia enterocolitica* infection in Hungary. Proceedings, Symposium
          on *Yersinia, Pasteurella* and *Francisella*. In Contributions in Microbiology and Im-
          munology. Vol. 2. S. Winblad, ed. Basel, Switœrland: Karger.
Tatini, S., D. G. Hoover, and R.V.F. Lachica
  1984   Methods for the isolation and enumeration of *Staphylococcus aureus*. In Compendium
          of Methods for the Microbiological Examination of Foods. 2nd Ed. M. L. Speck,
          ed. Washington, D.C.: American Public Health Association.
Twedt, R. M., J. M. Madden, and R. R. Colwell
  1984   Vibrio. In Compendium of Methods for the Microbiological Examination of Foods.
          2nd Ed. M. L. Speck, ed. Washington, D.C.: American Public Health Association.
USDA (U.S. Department of Agriculture)
  1973   Treatment of pork products to destroy trichinae. Meat and Poultry Inspection Reg-
          ulation Part 318. 10:125–131. Washington, D.C.: USDA.
  1981a   Bovine Tuberculosis Eradication, Uniform Methods and Rules, effective Jan. 2, 1981.
          Animal and Plant Health Inspection Service. Washington, D.C.: USDA.
  1981b   Labeling policy book. Food Safety and Inspection Service: 53. Washington,
          D.C.: USDA.
  1982   Brucellosis Uniform Methods and Rules and Amendment of May, 1982. Animal and
          Plant Health Inspection Service. Washington, D.C.: USDA.
USDHEW (U.S. Department of Health, Education and Welfare)
  1965   National Shellfish Sanitation Program, Manual of Operations, Part 1, Sanitation of
          shellfish growing areas, 1965 revision. Washington, D.C.: Superintendent of Doc-
          uments.
USPHS/FDA (U.S. Public Health Service/Food and Drug Administration)
  1978   Grade A Pasteurized Milk Ordinance. 1978 Recommendations. USPHS/FDA Publ.
          No. 229. Washington, D.C.: U.S. Government Printing Office.
Vernon, E.
  1977   Food Poisoning and *Salmonella* infections in England and Wales, 1973–1975. Public
          Health (UK) 91:225–235.

Veron, M., and R. Chatelain
  1973   Taxonomic study of the genus *Campylobacter* Sebald and Veron and designation of the neotype strain for the type species *Campylobacter fetus* (Smith and Taylor) Sebald and Veron. Int. J. Syst. Bacteriol. 23:122–134.
Voigt, M. N., and R. R. Eitenmiller
  1978   Role of histidine and tyrosine decarboxylases and mono- and diamine oxidases in amine build-up in cheese. J. Food Prot. 41:182–186.
Voigt, M. N., R. R. Eitenmiller, P. E. Koehler, and M. K. Hamdy
  1974   Tyramine, histamine and tryptamine content of cheese. J. Milk Food Technol. 37:377–381.
Wells, J. G., B. R. Davis, I. K. Wachsmuth, L. W. Riley, R. S. Remis, R. Solokow, and G. K. Morris
  1983   Laboratory investigation of hemorrhagic colitis outbreaks associated with a rare *Escherichia coli* serotype. J. Clin. Microbiol. 18:512–520.
WHO (World Health Organization)
  1976   Microbiological aspects of food hygiene. Report on a WHO Expert Committee with participation of FAO. Technical Report Series 578. Geneva, Switzerland: World Health Organization.
Withers, N.
  1982   Ciguatera fish poisoning. Am. Rev. Med. 33:97–111.

5

Selection of Indicator Organisms and Agents as Components of Microbiological Criteria

Regulatory agencies and industrial quality assurance personnel regularly examine foods or ingredients for microorganisms or their metabolic products that may indicate (1) the possible presence of a pathogen or harmful toxin, (2) the possibility that faulty practices occurred during production, processing, storage, and distribution, and/or (3) the suitability of a food or ingredient for a desired purpose.

The indicator organisms and agents discussed in this chapter are divided into four categories: (1) those that assess numbers of microorganisms and/or microbial activity, (2) indicators of potential human or fecal contamination or possible presence of pathogens, (3) indicators of post-heat processing contamination, and (4) metabolic products of pathogens that indicate a health hazard.

The section on assessment of numbers of microorganisms and/or microbial activity includes (1) the aerobic plate count, thermoduric, psychrotrophic, thermophilic, proteolytic, and lipolytic counts; the direct microscopic count; Howard mold count; rot fragment count; "machinery mold"; yeast and mold count; heat-resistant molds and thermophilic spore count; and (2) examination for metabolic products such as by organoleptic examination, dye or indicator reduction time, pH, trimethylamine (TMA), total volatile nitrogen (TVN), indole, ethanol, diacetyl, histamine, endotoxins (*Limulus* amoebocyte lysate test), extract release volume, and adenosine triphosphate.

Indicators of potential human or fecal contamination or of possible presence of pathogens include staphylococci, *Escherichia coli*, fecal coliforms, enterococci (fecal streptococci, group D streptococci), and *Pseudomonas aeruginosa*. Indicators of post-heat processing contamination include coliform bacteria and *Enterobacteriaceae*. Thermonuclease and U.V. light examination of grains are discussed in a section on metabolic products of pathogens that indicate a potential health hazard. The significance of the presence of phosphatase in certain dairy products is also discussed. Metabolic products such as tested for by organoleptic evaluation, pH, TMA, TVN, indole, ethanol, and diacetyl are not commonly used as components of microbiological criteria as are microorganisms. They are included in this chapter because they result from microbial activity and are intended as an adjunct or substitute for microbiological testing for one or more reasons such as convenience, economy, or effectiveness.

Each of these indicators (organisms, group of organisms, or agents) will be discussed in reference to (1) its relative importance, (2) status and limitations of method for detection or enumeration, and (3) suitability as part of a microbiological criterion. Recommended uses of these indicators as part of microbiological criteria for foods are given in Chapter 9.

ASSESSMENT OF NUMBERS OF MICROORGANISMS AND/OR MICROBIAL ACTIVITY

Estimating Numbers of Microorganisms

Aerobic Plate Count

The aerobic plate count (APC) is used as part of a microbiological standard for raw and pasteurized milk and many other dairy products, and for shellfish at the wholesale level (see Chapters 8 and 9). It is also used (1) to monitor a large number of other foods for compliance with standards or guidelines set by various regulatory agencies, (2) to monitor foods for compliance with purchase specifications, and (3) to monitor adherence to good manufacturing practices. The test is based on the assumption that each microbial cell, pair of cells, chain of cells, or clump or cluster of cells present in an analytical unit (which is mixed with agar containing appropriate nutrients) forms visible, separate colonies when incubated for a sufficient period of time in an aerobic atmosphere and at a temperature suitable for growth.

While the APC is the most popular method for estimating the number of viable microorganisms, it is often misused. Contrary to some assumptions, the APC does not measure the size of the total bacterial population in a sample of food. Instead it measures only that fraction of the microbial flora that is able to produce colonies in the medium used under the prevailing conditions of plate incubation. Alterations in medium or environmental conditions change the fraction of the organisms that can grow.

Hence, rigid adherence to standardized test conditions is required if the APC is to be part of a microbiological criterion.

The value of total counts as indexes of sanitary quality, organoleptic quality, safety, and utility of foods was reviewed by Silliker (1963). The APC of refrigerated perishable foods such as milk, meat, poultry, and fish may reflect conditions such as the microbial content of the raw materials and ingredients, the effectiveness of the processing procedure(s), the sanitary condition of equipment and utensils, and the time-temperature profile of storage and distribution. Specific causes of unexpected high counts can be identified by examination of samples at critical control points and by plant inspection. However, even perishable foods prepared from wholesome raw materials and properly processed, packaged, and stored develop high counts, lose quality, and ultimately spoil if held for long periods. Under these conditions, the APC reflects not sanitary quality but continued growth of psychrotrophic bacteria that were already present in the food. Thus, the usefulness of the APC depends to a great extent on the point in the process or distribution at which the sample was taken.

The APC of shelf-stable foods reflects the same conditions as listed for perishable foods except that certain attributes of the shelf-stable food (a_w, pH, heat treatment, frozen state) prevent further growth of contaminating bacteria. In the use or interpretation of the APC, additional factors need to be considered: (1) the APC measures only living microbial cells. Processing procedures, for example a heat treatment, can mask high-count raw materials or insanitary conditions. In addition, continued storage of a food in the frozen or dried state or at low pH values results in death and thus in decreases in count; (2) the APC is of little value in assessing the existing organoleptic quality of foods. Perceptible changes in quality characteristics of foods because of microbial activity do not occur until very high viable counts (10^6-10^7 per g or ml) have developed. Bacteriological analysis will then only confirm the results of an organoleptic examination; (3) the APC does not differentiate types of bacteria. Thus, even if numbers are approximately the same, biochemical activities leading to changes in a food may be different because of differences in microbial types or in composition of the food. In addition, high counts resulting from microbial growth are more likely to cause defects in foods than are similar levels resulting from massive contamination.

For some foods, the APC can be used successfully to estimate potential shelf-life. For example, a standard plate count (SPC) on freshly pasteurized milk that was subsequently held at 7°C (44.6°F) for 5 days can provide an estimate of the potential shelf-life of this food (APHA, 1978). This application of the APC requires an intimate knowledge of the association between count and shelf-life of a food.

The APC may or may not be useful as a measure of the utility of an ingredient for a food. In many cases, it may be necessary to analyze the ingredient for the presence of specific organisms known to be of importance for the stability of the final product. APCs have little if any relationship to safety of foods. Also, APCs of fermented or retorted foods are of little value.

Thermoduric, Psychrotrophic, Thermophilic, Proteolytic, and Lipolytic Counts

Minor modifications of the APC can be applied to enumerate specific groups of microorganisms such as thermoduric, psychrotrophic, thermophilic, proteolytic, or lipolytic bacteria. The thermoduric or laboratory pasteurization count (APHA, 1978) is used in the milk industry to check individual producer milk in order to identify samples with excessive numbers of these organisms. Thermoduric organisms survive pasteurization of milk and thus may contribute to high SPCs on pasteurized milk. High thermoduric counts are closely associated with persistent improper cleaning and sanitizing of equipment at the producer farm or at the processing plant.

From a quality control point of view, psychrotrophic microorganisms are of great significance in refrigerated perishable foods because they grow, although not at optimum rate, at refrigeration temperatures. Some of these psychrotrophs can cause serious off-tastes, off-odors, or sliminess of foods when numbers are allowed to increase to 10^6-10^8 cells per g or ml. Although the initial number of psychrotrophs in a refrigerated perishable food may be low, it can increase to large numbers during storage, the time depending upon factors such as the initial level of contamination and the temperature. Shelf-life of such foods will be severely impaired when initial numbers are high, particularly when foods are held at marginal refrigeration temperatures. Unless consumed prior to this event, high microbial counts will definitely occur in perishable foods even when these foods are prepared from wholesome materials and are properly processed and stored. Psychrotrophic bacteria are often sources of heat-resistant proteolytic and lipolytic enzymes that may affect adversely the quality of foods during long-term storage after heat processing (Griffiths et al., 1981).

Proteolytic and lipolytic microorganisms can be responsible for a variety of odor and flavor problems in foods. Some of the common psychrotrophic bacteria are strongly proteolytic and/or lipolytic and cause serious defects in dairy, meat, poultry, and seafood products when high counts (10^6 per g or ml or above) are reached during refrigerated storage. The proteolytic count (Chapter 8, Table 8-4) is part of a microbiological criterion for butter and whipped butter. The proteolytic count and lipolytic count of butter can be helpful in drawing attention to unsatisfactory manufacturing practices.

In addition to the APC (AOAC, 1980) and SPC (APHA, 1978), there are alternative procedures for determining viable bacterial counts such as the surface or spread plate method, plate loop, oval tube or bottle culture, drop plate, membrane filter, and spiral plate (AOAC, 1980; APHA, 1976, 1978, 1984).

Reliable interpretation of the APC of a food depends upon an intimate knowledge of the expected microbial population at the point in a process or distribution at which the sample was collected. Higher than expected counts can serve as an alerting mechanism to investigate the potential cause(s) of this event. The two most widely used APC methods are the AOAC method (AOAC, 1980) and the standard plate count (SPC) method as described in *Standard Methods for the Examination of Dairy Products* (APHA, 1978). These reliable methods are used routinely to determine APC as part of many microbiological criteria. With due consideration of the precautions and limitations discussed in this section, the APC can be a useful component of microbiological criteria of many foods. Specific applications of the APC in microbiological criteria for foods are given in Chapter 9.

Direct Microscopic Count

The direct microscopic count (DMC) is used as a component of microbiological criteria (standards) of raw (non-Grade A) milk, dried milks, liquid and frozen eggs, and dried eggs. The DMC gives an estimate of the total number of microorganisms, viable and nonviable, in a sample. The DMC is rapid, requires a minimum amount of equipment, and provides information about the morphological characteristics of the cells. The DMC is also used to count the number of leucocytes in raw milk and thereby detect mastitic milk. Disadvantages of the method are that it is suitable only for foods containing relatively large numbers of microorganisms (10^5-10^6 per ml) and that the small quantity of sample (0.01 ml) examined limits precision. The lower limit of precision for the DMC is dictated by the Microscopic Factor and the number of fields examined. Separation of viable and nonviable cells by this method is not possible, and consequently counts may exceed corresponding agar plate counts many times. For these reasons the use of the DMC as part of microbiological criteria is very limited and applicable only when fairly high microbial populations (viable, nonviable, or both) are expected and information on the microbial history of the product (such as dried milk) can be useful in quality control programs. Rapid standardized methods (AOAC, 1980; APHA, 1976, 1978, 1984) are available and are satisfactory for use in microbiological criteria.

Other applications of the DMC use counting chambers such as the Petroff-Hauser slide or the haemocytometer. These counting chambers are used to determine populations of yeasts and other microorganisms in foods such as fruit juice concentrates.

Microscopic Mold Counts

Microscopic mold counts are used to assess the soundness of raw horticultural products and the sanitary conditions of processing lines. The Howard mold count and rot fragment count are used for regulatory purposes (see Chapter 9).

Howard Mold Count. The Howard mold count, one of the oldest microbiological criteria, is widely used to detect introduction of moldy, decomposed fruits and vegetables into processed foods. It is used to monitor both raw products and sorting and trimming operations. The test was originally developed for tomato products. It is also applied to foods such as apple butter, drupelet berries, citrus and pineapple juices, cranberry sauce, strawberries, pureed infant food, and garlic powder and other spices. Microbiological criteria (see APHA, 1976, 1984) vary with the type of food being evaluated.

Rot Fragment Count. The rot fragment count is applied mainly to tomato products such as catsup and sauce. This test, a count of tomato cellular materials that exhibit mold filaments, is used mainly to evaluate whether or not a food was prepared from sound raw produce. Practical methods for these mold counts are applicable for microbiological criteria (AOAC, 1980; APHA, 1976, 1984). There is a sufficiently close relationship between the Howard mold and rot fragment counts and the amount of decayed tissue present for the counts to serve as useful microbiological criteria for certain fruits and vegetable products and to be an index of manufacturing practices. However, processing conditions such as milling and homogenization can affect microscopic mold counts.

"Machinery Mold." *Geotrichum candidum* is the predominant mold on tomato processing equipment and can be responsible for the slime that accumulates on this equipment. It has been referred to as ''machinery mold.'' *Geotrichum* filaments have also been recovered from a variety of

fruits and vegetables at different stages of processing. Careful cleaning of processing equipment results in a marked reduction in the *Geotrichum* count. Methods to determine *G. candidum* for purposes of microbiological criteria are adequate (AOAC, 1980; APHA, 1976, 1984). *G. candidum* is used as a microbiological criterion to check sanitation of equipment in fruit and vegetable processing plants and in bottling works.

Yeast and Mold Counts

Yeast and mold counts are used as part of microbiological standards of various dairy products, for example cottage cheese (Chapter 8, Table 8-4) and sugar (National Soft Drink Association, 1975).

Yeasts and molds are widely distributed in the environment and can enter foods through inadequately sanitized equipment or as airborne contaminants. Yeasts and molds frequently become predominant on foods when conditions for bacterial growth are less favorable, e.g., foods with low a_w, low pH, high salt, or high sugar content. Therefore, they become a problem in fermented dairy products, fruits, fruit beverages and soft drinks. They manifest themselves by producing undesirable odors, flavors, appearance (discoloration), gas, and sediment. Satisfactory methods are available for yeast and mold counts that are applicable for purposes of microbiological criteria. These methods use either acidified agars or agar media with added antibiotics to inhibit bacterial growth (APHA, 1976, 1978, 1984). Methods for osmophilic yeasts are available (APHA, 1984).

Heat-resistant Molds

A few molds such as *Byssochlamys fulva* and *Aspergillus fisheri* produce ascospores that are sufficiently heat resistant to survive the thermal processes applied to fruit and fruit products. Food processors sometimes set limits for these molds in purchase specifications for ingredients such as fruit concentrates and tapioca starch. Satisfactory methods for isolation and enumeration of these molds applicable for microbiological criteria are available (APHA, 1976, 1984).

Thermophilic Spore Count

Various types of sporeformers are used as part of the microbiological criteria, primarily specifications, by the canning industry to monitor the quality of ingredients such as sugar, starch, flour, spices, mushrooms, nonfat dry milk, and cereals that are intended for low-acid heat processed foods. National Food Processors Association criteria (NCA, 1968) for

sugar and starch to be used for this purpose include limits for total thermophilic spore count, flat sour spores, thermophilic anaerobic spores, and
sulfide spoilage spores.

Concern for thermophilic spores in these ingredients is related to their
high heat resistance and their ability to cause defects in foods held at
elevated temperatures because of inadequate cooling and/or storage at too
high temperatures. Examination of equipment surfaces, product in process,
or finished product is in some cases useful for location of foci of spore
buildup. Methods to determine these spores (AOAC, 1980; APHA, 1976,
1984; NCA, 1968) are adequate for application in microbiological criteria.
Microbiological criteria involving thermophilic spore counts have been
useful as purchase specifications to specify quality of or check ingredients
intended for use in low-acid heat processed foods (see sections of Chapter 9
that apply).

Measuring Metabolic Products

Metabolic products produced during growth of microorganisms have
been used to estimate bacterial populations and to express quantitatively
the effect of microbial activity on the quality of foods.

Organoleptic Examination

Organoleptic examinations of foods are used extensively for evaluation
of quality attributes such as taste, odor, body and texture, color, and
appearance. The food industry uses these examinations to classify certain
foods into quality grades. For basic information about organoleptic evaluations of foods, see Amerine et al. (1965) and Larmond (1977).

Use of organoleptic examinations of foods to evaluate microbial activity
is limited, as the effect of microbes on organoleptic attributes varies.
Certain microorganisms act upon the constituents of a food and produce
marked changes in perceptible characteristics of the food; others are relatively inert biochemically and produce little change. The effect of certain
levels and/or types of microorganisms on perceptible characteristics in
foods varies with differences in food composition and physical-chemical
characteristics. For example, objectionable odors in a perishable food may
result from extensive microbial activity; on the other hand, large microbial
populations do not necessarily cause perceptible odor problems. In addition, alterations in packaging and distribution methods can interfere with
normal expected changes in quality characteristics of a perishable food
(see Chapter 1). Microbial types on meat, poultry, and fish stored under
refrigeration in vacuum packages or in modified gaseous atmospheres

differ considerably from those on products exposed to air.

Nevertheless, organoleptic examinations of certain foods can be useful in evaluation of microbial activity. For example, organoleptic examinations are used to evaluate the amount of acid and/or aroma compounds produced by various lactic acid bacteria in cultured dairy products. The organoleptic evaluation of cheese for typical flavor and body and texture, to a large extent, reflects the activities of desirable bacteria. Organoleptic examination is also used with some foods to evaluate the activity of spoilage bacteria that may lead to quality deterioration and subsequent spoilage of the food. In these cases, an attempt is made to relate the organoleptic trait, usually odor, to the level of activity of spoilage bacteria. Although organoleptic examinations for this purpose are used for many commodities such as raw milk, meat, and poultry, they are used extensively for fish and other seafoods (see Chapter 9). In general, seafoods are more perishable than are other high-protein meat foods, because many seafoods contain relatively large amounts of nonprotein nitrogen compounds that are readily available to support microbial growth. Also, seafoods harvested from cold waters contain microbes that are not as effectively inhibited by refrigeration. The information in Table 5-1 is an example of organoleptic changes in relation to chemical changes and bacterial counts of fish.

In recent years, FDA has used organoleptic examination to determine the degree of decomposition of imported shrimp. The shrimp are placed in one of three classes:

Class 1, passable: This class includes fishery products that range from very fresh to those that contain fishy or other odors characteristic of the product, but not definitely identifiable as odors of decomposition.

Class 2, decomposed (slight but definite): This is the first stage of definitely identifiable decomposition. An odor is present that is not really intense, but is persistent and readily perceptible to the experienced examiner as that of decomposition.

Class 3, decomposed (advanced): This class of products possesses a strong odor of decomposition that is persistent, distinct, and unmistakable.

Limits of acceptability of a lot are based on the number of shrimp in a sample that are placed in the three classes (Anonymous, 1979). In general, trained personnel could consistently place shrimp correctly in the appropriate class.

The presence of objectionable odors in raw seafood usually indicates that extensive microbial activity has taken place. When such changes are perceptible, bacterial numbers exceed 10^6 per gram.

Successful application of organoleptic examination of fish and other foods to determine the degree of decomposition by microbial and tissue enzyme activity requires well-trained personnel. The organoleptic examination of specific foods including milk, meat, and poultry, but particularly raw fish and other seafoods, can be a most valuable tool to determine the degree of quality deterioration by microbial activity. If off-odors of microbial origin are perceptible, then counts are high and the product should be rejected.

Dye or Indicator Reduction Time

Attempts have been made to use oxidation-reduction indicators (dyes) for estimating the microbial quality of various foods such as milk, meat, poultry, seafoods, and vegetables (Bush, 1970). Present use of these dyes is restricted to the milk industry where they are used for classifying certain manufacturing milks into grades (APHA, 1978) and in rapid tests to estimate the potential shelf-life of freshly pasteurized milk (Broitman et al., 1958; Parmelee, 1974). The application of dye reduction tests to foods other than milk usually has not been successful because naturally present reducing enzymes and agents interfere with the dye reduction pattern. Comparisons of reduction times in milk with estimates of bacterial populations by the agar plate method and other tests have demonstrated that reduction times are, in general, inversely related to the initial bacterial content of the sample. Dye reduction tests provide only estimates of bacterial activity, as reduction times are influenced not only by bacterial numbers but also by the growth phase of the bacteria at time of testing and by the types present. With improvements in milk quality resulting in lower bacterial counts, reduction tests have become less applicable for quality evaluation of raw milk. Results of oxidation-reduction tests on pasteurized milk can be used by the processor as guidelines for estimation of the potential shelf-life of freshly pasteurized milk. Simple, practical dye reduction methods are available (APHA, 1978).

pH

The pH of some foods changes as a result of microbial activity; consequently, pH measurements have been applied to determine the degree of quality deterioration. The pH of fish and shrimp increases during storage because of the production of ammonia and amines by microbial and tissue enzyme activity. The pH of molluscs, on the other hand, decreases during spoilage. Microbial activity results in the production of basic substances in refrigerated ground meat stored under aerobic conditions (Shelef and Jay, 1970). However, changes in pH because of microbial activity vary with conditions such as nature of the food (available substrate for microbial

TABLE 5-1 Stages in Fish Spoilage

Stage	Tissue Changes[a]	Organoleptic Changes	Bacterial Count	Chemical Changes[a]
Stage I (0–5 days in ice)	Rigor mortis ATP → inosine Slight increase, TMA Changes in bacterial types	Eyes bright Flesh firm Color good Gills bright Odor fresh	10^2–10^3/cm^2	TMA ≲ 1–1.5 mg% VRS ≲ 2–8 units
Stage II (5–10 days in ice)	Bacterial growth becomes apparent Inosine → hypoxanthine TMAO → TMA NH$_3$ increases	Eyes begin to dull Gill color fades Skin color fades Odor neutral to slightly fishy Texture softening	10^3–10^6/cm^2	TMA < 5 mg% VRS CA 5–10 units TBV ≲ 15 mg%
Stage III (10–14 days in ice)	Rapid bacterial growth Penetration of tissues Hypoxanthine → xanthine, uric acid, etc. TMA increases rapidly TVB and TVA increase	Eyes sunken Gills discolored and slimy Skin bleached Odor sour and fishy Texture soft	10^6–10^8/cm^2	TMA ~ 10 mg% VRS ~ 10–15 units TVB 20–30 mg% TVA 15–20 mg%

| Stage IV (over 14 days in ice) | Eyes opaque and sunken
Gills bleached and slimy
Skin very slimy
Texture very soft
Odor offensive | Bacterial numbers stationary
Some changes of species
General deterioration of flesh
TVB and TVA increase rapidly
TMA increases or levels off
Proteolysis begins
H$_2$S and other products formed | $\sim 10^8/cm^2$ | TMA > 10 mg%
VRS > 20 units
TVB > 30 mg%
TVA $\geq$ 60 mg%
H$_2$S, indole, etc. detectable |

[a]TMA: Trimethylamine expressed as mg/100 g fish; TVB: total volatile base expressed as mg/100 g fish; TVA: total volatile acids expressed as mg/100 g fish; VRS: volatile reducing substances expressed as mg/100 g fish.

SOURCE: ICMSF, 1980, p. 582.

activity), the type of microbial flora, and packaging conditions (gaseous atmosphere). Acidity as measured by pH has limited but important application in the monitoring of certain critical control points in the production of some foods. For example, voluntary guidelines were recommended (AMI, 1982) for the production of dry and semidry fermented sausages in which time-temperature relationships are given for reaching a meat mixture pH of 5.3 or less by the action of lactic acid producing bacteria. The goal of these voluntary guidelines is to provide an understanding of the critical control points in the fermentation stage of production of dry and semidry fermented sausages in order to minimize the opportunity for *Staphylococcus aureus* to develop. In the production of cultured milk products and cheeses, measurement of pH of the inoculated milk is also of great importance as it monitors the rate of development of lactic acid bacteria. Lack of acid production (starter failure) may result in the buildup of *S. aureus* and in the presence of toxins in the cheese (see Chapter 9, Part A). Monitoring the pH of mayonnaise and salad dressings (Chapter 9, Part N) and of acidified canned foods (Chapter 9, Part K) is important in assuring safety of these foods. Reliable routine methods for pH measurement are available (APHA, 1984).

Trimethylamine and Total Volatile Nitrogen

Trimethylamine (TMA) and total volatile nitrogen (TVN) have been used for evaluation of the quality of fish and seafoods. Volatile amines, primarily ammonia, are produced in fish and other seafoods from amino acids by bacteria. TMA results from the reduction of trimethylamine oxide (TMAO) by bacteria particularly in gadoid fish such as cod, haddock, and hake. According to Montgomery et al. (1970), for example, 5 mg TMA-N/100 g and 30 mg TVN-N/100 g are limits for acceptability for shrimp in Australia and Japan. Stansby (1963) lists TVN values for different degrees of freshness of fish as follows: fresh fish, 12 mg or less; slight decomposition, but edible, 12-20 mg; borderline edible, 20-25 mg; badly decomposed and inedible, >25 mg TVN-N/100 g. These grading scales are at the present mainly applied for research purposes. Little detailed information is available on the TMA and TVN contents of seafoods in United States wholesale and retail markets.

Information obtained with gadoid fish may not be applicable to other types of fish and other seafood. For example, TMA could not be detected in ice-stored shrimp until 8 days had elapsed, at which time the APC was approximately 10^8 per gram and the shrimp was judged of poor quality (Chang et al., 1983). During this storage period, TVN values decreased, probably because of the washing action of melting ice (Cobb et al., 1977). Cobb and coworkers (1977) also suggested that low TMA values in Gulf shrimp could have resulted from lack of substrate (TMAO). In another study (Oberlender et al., 1983), TMA values of swordfish steaks stored in CO_2-enriched atmospheres did not exceed recommended values for acceptability even when the steaks had spoiled. In this case, the lack of relationship between TMA content and sensory characteristics may have resulted from a shift in the composition of the microflora. Lactic acid bacteria were predominant on the fish stored under modified gaseous atmospheres, whereas gram-negative, aerobic rods usually predominated on samples exposed to air.

Reliable methods are available to determine TMA and TVN (AOAC, 1980; Cobb et al., 1973).

Quality deterioration and subsequent spoilage of fish and seafoods is a very complex process and is influenced by a great many variables, such as (1) fish species, (2) area of catch, (3) method of catch, (4) handling on board of vessel, and (5) processing techniques. For a limited number of marine species under certain conditions of handling, a relationship may exist between indicators, such as TMA and/or TVN, and microbial activity that influences acceptability of a product. If such indicators or criteria are applied, caution should be exercised not to include either other species for which this relationship has not yet been established or the same species when they are handled under different conditions. Because of these severe limitations, TMA and TVN by themselves should not be applied broadly in criteria to reflect microbial activity in fish and seafoods.

Indole

Indole has been proposed as an indicator of decomposition for shrimp and oysters since the 1940s (Beacham, 1946; Duggan, 1948; King and Flynn, 1945). According to McClennan (1952) and Salwin (1964), indole is a good index for differentiating between acceptable and unacceptable shrimp. Indole is formed by the action of certain bacteria (such as *Proteus* spp., *E. coli*, and others) on tryptophan present in shrimp and oyster tissue.

A study conducted by FDA (Duggan and Strasburger, 1946) reported a good correlation between indole concentration and sensory evaluation; the indole content increased as decomposition advanced. Fresh shrimp does not contain indole in excess of 1 μg/100 g. The FDA established a defect action level of 25 μg/100 g for indole in imported canned and cooked/frozen shrimp (FDA, 1981). Shrimp at or exceeding this indole level is not permitted to enter the United States. This action resulted from concern with *Salmonella*, decomposition, and filth in frozen raw imported shrimp. Subsequent canning or cooking masks the odor of decomposition. Duggan and Strasburger (1946), however, reported that when shrinkage due to moisture loss was taken into consideration, the indole level in cooked shrimp was nearly identical to that of the original raw shrimp. Chang et al. (1983) showed that indole levels of shrimp of acceptable quality remained stable during a 5-minute boil.

High indole levels indicate decomposition, but shrimp of poor or unacceptable quality may not necessarily contain indole (Chang et al., 1983; Staruszkiewicz, 1974). When shrimp was stored at 4°C (39°F) until it was severely decomposed, the indole level was lower than 25 μg/100 g, the defect action level by FDA (Chang et al., 1983). The APC of this shrimp exceeded 10^8/g and the TVN value had reached 56 mg TVN-N/100 g. At higher storage temperatures (12° and 22°C/53° and 72°F), rapid production of indole took place. This suggests that mesophilic bacteria are more significant in the production of indole in shrimp than are psychrotrophic species. Hence, indole alone is not a suitable index of acceptability for all types of fresh or frozen shrimp, but when used in conjunction with other quality tests it can be of value in assessing prior high-temperature abuse. Methods for the determination of indole for microbiological criteria (AOAC, 1980; Cheuk and Finne, 1981) are satisfactory.

Ethanol

Ethanol can be produced by various bacteria from carbohydrates through glycolysis and/or the deamination and decarboxylation of amino acids such as alanine. Present knowledge (Crosgrove, 1978; Hollingworth and Throm, 1982, 1983) indicates that ethanol alone might be a useful index of decomposition of canned salmon. Hollingworth and Throm (1982) reported a high correlation between the ethanol content (as determined by gas chromatography) of four species of canned salmon and the sensory classification of decomposition. Tentative ranges suggested were: class 1 (passable), 0-24 ppm ethanol; class 2 (decomposed, slight but definite), 25-74 ppm ethanol; and class 3 (decomposed, advanced), 75 ppm ethanol and above. If this relationship is confirmed in collaborative studies, the ethanol level should have practical application as part of a HACCP system to monitor the precanning and postcanning quality of this salmon. It may be applicable to other seafoods if a similar relationship between sensory characteristics and ethanol can be established. The present analytical method for the ethanol determination, although relatively simple and rapid, requires sophisticated laboratory equipment.

Diacetyl

The diacetyl test was developed in the citrus industry to indicate microbial activity in the early stages of multiple-stage, low-temperature evaporators. The low oxygen tension, moderate temperature, and 18-20% sugar content of the juice during early stages of evaporation are ideal conditions for the rapid growth of lactic acid bacteria (*Lactobacillus* and *Leuconostoc*). These microorganisms produce diacetyl and acetylmethylcarbinol resulting in an undesirable buttermilk-like flavor in the finished concentrate (Fields, 1964). Several varieties of oranges (particularly mature Valencias) contain acetylmethylcarbinol as a normal constituent. By determining the diacetyl and acetylmethylcarbinol content of juice prepared in the laboratory from normal fruit, the quantities generated by microbial growth in the processed product can be estimated. The diacetyl test is a simple colorimetric procedure that requires approximately 30 minutes. Diacetyl can be used as a parameter to monitor the condition of the fruit and the sanitary condition of orange and apple processing (APHA, 1984; Fields, 1964; Hill et al., 1954; Hill and Wenzel, 1957).

Histamine

The formation of toxic levels of histamine in foods such as certain types of fish and cheeses and the limits for tuna set by FDA have been discussed in Chapter 4. The presence of toxic levels of histamine in fish such as tuna indicates extensive growth of bacteria such as *Proteus* and *Klebsiella* spp., which are capable of producing histamine from histidine. The principal reason for this growth is lack of postharvest cooling. An official fluorometric method (AOAC, 1980) is available to measure histamine and is applicable for use in microbiological criteria (see Chapter 4). Problems in detecting this type of spoilage at the plant level include the facts that (1) odor and appearance do not reliably indicate this type of spoilage, (2) a broad range of spoilage exists among individual fish in a lot, and (3) the AOAC fluorometric method (AOAC, 1980) is a lengthy procedure not adaptable to the plant level. Recently, Lerke and coworkers (1983) reported a rapid screening method than can detect histamine in both raw and heat-processed tuna and mahi-mahi. In this procedure, histaminase acts on histamine, forming hydrogen peroxide which is then broken down by peroxidase with simultaneous formation of crystal violet from the oxidation of its leuco form. If further studies confirm that this test has satisfactory sensitivity, then it could be a valuable tool to monitor incoming scombroid fish for toxic levels of histamine (resulting from extensive microbial growth) and thus reduce the frequency of scombroid poisoning from fish.

Limulus Amoebocyte Lysate Test

Endotoxins of gram-negative bacteria can be detected in small quantities by the *Limulus* amoebocyte lysate test (LLT). This test has mainly been used in clinical and pharmaceutical microbiology, but has also been experimentally used for detection of endotoxins in foods (Haska and Nystrand, 1979; Jay, 1977; Sullivan et al., 1983). The LLT has been used experimentally as a simple, rapid (two hours) screening test to estimate the microbial quality of certain foods such as fresh beef and fish in which, under aerobic conditions of storage, gram-negative bacteria are responsible for quality deterioration. The LLT potentially could be used in the future as a test to estimate shelf-life of foods such as ground beef and fish. However, at present there is not enough information to judge whether or not the LLT may have practical application in criteria to evaluate the microbiological condition of foods.

Extract Release Volume

Several reports relate extract release volume (ERV) to degree of microbial deterioration of fresh meats (Jay, 1978). As meat deteriorates, the amount of water retained increases and ERV decreases. According to Jay (1978) this technique is of value in determining incipient spoilage in meats as well as in predicting refrigerator shelf-life. At the present, ERV is used for research and investigational purposes only and has no application as a parameter to evaluate the microbiological condition of foods.

Adenosine Triphosphate

Determination of bacterial adenosine triphosphate (ATP) in foods is based on the fact that all terrestrial life forms contain ATP. Experimental data indicate that microorganisms can be detected in foods by this method (Sharpe, 1973; Wood and Gibbs, 1982). At the present no practical routine methods exist to apply ATP as a parameter to evaluate the microbiological condition of foods.

ASSESSMENT OF INDICATORS

Indicators of Potential Human or Fecal Contamination or Possible Presence of Pathogens

Staphylococci

Staphylococci originate from the nasal passages, skin, and lesions of man and other mammals. They are applicable as part of microbiological criteria for cooked foods, various other food products that are commonly handled after heat processing, and foods that are handled extensively in preparation.

Staphylococci are usually killed during heat processing. Their reappearance on heat-processed foods is due to handling by workers or, less commonly, by contact with contaminated equipment or air. Small numbers of *S. aureus* are to be expected in foods that have been exposed to or handled by food workers. Large numbers (the number depending on the type of product) usually result from growth and almost invariably occur in foods that have been heat processed to eliminate competing organisms. Temperature abuse then sets the stage for growth. The presence of *S. aureus* can indicate a potential health hazard (see Chapter 4).

Large numbers of staphylococci may be indicative of the presence of toxins, although small numbers do not mean absence of toxin since large populations may have been reduced to smaller ones by a processing step, e.g., heating or fermentation. Methods for the detection and enumeration of *S. aureus* are adequate for their use in microbiological criteria (AOAC, 1980; APHA, 1984). The AOAC procedure was originally designed to increase the sensitivity of the plating procedure but unfortunately is inhibitory to injured cells. The direct plating method employing Baird-Parker agar effectively recovers both injured and noninjured *S. aureus* (Rayman et al., 1978). *S. aureus* counts are useful as part of microbiological criteria for foods that are handled after heat processing.

Escherichia coli

E. coli conforms to the definitions of *Enterobacteriaceae*, coliforms, and fecal coliforms, but is further identified by an IMViC (indole, methyl red, Voges-Proskauer, citrate utilization) pattern of $+ + - -$ or $- + - -$. Its natural habitat is the intestines of vertebrate animals. Thus, the presence of *E. coli* in a food indicates the possibility that fecal contamination has occurred and that other microorganisms of fecal origin, including pathogens, may be present. At present, *E. coli* is the best indicator of fecal contamination among the commonly used fecal-indicator organisms. In evaluating foods for safety, the presence of *E. coli* signifies a more positive assumption of hazard than the presence of other coliform bacteria. The failure to detect *E. coli* in a food, however, does not assure the absence of enteric pathogens (Mossel, 1967; Silliker and Gabis, 1976).

In many raw foods of animal origin, small numbers of *E. coli* can be expected because of the close association of these foods with the animal environment and the likelihood of contamination of carcasses from fecal material, hides, or feathers during slaughter-dressing procedures. These organisms are easily destroyed by heat processing of foods. Thus, the presence of *E. coli* in a heat-processed food means either process failure or, more commonly, postprocessing contamination from equipment or employees or from contact with contaminated raw foods. If the objective is to check for postprocessing contamination, then coliforms, rather than *E. coli*, should be the target organisms. Large numbers of *E. coli* in some foods (soft cheese, for example) may be the result of growth in the product or buildup on the equipment.

Routine methods for the detection and enumeration of *E. coli* (AOAC, 1980; APHA, 1984) are applicable for use in microbiological criteria. However, the MPN procedures for the enumeration of *E. coli* in foods are time-consuming, costly, inhibitory to injured cells, and lacking in precision. A direct plating procedure is now available (Anderson and Baird-Parker, 1975; Holbrook et al., 1980). A comparative study showed that the direct plating procedure was preferable to the MPN method for enumerating *E. coli* in meats, because of its lower variability, better recovery of *E. coli* from frozen samples, rapidity (24 hours vs. 8 days), decreased requirements for media, and decreased cost of analysts' time (Rayman et al., 1979). In addition, Anderson and Baird-Parker (1975) considered indole production, the index in the direct plating method—a more reliable characteristic of *E. coli* from foods than gas production from lactose.

Microbiological criteria involving *E. coli* are useful in those cases where it is desirable to determine if fecal contamination may have occurred. Contamination of a food with *E. coli* implies a risk that one or more of a wide diversity of enteric pathogens may have gained access to the food and introduced a health hazard.

Fecal Coliforms

Fecal coliform bacteria are used as a component of microbiological standards to monitor the wholesomeness of shellfish and the quality of shellfish growing waters (USDHEW, 1965). The term fecal coliform has arisen from attempts to find rapid, dependable methods to establish the presence of *E. coli* without isolation and purification of cultures and application of the lengthy and costly IMViC tests. The fecal coliforms are a group of organisms selected by incubating an inoculum derived from a coliform enrichment broth at higher temperatures (44° to 45.5°C/111° to 114°F) than used for incubating coliforms. Such preparations usually contain a high proportion of *E. coli* and are thus useful for indication of a probable fecal source. The fecal coliforms have a higher probability of containing organisms of fecal origin and hence of indicating fecal contamination than do coliforms that have received no further differential tests.

The fecal coliforms comprise a population presumed to contain a high proportion of *E. coli* but without the actual proportion of *E. coli* being positively established. In many foods, most fecal coliforms are *E. coli*, but some strains of *Enterobacter* and *Klebsiella* are included. In some foods, frozen vegetables for example, the composition may be different. Thus, if fecal coliforms in a food are used as an index of *E. coli* and therefore as an index of fecal contamination, this population's proportions must be established first. Fecal coliforms can become established on equipment and utensils in the food processing and handling environment and contaminate processed foods. They are easily destroyed by heat and are injured sublethally or may die during freezing and frozen storage of foods.

Routine MPN procedures applicable for use in microbiological criteria are well established (AOAC, 1980; APHA, 1976, 1981, 1984). These MPN procedures are subject to limitations similar to those mentioned for *E. coli* MPN methods.

The fecal coliform test is a useful part of the microbiological standard to evaluate the quality of shellfish growing waters. Its purpose is to reduce the risk of harvesting shellfish from waters polluted with fecal material. Because rapid, direct plating methods for *E. coli* (Anderson and Baird-Parker, 1975; Holbrook et al., 1980), including provisions for resuscitation of injured cells, are now available it may be advantageous to use *E. coli* rather than fecal coliforms as a component of microbiological criteria for foods.

Enterococci

Enterococci have certain features that make them unique as indicator organisms. Most are quite salt-tolerant (grow in the presence of 6.5% NaCl). All are facultatively anaerobic and grow well at 45°C (113°F). Except for *Streptococcus bovis* and *Streptococcus equinus*, they can grow at 7-10°C (44.6°-50°F). Unlike *E. coli*, they are relatively resistant to freezing. *Streptococcus faecalis* and *Streptococcus faecium*, the most common enterococci of foods, are relatively heat-resistant and may survive usual milk pasteurization procedures. *S. faecium* may survive and cause defects in marginally pasteurized canned cured meats.

Enterococci may be of fecal origin from both warm-blooded and cold-blooded animals; they also can establish an epiphytic relationship with growing plants (Mundt, 1970). They are often associated with insects and are thus a part of the natural microflora of many foods. In addition, they can establish themselves and persist in the food processing establishment long after their introduction.

Many foods normally contain small to large numbers of enterococci, especially *S. faecalis* and *S. faecium*. For instance, certain cheeses and some fermented sausages may contain more than 10^6 enterococci per gram. A wide variety of other foods such as raw meats, poultry, and raw vegetables may have relatively low levels (10^1-10^3 per gram). It is well established that enterococci counts of foods are not a reliable index of fecal contamination. A thorough understanding of the role and significance of enterococci in a food is required before any meaning can be attached to their presence and population numbers.

Many media have been proposed (APHA, 1976, 1984; ICMSF, 1978) for the selective isolation and/or enumeration of enterococci. Present methods have definite shortcomings relative to the degree of selectivity, quantitative recovery or differential ability (APHA, 1984). Enterococci counts have little useful application in microbiological criteria for foods. If they are used in specific cases to identify poor manufacturing practices, it is necessary to first establish the normal population levels at different stages of processing and handling with a standardized test procedure.

Pseudomonas aeruginosa

P. aeruginosa is a frequent contaminant of the environment (including water) and enters the environment with fecal wastes of human or of animals associated with humans (Hoadley, 1976). It is an opportunistic pathogen and, in some countries, is of particular concern for infants who may become infected when contaminated water or equipment is used to make infant formulas. This organism has been used in Europe as an indicator of contamination of bottled mineral water. It is oligocarbo-tolerant; therefore, after a period of adaptation, it can multiply in water of low nutrient level. Although there is not an acceptable standard method of detection of *P. aeruginosa*, methods are given in APHA (1981) and by Mossel et al. (1976). Most other test procedures, except for incubation at 42°C (107.6°F), are of little value in detecting *P. aeruginosa*. At the present time, *P. aeruginosa* has no application in microbiological criteria for water in the United States.

Indicators of Post-Heat Processing Contamination

Coliform Bacteria

Coliform bacteria are members of the *Enterobacteriaceae* that are capable of fermenting lactose with the production of acid and gas within 48 hours at 35°C (95°F); for dairy products some workers specify 32°C (89.6°F). Some coliforms (*E. coli*) are common in feces of man and other animals, but others (*Enterobacter, Klebsiella, Serratia, Erwinia,* and

Aeromonas) are commonly found in soil, water, and grains.

Small numbers of coliform bacteria are usually present in raw milk, vegetables, meat, poultry, and many other raw foods. Therefore, they are of little, if any, value in monitoring raw foods. These organisms are easily killed by heat; hence, their presence in heat-processed foods suggests post-heat contamination or, possibly, process failure. To locate the source and/or mode of entry of coliform bacteria into a food may require the examination of line samples. When large numbers are present in a heat-processed food, growth most likely occurred because of a lack of or improper refrigeration. Coliform bacteria are easily sublethally stressed by freezing, so coliform counts of frozen foods should be interpreted cautiously. Special resuscitation procedures are recommended (APHA, 1976, 1984) for their detection and enumeration from frozen foods.

From their original fecal, soil, water, or plant environment, coliform bacteria can reach the food processing plant, food service establishment, or home environment, where they may be spread via equipment and utensil surfaces or by employees. The presence of coliforms in food does not necessarily mean that there was fecal contamination or that pathogens are present. Their significance in foods depends upon the circumstances to which the food has been exposed. The fecal connotation of *E. coli*, a member of the coliform group, is often inappropriately linked to foods in which coliform bacteria are found. Further examination (see sections on fecal coliform bacteria and *E. coli*, above) is required to establish potential fecal association. The use of coliform bacteria as an index of contamination after heat processing of foods requires a thorough understanding of the production, processing, and distribution practices to which a food is subjected and the effect of these practices on coliform bacteria. Methods for the enumeration of coliforms are adequate for purpose of use in microbiological criteria (AOAC, 1980; APHA, 1978, 1984; ICMSF, 1978).

Coliform bacteria are particularly useful as part of microbiological criteria to indicate postprocessing contamination of foods that have been processed (heating, irradiation, or chlorination) for safety. They are also useful indicators in guidelines at critical control points, particularly after heat processing.

Enterobacteriaceae

Enterobacteriaceae counts are not a component of microbiological criteria for foods in the United States; they are, however, used in Europe for this purpose. The enrichment-plating procedure, which employs violet-red bile agar with 1% glucose, allows colony formation by a greater spectrum of members of the *Enterobacteriaceae* than the usual procedures, which select for the lactose-positive members only (Mossel, 1967; Mossel et al., 1963). The *Enterobacteriaceae* test, like the coliform test, is useful to indicate postprocessing contamination in foods, but the presence of either group does not imply fecal contamination. Whether or not the *Enterobacteriaceae* count should supplant the coliform count in microbiological criteria is a debatable question.

TESTS FOR OTHER COMPONENTS

Tests for Metabolic Products of Pathogens That Indicate a Health Hazard

In a number of circumstances, tests for metabolic products of pathogens are preferred to tests for pathogens (see Chapter 4) to indicate the presence of pathogens or their toxins.

Thermonuclease Test for Evidence of Growth of Staphylococci and Presence of Enterotoxins

When large numbers ($\geq 10^6$/g or ml) of *S. aureus* are present or suspected in processed foods, actual testing for enterotoxins is desirable, but the procedure is time-consuming and expensive. Furthermore, not all food laboratories have the capability to perform the test (see Chapter 9, Part A). Low counts of *S. aureus* in reheated or fermented foods may be misleading because the number of viable cells of *S. aureus* may be the remainder of larger populations, whereas enterotoxins may be present. *S. aureus* produces thermostable deoxyribonuclease (TNase), which has been used as a rapid and inexpensive procedure for screening foods for indication of extensive staphylococcal growth and possible presence of enterotoxin (APHA, 1984). The method is adequate for application in microbiological criteria. The TNase test has been recommended for testing foods such as cheeses and sausages when conditions such as improper lactic starter performance may have been responsible for the presence of significant levels of coagulase-positive *S. aureus* (Emswiler-Rose et al., 1980; Todd et al., 1981. See also Chapter 9, Part A). TNase can be a useful indicator because it can almost always be detected in foods whenever enterotoxins can be detected (Tatini, 1981). TNase-positive samples, whenever possible, should be tested for enterotoxin.

Aflatoxin Detection by Ultraviolet Light

Long-wave ultraviolet (black) light (U.V.) has been used to detect the presence of *Aspergillus flavus* and *Aspergillus parasiticus* in corn (Shotwell and Hesseltine, 1981). When corn viewed under U.V. light displays a bright greenish-yellow fluorescence (BGYF), it is probable that aflatoxin may be present. Detection procedures for aflatoxins are given in AOAC (1980). Because of the association of BGYF with the potential occurrence of aflatoxins, the examination of corn and other grains with U.V. light as a rapid screening procedure has been adopted by industry. This examination is utilized only as a presumptive test; the occurrence of BGYF is indicative that more sophisticated testing for the presence of aflatoxin, e.g., by high-pressure liquid chromatography, is needed. The use of U.V. examination as a component of microbiological criteria is limited to purchase specifications or guidelines.

Test for Phosphatase

The phosphatase test is part of a criterion for certain milk and milk products to determine whether the product in question was pasteurized properly and also to detect the possible addition of raw milk to pasteurized milk (APHA, 1978; USPHS/FDA 1978). Methods, limitations, and interpretation of test results are presented in detail in *Standard Methods for the Examination of Dairy Products* (APHA, 1978). Routine methods for the detection of phosphatase are well established and applicable to evaluate the acceptability of pasteurized milk and milk products.

REFERENCES

Amerine, M. A., R. M. Pangborn, and E. B. Roessler
    1965   Principles of Sensory Evaluation of Food. New York: Academic Press.
AMI (American Meat Institute)
    1982   Good Manufacturing Practices. I. Voluntary Guidelines for the Production of Dry Fermented Sausage; II. Voluntary Guidelines for the Production of Semi-dry Fermented Sausage. Washington, D.C.: AMI. 10 pp.
Anderson, J. M., and A. C. Baird-Parker
    1975   A rapid and direct plate method for enumerating *Escherichia coli* biotype 1 in food. J. Appl. Bacteriol. 39:111–117.
Anonymous
    1979   Shrimp Decomposition Workshop. National Shrimp Breaders and Processors Association, National Fisheries Institute and FDA, Tampa, Florida.
AOAC (Association of Official Analytical Chemists)
    1980   Official Methods of Analysis of the Association of Official Analytical Chemists. 13th Ed. W. Horwitz, ed. Washington, D.C.: AOAC.
APHA (American Public Health Association)
    1976   Compendium of Methods for the Microbiological Examination of Foods. M. L. Speck, ed. Washington, D.C.: APHA.
    1978   Standard Methods for the Examination of Dairy Products. 14th Ed. E. H. Marth, ed. Washington, D.C.: APHA.
    1981   Standard Methods for the Examination of Water and Wastewater. 15th Ed. A. E.

Greenburg, J. J. Conners, D. Jenkins, and M. A. H. Franson, eds. Washington, D.C.: APHA.

1984   Compendium of Methods for the Microbiological Examination of Foods. 2nd Ed. M. L. Speck, ed. Washington, D.C.: APHA.

Beacham, L. M.
1946   A study of decomposition in canned oysters and clams. J. Assoc. Off. Agric. Chem. 29:89–99.

Broitman, S., W. L. Mallmann, and G. M. Trout
1958   A simple test for detecting keeping quality for milk. J. Milk Food Technol. 21:280–284.

Bush, J. C.
1970   The Use of Oxidation-Reduction Dyes in the Determination of the Shelf Life of Meats. M.S. thesis. College Station: Texas A&M University.

Chang, O., W. L. Cheuk, R. Nickelson, R. Martin, and G. Finne
1983   Indole in shrimp: effect of fresh storage temperature, freezing and boiling. J. Food Sci. 48:813–816.

Cheuk, W. L., and G. Finne
1981   Modified colorimetric method for determining indole in shrimp. J. Assoc. Off. Anal. Chem. 64:783–785.

Cobb, B. F., I. Alaniz, and C. A. Thompson, Jr.
1973   Biochemical and microbial studies on shrimp. Volatile nitrogen and amino nitrogen analysis. J. Food Sci. 38:431–436.

Cobb, B. F., III., C. S. Yeh, F. Christopher, and Carl Vanderzant
1977   Organoleptic, bacterial and chemical characteristics of penaeid shrimp subjected to short-term high-temperature holding. J. Food Prot. 40:256–260.

Crosgrove, D. M.
1978   A rapid method for estimating ethanol in canned salmon. J. Food Sci. 43:641–643.

Duggan, R. E.
1948   Report on decomposition in shellfish—indole in shrimp, oysters and crabmeat. J. Assoc. Off. Agric. Chem. 31:507–510.

Duggan, R. E., and L. W. Strasburger
1946   Indole in shrimp. J. Assoc. Off. Agric. Chem. 29:177–188.

Emswiler-Rose, B. S., R. W. Johnston, M. E. Harris, and W. H. Lee
1980   Rapid detection of staphylococcal thermonuclease on casings of naturally contaminated fermented sausages. Appl. Environ. Microbiol. 40:13–18.

FDA (Food and Drug Administration)
1981   Defect action level for decomposition in imported canned and cooked frozen shrimp; availability of guide. Federal Register 46:39221.

Fields, M. L.
1964   Acetylmethylcarbinol and diacetyl as chemical indexes of microbial quality of apple juice. Food Technol. 18:1224–1238.

Griffiths, M. W., J. D. Phillips, and D. D. Muir
1981   Thermostability of proteases and lipases from a number of species of psychrotrophic bacteria of dairy origin. J. Appl. Bacteriol. 50:289–303.

Haska, G., and R. Nystrand
1979   Determination of endotoxins in sugar with the Limulus test. Appl. Environ. Microbiol. 38:1078–1080.

Hill, E. C., and F. W. Wenzel
1957   The diacetyl test as an aid for quality control of citrus products. 1. Detection of bacterial growth in orange juice during concentration. Food Technol. 11:240–243.

Hill, E. C., F. W. Wenzel, and A. Barreto
1954 Colorimetric method for detection of microbiological spoilage in citrus juices. Food Technol. 8:168–171.

Hoadley, A. W.
1976 Potential health hazards associated with *Pseudomonas aeruginosa* in water. Pp. 80–114 in Bacterial Indicators/Health Hazards Associated with Water. A. W. Hoadley and B. J. Dutka, eds. Philadelphia: American Society for Testing Materials.

Holbrook, R., J. M. Anderson, and A. C. Baird-Parker
1980 Modified direct plate method for counting *Escherichia coli* in foods. Food Technol. Austral. 32:78–83.

Hollingworth, T. A., Jr., and H. R. Throm
1982 Correlation of ethanol concentration with sensory classification of decomposition in canned salmon. J. Food Sci. 47:1315–1317.
1983 A headspace gas chromatographic method for the rapid analysis of ethanol in canned salmon. J. Food Sci. 48:290–291.

ICMSF (International Commission on Microbiological Specifications for Foods)
1978 Microorganisms in Foods. 1. Their significance and methods of enumeration. Toronto: University of Toronto Press.
1980 Fish and shellfish and their products. Pp. 567–605 in Microbial Ecology of Foods. Vol. 2. Food Commodities. New York: Academic Press.

Jay, J. M.
1977 The *Limulus* lysate endotoxin assay as a test of microbial quality of ground beef. J. Appl. Bacteriol. 43:99–109.
1978 Modern Food Microbiology. 2nd Ed. New York: D. Van Nostrand.

King, W. H., and F. F. Flynn
1945 Experimental studies on decomposition of oysters used for canning. J. Assoc. Off. Agric. Chem. 28:385–398.

Larmond, E.
1977 Laboratory Methods for Sensory Evaluation of Food. Research Branch. Canada Dept. of Agric. Pub. No. 1637.

Lerke, P. A., M. N. Porcuna, and H. B. Chin
1983 Screening test for histamine in fish. J. Food Sci. 48:155–157.

McClellan, G.
1952 Report on chemical indices to decomposition in shellfish. J. Assoc. Off. Agric. Chem. 35:524–525.

Montgomery, W. A., G. S. Sidhu, and G. L. Vale
1970 The Australian prawn industry. 1. Natural resources and quality aspects of whole cooked fresh prawns and frozen prawn meat. CSIRO Food Preserv. Quart. 30(2):21.

Mossel, D. A. A.
1967 Ecological principles and methodological aspects of the examination of foods and feeds for indicator microorganisms. J. Assoc. Off. Agric. Chem. 50:91–104.

Mossel, D. A. A., M. Visser, and A. M. R. Cornelissen
1963 The examination of foods for *Enterobacteriaceae* using a test of the type generally adopted for the detection of salmonellae. J. Appl. Bacteriol. 26:444–452.

Mossel, D. A. A., H. DeVor, and I. Eelderink
1976 A further simplified procedure for the detection of *Pseudomonas aeruginosa* in contaminated aqueous substrata. J. Appl. Bacteriol. 41:307–309.

Mundt, J. O.
1970 Lactic acid bacteria associated with raw plant food materials. J. Milk Food Technol. 33:550–553.

National Soft Drink Association
  1975   Quality Specifications and Test Procedures for "Bottler's Granulated and Liquid
            Sugar." Washington, D.C.: Natl. Soft Drink Assoc.
NCA (National Canners Association Research Laboratories)
  1968   Laboratory Manual for Food Canners and Processors. Vol. 1. Microbiology and
            Processing. Westport, Conn.: AVI Publishing.
Oberlender, V., M. O. Hanna, R. Miget, C. Vanderzant, and G. Finne
  1983   Storage characteristics of fresh swordfish steaks stored in carbon dioxide enriched
            controlled (flow-through) atmospheres. J. Food Prot. 46:434–440.
Parmelee, C. E.
  1974   Early detection of psychrotrophs in pasteurized milk. Dairy and Ice Cream Field
            157(8):38.
Rayman, M. K., J. J. Devoyod, U. Purvis, D. Kusch, J. Lanier, R. J. Gilbert, D. G. Till, and
G. A. Jarvis
  1978   ICMSF Methods Studies. X. An international comparative study of four media for
            the enumeration of *Staphylococcus aureus* in foods. Can. J. Microbiol. 24:274–281.
Rayman, M. K., G. A. Jarvis, C. M. Davidson, S. Long, J. M. Allen, T. Tong, P. Dodsworth,
S. McLaughlin, S. Greenburg, B. G. Shaw, H. J. Beckers, S. Qvist, P. M. Nottingham, and
B. J. Stewart
  1979   ICMSF Methods Studies. XIII. An international comparative study of the MPN pro-
            cedure and the Anderson-Baird-Parker direct plating method for the enumeration of
            Escherichia coli biotype 1 in raw meats. Can. J. Microbiol. 25:1321–1327.
Salwin, H.
  1964   Report on decomposition and filth in foods (Chemical indexes). J. Assoc. Off. Agric.
            Chem. 47:57–58.
Sharpe, A. N.
  1973   Automation and instrumentation developments for the bacteriology laboratory. Pp. 197–
            232 in Sampling—Microbiological Monitoring of Environments. R. G. Board and
            D. W. Lovelock, eds. London: Academic Press.
Shelef, L. A., and J. M. Jay
  1970   Use of a titrimetric method to assess the bacterial spoilage of fresh beef. Appl.
            Microbiol. 19:902–905.
Shotwell, O. L., and C. W. Hesseltine
  1981   Use of bright greenish-yellow fluorescence as a presumptive test for aflatoxin in corn.
            Cereal Chem. 58:124–127.
Silliker, J. H.
  1963   Total counts as indexes of food quality. Pp. 102–112 in Microbiological Quality of
            Foods. L. W. Slanetz, C. O. Chichester, A. R. Gaufin, and Z. J. Ordal, eds. New
            York: Academic Press.
Silliker, J. H., and D. A. Gabis
  1976   ICMSF Methods Studies. VII. Indicator tests as substitutes for direct testing of dried
            foods and feeds for *Salmonella*. Can. J. Microbiol. 22:971–974.
Stansby, M. E.
  1963   Analytical methods. Pp. 367–373 in Industrial Fishery Technology. M. E. Stansby,
            ed. Huntington, N.Y.: Robert E. Krieger.
Staruszkiewicz, W. F.
  1974   Collaborative study of the gas-liquid chromatographic determination of indole in
            shrimp. J. Assoc. Off. Anal. Chem. 57:813–818.
Sullivan, J. D. Jr., P. C. Ellis, R. G. Lee, W. S. Combs, Jr., and S. W. Watson
  1983   Comparison of the *Limulus* amoebocyte lysate test with plate counts and chemical

analyses for assessment of the quality of lean fish. Appl. Environ. Microbiol. 45:720–722.

Tatini, S. R.
  1981   Thermonuclease as an indicator of staphylococcal enterotoxins in food. Pp. 53–75 in Antinutrients and Natural Toxicants in Foods. R. L. Ory, ed. Westport, Conn.: Food and Nutrition Press.

Todd, E., R. Szabo, H. Robern, T. Gleeson, C. Park, and D. S. Clark
  1981   Variation in counts, enterotoxin levels and TNase in Swiss-type cheese contaminated with *Staphylococcus aureus*. J. Food Prot. 44:839–848.

USDHEW (U.S. Department of Health, Education and Welfare)
  1965   National Shellfish Sanitation Program, Manual of Operations. Part 1. Sanitation of shellfish growing areas. Washington, D.C.: U.S. Government Printing Office.

USPHS/FDA (U.S. Public Health Service/Food and Drug Administration)
  1978   Grade A Pasteurized Milk Ordinance. 1978 Recommendations. USPHS/FDA Publ. No. 229. Washington, D.C.: U.S. Government Printing Office.

Wood, J. M., and P. A. Gibbs
  1982   New developments in the rapid estimation of microbial populations in foods. Pp. 183–214 in Developments in Food Microbiology-1. R. Davies, ed. Englewood, N.J.: Applied Science.

6

Consideration of Sampling Associated With a Criterion

An effective sampling plan is one of the essential components of a microbiological criterion. The purpose of this chapter is to discuss the most common sampling plans applicable to microbiological criteria for foods. For more detailed information regarding statistical concepts of population probabilities and sampling, choice of sampling procedures, decision criteria, and practical aspects of application, the reader is referred to publications such as those by the ICMSF (1974); Kilsby (1982); Kilsby and Baird-Parker (1983); Kramer and Twigg (1970); Puri et al. (1979); and Puri and Mullen (1980). The ICMSF publication is especially useful because it deals with statistically based sampling plans as applied to microorganisms in foods.

It is important to establish a sampling plan that can effectively discriminate between good and bad lots. A lot in this case is defined as the quantity of goods that has been produced, handled, and stored within a limited period of time under uniform conditions. For example, the same goods produced on a single line or processed in a day or during one shift can be considered a lot. A lot is made up of sample units whose microbiological quality can be assessed. Sampling procedures and decision criteria should be based on sound statistical concepts in order to achieve a high degree of confidence in decisions relative to the acceptability of a lot. A company may at times rely on a sampling plan in which the experience of its quality control personnel is used to select the location of sampling, the number of sample units withdrawn from the lot, and the limit(s) for acceptance or rejection. Such procedures are often used in investigations of rejected lots. Validity of the conclusion reached depends on the ability of personnel to choose a representative sample. Only with

132

a well-defined probability sample is the investigator guaranteed that the sampling plan used has the stated properties, i.e., that it rejects inferior batches with the stated frequency.

Many reviews regarding microbiological criteria deal with the problems of sampling and decision criteria and recognize that reliable microbiological criteria are not possible without a carefully chosen sampling plan (Bartrum and Slocum, 1964; Charles, 1979; Corlett, 1974; Dyett, 1970; Hobbs and Gilbert, 1970; Leininger et al., 1971; Shuffman and Kronick, 1963). Useful historical data on sampling and rejection criteria have resulted from such studies. Factors to be considered in choosing a sampling plan, as outlined by Kramer and Twigg (1970) include:

- purpose of inspection
- nature of product
- nature of the sampling and analytical procedure
- nature of the lots being examined

A common purpose of inspection and analysis of food, including microbiological testing, is to obtain information upon which to base a decision to either accept or reject the food. The acceptability of a lot is determined by selecting a suitable property or attribute, in this context, whether or not some particular organism or group of organisms occurs in number above a specified level.

The type of plan chosen for this purpose is termed an acceptance sampling plan. The product type, its microbiological history, and its intended use will influence the selection of the sampling plan. Difficulties in the application of acceptance sampling plans that test for microbial levels in foods have been outlined by a number of sources (Clark, 1978; Cowell and Morisetti, 1969; Ingram and Kitchell, 1970; Kilsby et al., 1979; Wodicka, 1973). The first difficulty arises in sampling because the microorganisms in many foods are often unevenly distributed within a lot, e.g., *Salmonella* in dried milk powder. A second difficulty is related to the errors inherent in the methods used to detect and enumerate microorganisms. (See Chapters 4 and 5.)

The International Commission on Microbiological Specifications for Foods (ICMSF, 1974) has recognized many of these considerations by relating the stringency of the sampling plan to the degree and type of hazard of the food (Table 6-1). The stringency of sampling increases with the hazard, from a condition of no health hazard but only of utility (shelf-life) through a low indirect health hazard to direct health hazards related to diseases of moderate or severe implication. For example, foods in the "case 1" category present no direct health hazard. By contrast, foods in the "case 15" category present a severe, direct health hazard where conditions of handling and use after sampling may increase the hazard. Clinical severity of a foodborne disease, available epidemiological information, processing conditions, handling and ultimate use of the food are built into these "case" numbers. A similar approach for selection of sampling plans was adopted by the Committee on Evaluation of the *Salmonella* Problem (NRC, 1969). The sampling plans proposed by this committee were recommended not for routine use but for application where a *Salmonella* problem had been defined.

2-CLASS ATTRIBUTES SAMPLING PLANS

The 2-class attributes sampling plan simply classifies each sample unit as acceptable (nondefective) or unacceptable (defective). In some plans, the presence of any organism of a particular type, e.g., *Salmonella*, would be unacceptable; in others, a limited number of organisms may be acceptable, e.g., *Vibrio parahaemolyticus*. In the latter, a boundary is chosen, denoted by m, which divides an acceptable count from an unacceptable count. The 2-class plan rejects a lot if more than "c" out of the "n" sample units tested were unacceptable.[1] For example, a typical 2-class plan with n = 5 and c = 0 requires that five sample units be tested and specifies a c value of 0 (see Table 6-1, case 10). The lot would be rejected if any one of the five sample units tested was defective. Such plans are used for *Salmonella*. The choice of n and c varies with the desired stringency of the plan. By appropriate calculations the probability of acceptance can be determined for a lot of a given quality for any specified sampling plan (see section below on operating characteristic curves). These sampling plans are valid regardless of the statistical distributions of the microbiological counts provided that an appropriate probability sampling scheme has been used to select the units to be tested.

Military Standard 105D (DOD, 1963), which was developed to meet mass-production quality requirements during World War II, is a prime example of statistically designed single and multiple 2-class attributes

---

[1] n = number of sample units analyzed which are chosen separately and independently.

c = maximum allowable number of sample units yielding unsatisfactory test results, e.g., the presence of the organism, or a count above m.

m = a microbiological criterion that in a 2-class plan separates good quality from defective quality; or in a 3-class plan separates good quality from marginally acceptable quality.

M = a microbiological criterion that in a 3-class plan separates marginally acceptable quality from defective quality. Values at or above M are unacceptable.

case = a set of circumstances related to the nature and treatment of a food, categorized into 15 such sets which influence the anticipated hazard from the presence of specified bacterial species or groups within a food (ICMSF, 1974).

TABLE 6-1 Suggested Sampling Plans for Combinations of Degrees of Health Hazard and Conditions of Use (i.e., the 15 'Cases')

Degree of Concern Relative to Utility and Health Hazard	Conditions in Which Food is Expected to be Handled and Consumed After Sampling, in the Usual Course of Events[a]		
	Conditions Reduce Degree of Concern	Conditions Cause No Change in Concern	Conditions May Increase Concern
No direct health hazard Utility, e.g. shelf-life and spoilage	Increase shelf-life Case 1 3-class $n = 5$, $c = 3$	No change Case 2 3-class $n = 5$, $c = 2$	Reduce shelf life Case 3 3-class $n = 5$, $c = 1$
Health hazard Low, indirect (indicator)	Reduce hazard Case 4 3-class $n = 5$, $c = 3$	No change Case 5 3-class $n = 5$, $c = 2$	Increase hazard Case 6 3-class $n = 5$, $c = 1$
Moderate, direct, limited spread	Case 7 3-class $n = 5$, $c = 2$	Case 8 3-class $n = 5$, $c = 1$	Case 9 3-class $n = 10$, $c = 1$
Moderate, direct, potentially extensive spread	Case 10 2-class $n = 5$, $c = 0$	Case 11 2-class $n = 10$, $c = 0$	Case 12 2-class $n = 20$, $c = 0$
Severe, direct	Case 13 2-class $n = 15$, $c = 0$	Case 14 2-class $n = 30$, $c = 0$	Case 15 2-class $n = 60$, $c = 0$

[a]More stringent sampling plans would generally be used for sensitive foods destined for susceptible populations.

SOURCE: ICMSF, 1974, p. 60. © University of Toronto Press, 1974.

sampling plans. These concepts were used also in sampling plans for *Salmonella* by the committee evaluating the *Salmonella* problem (NRC, 1969).

3-CLASS ATTRIBUTES SAMPLING PLANS

Because the choice of a boundary between an acceptable count and an unacceptable count is rather arbitrary, Bray et al. (1973) introduced the concept of a 3-class plan. Sample units with a count of less than m are of acceptable or good quality. Units with a count between m and M (see footnote 1) are judged to be of marginal quality, and units whose counts are greater than M are of unacceptable or bad quality. A random sample of n sample units would be chosen from the lot and the lot would be rejected if any of the sample units had a count above M and/or if more than c of the units had a count above m. For example, a typical 3-class plan is characterized by $n = 5$, $c = 2$, $m = 10^5/g$, $M = 10^7/g$. Thus five sample units ($n = 5$) are analyzed. The lot will be rejected if any sample unit exceeds a count of $10^7/g$ and/or if three or more sample units exceed a count of $10^5/g$. The lot will be accepted if all units have counts of less than $10^7/g$ and if no more than two units have counts greater than $10^5/g$.

The 3-class plan makes no assumption about the distribution of counts in the lot. It assumes only that an appropriate probability sampling procedure was used to select the sample units. As with 2-class plans, the choice of n and c varies with the desired stringency of the plan. The ICMSF (1974) has applied 2- and 3-class attributes sampling plans to assess microbiological safety or quality for a variety of foods involved in international trade.

VARIABLES SAMPLING PLANS

As stated previously, for the 2-class attributes sampling plan, no assumption is necessary regarding the distribution of counts in the population of sample units from which the sample is taken. When the distribution of counts is known, this additional information can be used to increase the chance of making a correct decision or equivalently to reduce the sample size while maintaining the same probability of a correct decision.

Frequently it is assumed that the log of the count follows a normal distribution. Kilsby and coworkers (Kilsby, 1982; Kilsby and Pugh, 1981; Kilsby et al., 1979) have stated that this assumption is reasonable when the food comes from a common source and is processed under uniform conditions. The variables plan is chosen so as to reject a lot with probability

P if the proportion of unacceptable sample units (as defined in the 2-class attributes plan) exceeds p (a proportion). For example, if more than 10% of the sample units are unacceptable, the goal is to reject the lot with 80% probability. The rule for deciding whether to reject a lot is the following: reject the lot if $\bar{x} + ks > m$ where $\bar{x}$ and s are the sample mean and standard deviation of the log counts from a sample of size n. The value m is some microbiological concentration that is critical. The value k is determined from the noncentral t-distribution (Johnson and Welch, 1940).

OPERATING CHARACTERISTIC CURVES

In general, it is necessary to balance the probabilities of two risks in acceptance sampling. The acceptance quality level is defined as the maximum proportion of unacceptable sample units that a lot can possess and still be acceptable. Some larger proportion of defective units, judged to be the minimum proportion of defective units for which the lot is entirely unacceptable might be termed the defective quality level. For example, a lot with fewer than 5% defective units might be judged entirely acceptable but with more than 10% defective units might be judged entirely unacceptable. The zone between 5% and 10% defective units might be termed a zone of indifference. The acceptable quality level is 5% and the defective quality level is 10%. The vendors' or producers' risk is the probability that a lot of acceptable quality level is rejected. The consumers' or buyers' risk is the probability that a lot of defective quality level is accepted. The operating characteristic (OC) curve provides the information necessary to evaluate these risks. For a 2-class attributes sampling plan, the OC curve is simply the probability of accepting the lot, plotted as a function of the true proportion of defectives in the lot.

Figure 6-1 gives the OC curve for an attributes sampling plan in which n = 10 and c = 2. The lot is rejected if more than two samples are found to be defective. A lot with 20% defective sample units would be accepted 68% of the time and rejected 32% of the time. With 40% defective units, the lot would be accepted 17% of the time, and with only 10% defective units, the lot would be accepted 93% of the time. With this information, it is possible to judge whether both the consumers' and the producers' interests are being met.

The influence of the c value on the OC curve can be seen in Figure 6-2. Increasing c but holding n at a fixed value causes a lot with a larger proportion of defective units to be accepted. Increasing n but holding the c/n constant (i.e., the maximum proportion of defectives tolerated) causes the OC curve to become steeper (Figure 6-3). This means that the ability to discriminate between acceptable and unacceptable lots has been increased. For example, with a sample size of n = 5 and c = 1, there is a 0.20 probability of rejecting a lot with 17% defective units and a 0.20 probability of accepting a lot with 49% defective units. With a sample size of n = 10 and c = 2, there is a 0.20 probability of rejecting a lot with 16% defective units and a 0.20 probability of accepting a lot with 38% defective units. For n = 20 and c = 4, these percentages become 16 and 29.6, respectively. It is apparent from these examples that as the sample size increases, the difference between producers' and consumers' risks can be made smaller. In fact, one can calculate the minimum sample size required to satisfy prescribed producers' and consumers' risks. Alternatively, if the sample size and one of the risks is specified, the other risk is determined and can be calculated.

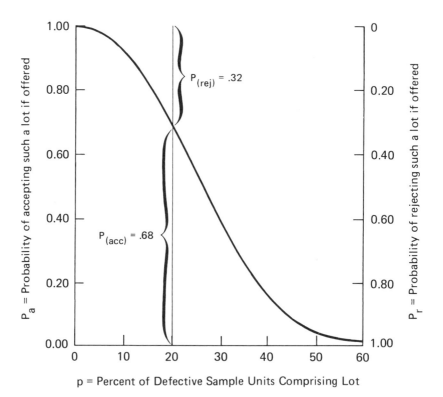

FIGURE 6-1   The operating characteristic curve for $n = 10$, $c = 2$, i.e., the probability of accepting lots, in relation to the proportion defective among the sample units comprising the lots.

SOURCE: ICMSF, 1974, p. 7. Copyright © 1974 by University of Toronto Press.

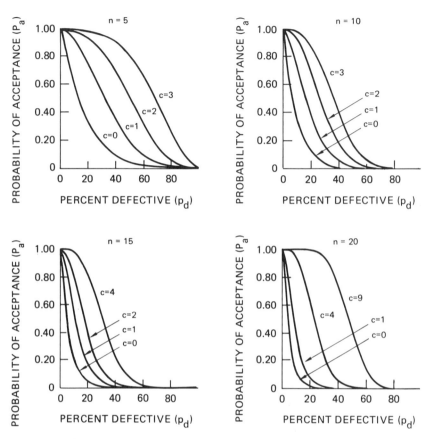

FIGURE 6-2   Operating characteristic curves for different sample sizes (*n*) and different criteria of acceptance (*c*) for 2-class attributes plan.

SOURCE: ICMSF, 1974, p. 24. Copyright © 1974 by University of Toronto Press.

It is important to note that unless the proportion of the lot sampled is greater than 10%, the size of the lot has very little effect on the probability of acceptance. In fact, OC curves for attributes plans are normally computed assuming an infinite lot size and using the binomial distribution. When the sample size exceeds 10% of the lot size, the binomial distribution should be replaced by the hypergeometric distribution for computing probabilities of acceptance (Puri and Mullen, 1980).

In the 3-class plans the OC curve is replaced by an OC surface. For these plans the probability of accepting the lot is plotted as a function of the proportion of defective or unacceptable sample units and the proportion

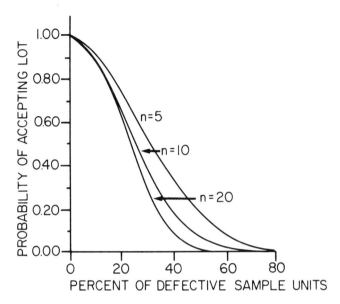

FIGURE 6-3   Operating characteristic curves for different sample sizes n keeping
*c/n constant for two-class attributes plan (*c = criteria for acceptance).

of marginally acceptable sample units. The ICMSF (1974) publication
contains tables giving the probability of acceptance for various proportions
of defective and marginally acceptable sample units for commonly used
3-class attributes plans.

Sampling plans for use in the microbiological examination of foods are
usually by necessity single sampling plans based on one sample size with
a number of sample units, because the analytical procedures are frequently
destructive and time-consuming. Such conditions generally make double
or sequential sampling plans uneconomical for frequent application in
microbiological criteria. Sequential sampling plans are used, however, in
visual nondestructive examination of canned foods for physical defects
such as dents or overall seam measurement.

ESTABLISHING LIMITS

Limits expressed in sampling plans can be determined in two ways.
One method is to use data generated by surveys. When using appropriate
probability sampling techniques, results from surveys can produce un-
biased estimates of the mean and standard deviation of the distribution of
the desired microbiological parameter (Puri and Mullen, 1980; Sukhatme

and Sukhatme, 1970). It may be appropriate to first transform the scale of measurement of the desired parameter. For example, frequently the logs of the microbiological counts follow a normal distribution more closely than the counts themselves. Collins-Thompson et al. (1978) chose m to be $\bar{x} + 2s$ where $\bar{x}$ and s are the sample mean and sample standard deviation based on a national survey. If the microbiological parameters under consideration follow a normal distribution, then approximately 2.5% of the sample units would exceed m. Hence this approach implicitly assumes that at the time of the survey only 2.5% of sample units are unacceptable.

Corlett (1974) described the process of determining limits by judging count levels consistent with Good Manufacturing Practices (GMP). For example, if a product consistently yielded counts of less than, say, 10 coliforms per gram under good processing controls, then this level would be used as a limit. This approach to selection of limits appears to be common and practical. A further approach to judgment limits was suggested by Davis (1969). Since there are inherent errors in microbiological testing, he proposed a 3-tier system of limits that differs by multiples of 10. Using his example, raw meat for pies would be declared satisfactory (S) when total counts were under 10^6/g, doubtful (D) when counts ranged between 10^6 and 10^7/g and unsatisfactory (U) when counts exceeded 10^7/g. This SDU system is somewhat analogous to the 3-class ICMSF sampling plan (ICMSF, 1974) where a m value represents levels consistent with GMP and the M value is the smallest value that poses a health hazard, spoilage, or an overt sanitation problem. The M value should not be used to reflect GMP nor should it be set at some arbitrary level, for example, where 98% of the lots can meet it. This is a misuse of the philosophy behind the establishment of this value. The M value should be chosen based on expert judgment and historical data. The establishment of limits for variables sampling plans for commodities such as meat has been described by Kilsby (1982) and Brown and Baird-Parker (1982).

RESAMPLING

No discussion about sampling plans is complete without discussing the problem of resampling. This problem, described by Pitt (1978) as the resampling syndrome, is a common practice when the first set of analyses yields unfavorable results. By resampling, we mean that when the initial sample yields results that are unacceptable, a second sample may be taken. If the test results on this sample are favorable, the lot is then accepted. (Pitt [1978] further associates this situation to ancient times when messengers who brought bad news were killed or made to repeat the journey until glad tidings were delivered.) Resampling changes the characteristics of the sampling plan, for example, by increasing the probability of accepting lots of poor quality. This becomes a problem if the investigator believes that the operating characteristic curve associated with the original 1-stage sampling plan is still valid. It is not! For example, in sampling a lot with 20% defective units, a 2-class attributes sampling plan (n = 5, c = 0) will accept the lot only 33% of the time. If resampling is allowed when one unacceptable unit is detected and the lot is accepted if no further unacceptable units occur in the next five units sampled, then the probability of accepting the lot increases to 46%. Decision criteria based upon an undetermined OC curve can lead to incorrect decisions about the acceptability of the lot. This situation is aggravated because resampling is undertaken only on selective occasions when lots have been rejected. (For additional information see Appendix A-I and ICMSF, 1974, p. 71).

This is not to say that resampling is always wrong since there are occasions when testing for pathogens such as *Salmonella* may produce a false-positive result and retesting is necessary. The *Salmonella* committee offered a corresponding solution to this problem (NRC, 1969) when it proposed a 2-stage sampling plan to avoid rejection on the basis of a single positive test. Thus, the acceptance criteria for a lot are based on a 2-stage sampling plan with determined probabilities. Two-stage sampling plans, when properly used, can reduce the average sample size necessary to achieve adequate protection because, with badly contaminated lots, a small first-stage sample may be sufficient to reject the lot. A second-stage sample is then needed only for doubtful cases.

When resampling is required the consequences of this procedure should be included in the final decision criterion. Resampling is useful during investigational proceedings. When it is established that a lot is unacceptable, one may wish to reexamine it to determine selective salvage or corrective measures (see Chapter 7). This increase in data generated by resampling can prove to be beneficial in reaching sensible and realistic decisions.

APPLICATIONS

There are two prime reasons for microbiological sampling. The first is to enable a decision to be reached on the suitability of a food or ingredient for its intended purpose. The ICMSF 2- and 3-class attributes sampling plans are appropriate for this purpose. These plans are used in Canada on a national basis and are incorporated in legislative programs (see Chapter 8). The second reason for microbiological sampling is to monitor performance relative to accepted Good Manufacturing Practices. Attributes sampling may also be applicable when sample units can be appropriately drawn at critical control points (including end product). On the other hand, sampling may be required to detect faulty cleaning or some other neglectful practice by, for example, analyzing for "indicator organisms." It is also likely that samples would be taken at critical control points to detect an unusual change in the extent of contamination or growth.

In many instances, including the preceding examples, attributes sampling may not be applicable because there may be no defined lot and random sampling may not be possible. Nevertheless, the analytical results may be used by experienced personnel to assess the performance of the critical control point.

There are other statistically based systems by which analytical results can be assessed as to validity in reaching a decision, e.g., variables sampling (Kilsby and Baird-Parker, 1983). Additional studies are needed to determine the extent to which these systems are suitable for foods.

REFERENCES

Bartram, M. T., and G. G. Slocum
  1964   Microbiological criteria for foods. IV. Problems of sampling and interpretation of bacteriological results on frozen foods. J. Assoc. Food Drug Off. of the U.S. Quart. Bull. 30(1):14-17.
Bray, D. F., D. A. Lyon, and I. Burr
  1973   Three-class attributes plans in acceptance sampling. Technometrics 15:575.
Brown, M. H., and A. C. Baird-Parker
  1982   The microbiological examination of meat. In Meat Microbiology. M. H. Brown, ed. London: Applied Science. Pp. 423–509.
Charles, R.H.G.
  1979   Microbiological standards for foodstuffs. Health Trends 11:1–4.
Clark, D. S.
  1978   The International Commission on Microbiological Specifications for Foods. Food Technol. 32(1):51–54, 67.
Collins-Thompson, D. L., K. F. Weiss, G. W. Riedel, and S. Charbonneau
  1978   Sampling plans and guidelines for domestic and imported cocoa from a Canadian national microbiological survey. Can. Inst. Food Sci. Technol. J. 11:177–179.
Corlett, D. A., Jr.
  1974   Setting microbial limits in the food industry. Food Technol. 28(10):34–40.
Cowell, N. D., and M. D. Morisetti
  1969   Microbiological techniques—some statistical aspects. J. Sci. Food Agric. 20:573–579.
Davis, J. G.
  1969   Microbiological standards for foods. Part 2. Lab. Practice 18:839–845.
DOD (U.S. Department of Defense)
  1963   Military Standard 105D. Sampling procedures and tables for inspection by attributes. Washington, D.C.: DOD.
Dyett, E. J.
  1970   Microbiological standards applicable in the food factory. Chem. and Ind. 189–192.

Hobbs, B. C., and R. J. Gilbert
1970   Microbiological standards for food: public health aspects. Chem. and Ind. 215–219.
ICMSF (International Commission on Microbiological Specifications for Foods)
1974   Microorganisms in Foods. 2. Sampling for microbiological analysis: Principles and specific applications. Toronto: University of Toronto Press.
Ingram, M., and A. G. Kitchell
1970   Symposium on microbiological standards for foods. Chem. and Ind. 186–188.
Johnson, N. L., and B. L. Welch
1940   Applications of the non-central t-distribution. Biometrika 31:362–389.
Kilsby, D. C.
1982   Sampling schemes and limits. In Meat Microbiology. M. H. Brown, ed. London: Applied Science. Pp. 387–421.
Kilsby, D. C., and A. C. Baird-Parker
1983   Sampling programs for the microbiological analysis of foods. In Food Microbiology: Advances and Prospects. T. A. Roberts and F. A. Skinner, eds. London and New York: Academic Press.
Kilsby, D. C., and M. E. Pugh
1981   The relevance of the distribution of microorganisms within batches of food to the control of microbiological hazards from food. J. Appl. Bacteriol. 51:345–354.
Kilsby, D. C., L. J. Aspinall, and A. C. Baird-Parker
1979   A system for setting numerical microbiological specifications for foods. J. Appl. Bacteriol. 46:591–599.
Kramer, A., and B. A. Twigg
1970   Quality Control in the Food Industry. 3rd Ed. Vol. 1. Fundamentals. Westport, Conn.: AVI Publishing.
Leininger, H. V., L. R. Shelton, and K. H. Lewis
1971   Microbiology of frozen cream type pies, frozen cooked peeled shrimp and dry food grade gelatin. Food Technol. 25(3):28–30.
NRC (National Research Council)
1969   An Evaluation of the *Salmonella* Problem. Committee on *Salmonella*. Washington, D.C.: National Academy of Sciences.
Pitt, H.
1978   The resampling syndrome. Quality Progress 11(4):27–29.
Puri, S. C., and K. Mullen
1980   Applied Statistics for Food and Agricultural Scientists. Boston, Mass.: G. K. Hall and Co.
Puri, S. C., D. Ennis, and K. Mullen
1979   Statistical Quality Control for Food and Agricultural Scientists. Boston, Mass.: G. K. Hall and Co.
Shuffman, M. A., and D. Kronick
1963   The development of microbiological standards for foods. J. Milk Food Technol. 26:110–114.
Sukhatme, T. V., and B. V. Sukhatme
1970   Sampling Theory of Survey with Applications. 2nd Ed. Ames: Iowa State University Press.
Wodicka, V. O.
1973   The food regulatory agencies and industrial quality control. Food Technol. 27(10):52–58.

7

Consideration of Decision (Action) To Be Taken When a Criterion (Limit) Is Exceeded

In general, the decision taken when the limit in a microbiological criterion is exceeded relates to the purpose for which the criterion was established. Criterion limits are related to the acceptability of a raw material, the adequacy of sanitation measures, the possibility of environmental contamination, microbial buildup on equipment, or the acceptability of finished product.

In most cases, knowledge that a limit has been exceeded comes "after the fact." For example, the equipment was dirty at start-up; thermophilic anaerobe levels built up in the starch-holding vat feeding the canning line; lactobacilli that produce hydrogen peroxide reached excessive numbers on a stainless steel table where canned hams were emptied prior to slicing, thus posing the threat of discoloration if growth of these organisms continued in the finished product; or *Salmonella* was detected in the sifter tailings from a milk dryer. In each instance the facts became known days after the finished product was packaged, and in most cases after it had left the processing plant. If microbiological criteria for monitoring conditions such as these have been intelligently established, the retrospective findings are of value and should trigger appropriate action.

Certain finished products must be held until their compliance with established limits has been determined, e.g., infant formulas (Codex Alimentarius Commission, 1979). Embargoing finished product is costly and cumbersome; alternative actions should be sought and used wherever possible. For example, with low-acid canned foods, reliance is placed upon monitoring critical control points to give assurance that the process has been properly applied (FDA, 1973; see also Chapter 9, Part J). Other alternatives must be used with perishable foods. With fluid milk, for example, further sampling is undertaken when the standard plate count exceeds the limit. If the problem persists and three out of the last five analyses exceed the limit, a specified penalty provision is applied, one of which is permit suspension (USPHS/FDA, 1978). If shucked oysters exceed the fecal coliform MPN limit, the oysters are accepted on the condition that the state sanitation authority in the originating state makes immediate investigation of the producer's plant and operations and submits a report to the control agency in the market area. On the basis of this report, the control agency in the market area will accept or reject further shipments (USDHEW, 1965).

DECISION CATEGORIES

Evidence of Existence of a Direct Health Hazard

Whenever a product poses a direct hazard to health (see Chapter 4), an implied standard (see Chapter 1, p. 52, note 3) exists and the product is subject to seizure under the Food, Drug and Cosmetic Act (U.S. Congress, 1980). Examples would be the occurrence of *Salmonella* in dried milk and botulinal toxin in smoked fish. The products involved are generally voluntarily removed from the market by the processor, with the extent of the recall and the form of publicity being commensurate with the degree of hazard. If the processor or other responsible entity refuses voluntarily to recall the product, then the Food and Drug Administration may take legal action leading to seizure of the product. This is generally not necessary when a product poses a direct hazard to health, as the processor usually is willing to undertake a prompt recall.

The FDA may request recall of a product even if it does not pose a direct health hazard, i.e., if the food is adulterated under Section 402 (a) (3) and (4) of the Federal Food, Drug and Cosmetic Act (U.S. Congress, 1980). Examples are tree nuts contaminated with *Escherichia coli* and raw shrimp containing salmonellae. It is held that *E. coli* in tree nuts is evidence of the occurrence of filth (fecal material). Similarly, it is held that salmonellae in raw shrimp constitute an added substance that would not be present were the product prepared, packed, and held under sanitary conditions. In neither case is it claimed that a direct health hazard exists. Nevertheless, if recall is not voluntarily undertaken the FDA may take legal action resulting in seizure.

Most states have even broader powers than the FDA. For example, a state regulatory inspector may embargo a product without a court order; most commonly this occurs within a processing plant, but it may extend beyond the processing facility into wholesale or retail channels. A USDA inspector may similarly embargo a product without a court order.

The law provides alternatives to destruction, if the product can be rendered safe for sale. Reprocessing of the product is permitted and should be considered if the hazard can be eliminated, e.g., reconstitution and repasteurization of dried milk or eggs containing salmonellae. The material may be diverted into a product where the hazard is eliminated, e.g., dried milk or eggs containing *Salmonella* used as ingredients in retorted foods or dried egg yolk used as a component of mayonnaise.

In the case of products that are recalled or seized due to evidence of filth, as in the case of *E. coli* in tree nuts, elimination of the indicator of filth, ergo *E. coli*, by some physical or chemical treatment does not constitute a reconditioning process satisfactory to the FDA. The filth as well as the indicator of its presence must be eliminated. Thus, a washing procedure resulting in the elimination of *E. coli* would be satisfactory whereas soaking the product in a chlorine solution would not be satisfactory even if *E. coli* were eliminated by this treatment.

Frequently a product that is considered unfit for human consumption is diverted into animal feeds. It is common for condemned or inedible meat, poultry, dairy, and egg products to be used as ingredients in pet foods. Inedible meat, poultry, and fish are rendered and the resultant high-protein meals are used as components of animal feeds. These procedures are justifiable, but not if the diversion ultimately results in perpetuation of a problem in the human population. Blending of uncontaminated with contaminated products in order to comply with established limits has generally not been tolerated by regulatory authorities. In 1977, however, large amounts of corn produced in the southeastern United States were contaminated with aflatoxin. At that time, blending was permitted to bring the concentration of aflatoxin to levels below the maximum permitted for animal feed (FDA, 1978). A similar situation occurred with respect to the 1980 corn crop (FDA, 1981). It is to be expected, however, that blending will continue in the future.

Destruction of the food is frequently the only alternative. Though botulinal toxin is relatively heat labile, nothing short of destruction of a product containing this toxin is acceptable. Even though consumption of a food containing *Staphylococcus* enterotoxin does not produce the dire results associated with consumption of botulinal toxin, total destruction of food containing this enterotoxin is indicated since it is heat stable.

In considering decisions concerning the fate of foods posing a direct health hazard, careful consideration should be undertaken when alternatives other than total destruction are contemplated.

Evidence That a Direct Health Hazard Could Develop

Though virtually any low-acid perishable food poses a potential health hazard if mishandled, the potential for foodborne illness and the speed with which it will develop are related to the numbers and types of contaminants present. Though small numbers of *Staphylococcus aureus, Clostridium perfringens* and *Bacillus cereus* may be present in foods, they pose no direct health hazard. If, however, mishandling occurs, growth of any of these three organisms may lead to a direct health hazard. Large numbers of *B. cereus* or *S. aureus* may produce enterotoxin in food before it is consumed. Large numbers of *C. perfringens*, if present in food, may lead to the *in vivo* production of enterotoxin in the consumer. Since small numbers of *S. aureus, C. perfringens,* and *B. cereus* are frequently found in food produced under Good Manufacturing Practices, criteria relating to them usually recognize a tolerance, e.g., a few 100/g. Even if this tolerance is greatly exceeded, e.g., levels between 10,000 and 100,000/g are reached, a direct health hazard still may not exist. A hazard lies in the possibility that further mishandling or previous growth not reflected in such counts (preformed toxins) would create a direct health hazard (see Chapter 4). If tests for preformed toxins are negative, then under controlled circumstances foods of this type can be diverted to use under conditions where proper food handling is assured, thereby avoiding the risk of development of a direct hazard. Release to general distribution with all the vagaries inherent therein is not advisable. If tests for preformed toxins are positive, the food should be destroyed.

Indications That a Product Was Not Produced Under Conditions Assuring Safety

Considerations relating to the above conditions have been discussed previously with respect to the existing standards for fluid milk, water, shellfish, and other commodities. For these products, standards based upon the determination of indicator organisms have been established. The validity of these as measures of safe production practices has stood the test of time. For example, shellfish and shellfish growing waters with excessive numbers of coliforms and/or fecal coliforms pose the threat that pathogenic microorganisms may also be present. Similar relationships between indicator organisms and safety have not been widely applicable to other foods. For example, indicator tests cannot be substituted for direct determination of *Salmonella* in dried foods and feeds (Silliker and Gabis, 1976).

Mesophilic anaerobic sporeforming bacteria in low-acid canned foods have been used as indicators of unsafe processing conditions. Since *Clostridium botulinum* is one of the most heat-resistant mesophilic sporeforming bacteria, the occurrence of mesophilic sporeforming bacteria in low-acid canned foods purported to have received a botulinum cook suggests underprocessing. Such bacterial examinations would be used in the investigation of a spoilage outbreak, but examination for mesophilic anaerobic sporeformers in sound containers should not be routinely recommended.

Indications That a Raw Material May
Adversely Affect Shelf-life

With perishable raw materials such as raw meats, poultry, fish, and liquid eggs, off-condition may be detected by sensory evaluation. The consignment should be rejected when off-conditions are perceptible. The same raw materials may contain high numbers of microorganisms and be on the verge of spoilage (incipient spoilage) and yet show no overt evidence in a sensory evaluation. Microbiological testing will detect borderline raw materials of this type, but if sensory evaluation has been relied upon as the acceptance criterion, then the information derived from the microbiological tests is of retrospective value, i.e., it becomes the basis for decisions regarding suitability of suppliers. Frozen perishable raw products may be held pending the determination of their acceptability prior to use, in which case judgements may be made based upon either sensory evaluation or microbiological testing.

Nonperishable ingredients may be examined prior to use and, if they fail to meet the limit in an established criterion, may be rejected as unsuitable for their intended use. For example, sugar and starch destined to be components of retorted canned foods may be rejected if they contain excessive levels of thermophilic anaerobic sporeforming bacteria; spices destined to be used in cooked sausages may be rejected if they contain excessive levels of aerobic sporeforming bacteria (Silliker, 1963). Many such criteria exist as components of purchase specifications.

As a rule, a raw material that is judged unsatisfactory for one purpose, based upon failure to meet purchase specification limitations, may be quite useful for another purpose. The presence of excessive levels of anaerobic sporeforming bacteria in sugar may render it unsatisfactory as a raw ingredient for retorted canned products. This attribute is of no relevance, however, if the same sugar is to be used as a sweetening agent in coffee or baked goods.

Evidence That a Critical Control
Point Is Not Under Control

Evidence that a critical control point is not under control should trigger immediate action. Such evidence may relate to a raw ingredient, to the microbiological condition of processing equipment, to the effectiveness of a process, to the occurrence of undesirable microorganisms in a processing environment, or to the microbiological condition of a finished product. If it relates to a raw material, that ingredient should not be used. If the raw material has been used, then its influence on the safety and quality of the finished product must be assessed and appropriate measures based upon the findings must be taken. If the critical control point relates to equipment sanitation, the frequency and adequacy of cleaning procedures must be reviewed. If failures in these areas influence finished product safety or quality, appropriate decisions must be made with reference to product distribution. If environmental contamination, as for example with *Salmonella*, is indicated, then the source of such contamination must be determined; furthermore, more intensive finished product testing may be indicated. If failure of a processing step is indicated, the source of the failure must be determined and eliminated. If the quality or safety of the finished product is affected, appropriate steps must be taken with respect to its distribution. If the problem relates to the microbiological condition of the finished product, decisions must be made with respect to its distribution, and the reasons for the unsatisfactory condition of the finished product must be determined. If the HACCP system has been properly applied, the reasons for finished product failure should be evident from monitoring results on critical control points.

Finally, it should be mentioned that where the Food and Drug Administration is responsible for assuring that processing plants operate under Good Manufacturing Practices, failure of processors to control critical points might be grounds for regulatory action, even though the limits for these points were established by the processor.

REFERENCES

Codex Alimentarius Commission
   1979   Microbiological specifications for foods for infants and children. Alinorm 79:13, Appendix V.
FDA (Food and Drug Administration)
   1973   Thermally processed low-acid foods packaged in hermetically sealed containers. Part 128B (recodified as Part 113). Federal Register 38(16):2398–2410, Jan. 24.
   1978   Aflatoxin-contaminated corn. Limited exemption from blending prohibition. Federal Register 43(65):14122–14123. Apr. 4.
   1981   Aflatoxin-contaminated corn; limited exemptions from prohibition of interstate shipment and blending. Federal Register 46(15):7447–7449. Jan. 23.
Silliker, J. H.
   1963   Total counts as indexes of food quality. Pp. 102–112 in Microbiological Quality of Foods. L. W. Slanetz, C. O. Chichester, A. R. Gaufin, and Z. J. Ordal, eds. New York: Academic Press.

Silliker, J. H., and D. A. Gabis
  1976   ICMSF Methods Studies. VII. Indicator tests as substitutes for direct testing of dried
          foods and feeds for *Salmonella*. Can. J. Microbiol. 22:971–974.
USDHEW (U.S. Department of Health, Education and Welfare)
  1965   Bacteriological criteria for shucked oysters at the wholesale market level. Appendix A
          in National Shellfish Sanitation Program. Manual of Operations. PHS Pub. 33 (Re-
          vised 1965). Washington D.C.: U.S. Government Printing Office.
USPHS/FDA (U.S. Public Health Service/Food and Drug Administration)
  1978   Grade A Pasteurized Milk Ordinance. 1978 Recommendations. PHS/FDA Publication
          229. Washington, D.C.: U.S. Government Printing Office.
U.S. Congress
  1980   Federal Food, Drug and Cosmetic Act as amended. Washington, D.C.: U.S. Gov-
          ernment Printing Office.

8

Current Status of Microbiological Criteria and Legislative Bases

INTRODUCTION

Early Programs in the United States

Some of the initial intensive efforts directed at the control of bacteria in processing and storage were focused on fluid milk and other dairy products because of the role these foods played in foodborne disease transmission. The milk sanitation program is one of the oldest in the Public Health Service; the initial ordinance was developed in 1924 as a model regulation for voluntary adoption by state and local milk control agencies (USPHS, 1924). An accompanying code provided administrative and technical details on satisfactory compliance (USPHS, 1927). Microbiological criteria were included in these original regulations.

Periodic revisions followed as improvements in technology for the production and transport of raw milk and for the processing, packaging, and storage of pasteurized milk products occurred. Each of the revisions was developed with the assistance of milk sanitation and regulatory agencies at the federal, state, and local levels and with other segments of the dairy industry. These early efforts led to the current programs. The Grade A Pasteurized Milk Ordinance, 1978 Recommendations, of the U.S. Public Health Service, Food and Drug Administration (USPHS/FDA, 1978), the most recent revision, was produced with substantial assistance from the National Conference on Interstate Milk Shippers (NCIMS) and was implemented in 1980. The chemical, bacteriological, and temperature standards in this revision are presented in Table 8-1.

Recognition of the public health problems associated with shellfish in the United States in the early 1900s resulted in the establishment of a

152

TABLE 8-1 Chemical, Bacteriological, and Temperature Standards for Grade A Milk and Milk Products

Grade A raw milk for pasteurization (ultrapasteurization or aseptic processing):

Temperature	—	Cooled to 45°F (7°C) or less within two hours after milking: Provided that the blend temperature after the first and subsequent milkings does not exceed 50°F (10°C).
Bacterial limits	—	Individual producer milk not to exceed 100,000 per ml prior to comingling with other producer milk.
	—	Not to exceed 300,000 per ml as comingled milk prior to pasteurization.
Antibiotics	—	No zone equal to or greater than 16 mm with the *Bacillus stearothermophilus* disc assay method specified by NCIMS.
Somatic cell count	—	Individual producer milk: Not to exceed 1,500,000 per ml.

Grade A pasteurized milk and milk products:

Temperature	—	Cooled to 45°F (7°C) or less and maintained thereat.
Bacterial limits*	—	20,000 per ml.
Coliform	—	Not to exceed 10 per ml: Provided that, in the case of bulk milk transport tank shipments, shall not exceed 100 per ml.
Phosphatase	—	Less than 1 μg per ml by the Scharer Rapid Method or equivalent.
Antibiotics	—	No zone equal to or greater than 16 mm with the *Bacillus stearothermophilus* disc assay method specified by NCIMS.

Grade A aseptically processed milk and milk products:

Temperature	—	None
Bacterial limits	—	No growth by test specified in Section 6.
Antibiotics	—	No zone equal to or greater than 16 mm with the *Bacillus stearothermophilus* disc assay method specified by NCIMS.

*Not applicable to cultured products.

SOURCES: USPHS/FDA, 1978; FDA, 1983e (1979 NCIMS, Aseptic Processing, and 1981 Antibiotic Testing NCIMS Changes).

National Shellfish Sanitation Program (NSSP) (USPHS, 1925). The Public Health Service, the states, and the shellfish industry each accepted responsibilities for certain aspects of the program. The National Shellfish Sanitation Program, Manual of Operations, was last revised in 1965 (US-DHEW, 1965).

Current Levels of Concern and Application

Microbiologial criteria are applicable at the international, federal, state (both health and agriculture departments), and local (city-county) levels, as well as by the food industry. The types of criteria at each of these levels are influenced by the mission and responsibilities of the agency or organization involved.

INTERNATIONAL ACTIVITIES

Joint FAO/WHO Food Standards Program

Microbiological criteria for foods at the international level are applied primarily within the Joint FAO/WHO Food Standards Program as implemented by the Codex Alimentarius Commission (Olson, 1978). The history of international food standards is relatively short. In 1958 the governing bodies of the Food and Agriculture Organization (FAO) and the World Health Organization (WHO) established a joint food standards[1] program having the following purposes:

1. protect the health of the consumers and ensure fair practices in the food trade;

2. promote coordination of all food standards work undertaken by international, governmental, and nongovernmental organizations;

3. determine priorities and initiate and guide the preparation of drafts of standards through and with the aid of appropriate organizations;

4. finalize standards elaborated under (3) above and, after acceptance by governments, publish them in a *Codex Alimentarius* as either regional or worldwide standards, together with international standards already finalized by other bodies under (2) above, wherever this is practicable;

5. amend published standards, after appropriate survey in the light of developments.

The Codex Alimentarius Commission was created to implement the program through which international food standards for processed, semiprocessed, and raw foods are established. Membership in the commission is voluntary and is made up of member and associate member nations of FAO and WHO. At present, 121 nations are members (Kimbrell, 1982). Each member government is free to adopt each standard at any one of four levels of participation:

1. full acceptance of the standard and food(s) affected;

2. acceptance with specified deviations from the standard and food(s) affected;

---

[1]The term standard(s) as used by Codex has a different meaning than that defined in this report. The Codex meaning relates to requirements or provisions set forth in various documents and codes quite apart from microbiological criteria.

3. target acceptance of food products in anticipation of later approval of Codex Standard;

4. nonacceptance with free distribution of food(s) conforming to Codex Standard.

The specific objectives of the Codex program are:

1. to develop international food standards on a worldwide or regional basis;
2. to publish these standards in a food code (*Codex Alimentarius*);
3. to record acceptance and implementation of these standards by governments.

To date, 148 international standards have been adopted and 19 more are under development (Kimbrell, 1982). These Codex standards are very similar to standards of identity; microbiological criteria have seldom been included as part of a standard. They contain qualitative statements about hygiene and end-product specifications. Codex standards are intended to be mandatory and thus require government approval. The United States has completed action on 41 of the 148 standards; 14 more are in the rule-making process.

Other recommendations and provisions, including the codes of practice, are advisory in nature and do not require government approval. Subsidiary bodies (committees and expert groups) of the commission develop the standards and codes. Some committees deal with general subjects such as hygiene, analysis, or sampling applicable to all foods. Others, including the commodity committees, deal with specific foods.

The Codex Committee on Food Hygiene has the major responsibility for all provisions of food hygiene related to standards or codes of practices including microbiological criteria. In recent years, activities to establish microbiological criteria for foods in international trade that may present microbiological hazards have increased.

The First Joint FAO/WHO Expert Consultation on Microbiological Criteria for Foods (FAO/WHO, 1975) gave high priority to criteria for egg products, dried milks, precooked frozen seafoods, and frozen meat. A specific recommendation for establishment of microbiological specifications for egg products was forwarded to the Codex Committee on Food Hygiene. Specifications were quickly adopted; they became the first microbiological criteria for a food or food commodity group to be included in a Code of Hygienic Practice.

A second Joint FAO/WHO Expert Consultation (FAO/WHO, 1977) recommended that the Committee on Food Hygiene consider development of microbiological criteria for precooked shrimps and prawns, foods for infants and children, and ice mixes and edible ices. The consultation recommended that high priority be given to consideration of criteria for dried milk, cheese, precooked frozen crabmeat, desiccated coconut, and precooked frozen lobster. It assigned a lesser, yet strong, priority to consideration of criteria for cooked meat and poultry, fish and fishery products, dried soups and broths, dried fruits, enzymes, gelatin, protein concentrates, and low-acid salad dressing. This second expert consultation developed the statement on ''General Principles for the Establishment and Application of Microbiological Criteria for Foods'' for inclusion in the Codex Procedural Manual (see Appendix B).

As of 1978 a Code of Practice on General Principles of Food Hygiene and 12 Codes of Hygienic Practice for specific food commodities had been completed or were in the process of being developed (Olson, 1978); by 1982, 21 codes of hygienic or technological practice had been developed (Kimbrell, 1982). These codes apply to foods in the following commodity groups: canned fruit and vegetable products, dried fruits, desiccated coconut, dehydrated fruits and vegetables including edible fungi, tree nuts, processed poultry, egg products, molluscan shellfish, low-acid and acidified low-acid canned foods, foods for infants and children, peanuts, frog legs, dried milk, natural mineral waters, and salvaging of canned foods. Microbiological criteria are included in the codes of hygienic practice for egg products, food for infants and children, dried milk, and natural mineral waters. Other international microbiological specifications are listed in Appendix C.

European Economic Community

The interests of the European Economic Community (EEC) in microbiological criteria are based on the creation of a single common market for foods and feeds. The Common Market's attempts to eliminate technical barriers to trade include the consideration of the application of microbiological criteria to foods and feeds in order to protect the health of the consumer. A proposal based on the Codex Alimentarius General Principles for the Establishment and Application of Microbiological Criteria for Foods was developed by the Commission of the European Communities and submitted to the European Council of Ministers in September 1981 (B. Simonsen, Danish Ministry of Agriculture, 1982. Personal communication). A revised proposal was approved by the European Parliament in April 1982.

The EEC is a circumscribed version of Codex; it has fewer members, covers a much smaller geographic area, and encompasses less diverse cultures. Both groups depend on voluntary membership, but as the rulings of the EEC are binding, the compliance may ultimately be more stringent with EEC criteria than with Codex criteria.

International Commission on Microbiological Specifications for Foods (ICMSF)

The ICMSF (Clark, 1978) is a voluntary advisory body which was formed to:

1. assemble and evaluate evidence about the microbiologial quality of foods;
2. consider whether criteria are necessary for any particular food;
3. propose suitable criteria where necessary;
4. suggest appropriate methods of examination.

Functionally, the commission seeks to:

1. provide the bases for comparable standards for microbiological judgment of foods between countries;
2. foster safe movement of foods in international commerce;
3. overcome difficulties caused by differing microbiological standards and methods of analysis.

The ICMSF activities focus on microbiological methods for examination of food, comparative studies on suitability of media, sampling plans and acceptance criteria, interpretation of microbiological data, and control of food operations to assure safety and quality. Cooperative work on methods has been carried out with the International Dairy Federation, the International Standards Organization, and the Association of Official Analytical Chemists.

Classic work on sampling plans as related to foods has been published in the commission's book, *Microorganisms in Foods 2*, first published in 1974 and now in revision (ICMSF, 1974, 1985; see also Chapter 6).

Canadian Microbiological Standards for Foods

The Canadian regulations (Pivnick, 1978) apply to microbiological criteria at a national level where the production and processing conditions closely resemble those in the United States. The microbiological quality of food in Canada is governed by federal, provincial, and municipal jurisdictions. Provincial and municipal regulations may be more stringent than federal regulations. The Food and Drugs Act and Regulations cover all food sold in Canada regardless of place of production. The Canadian

Food and Drugs Act is similar to the U.S. Federal Food, Drug and Cosmetic Act. Sections 4, 5 and 7 are pertinent:

(4) No person shall sell an article of food that

(a) has in or upon it any poisonous or harmful substance;

(b) is unfit for human consumption;

(c) consists in whole or in part of any filthy, putrid, disgusting, rotten, decomposed or diseased animal or vegetable substance;

(d) is adulterated; or

(e) was manufactured, prepared, preserved, packaged or stored under unsanitary conditions.

(5) No person shall label, package, treat, process, sell or advertise any food in a manner that is false, misleading or deceptive or is likely to create an erroneous impression regarding its character, value, quantity, composition, merit or safety.

(7) No person shall manufacture, prepare, preserve, package or store for sale any food under unsanitary conditions.

To avoid the possibility of misinterpretation, numerous standards that include microbial limits have been established under the act.

However, differences do exist between the acts of the two nations. Whereas in the United States microbiological standards are usually established by a proposal, response, and hearing process, the Canadian law allows direct establishment of standards, with any product in violation of the standards being automatically illegal. The microbiological standards currently incorporated as regulations pursuant to the Canadian Food and Drugs Act are summarized in Appendix D. Sampling plans associated with each food or food commodity are included.

U.S. FEDERAL AGENCIES

Food and Drug Administration (FDA)

The basic mission of FDA is to protect the health and welfare of the consumer. The principal responsibility relative to foods is to ensure that they are safe and wholesome and are honestly and informatively labeled. The legislative basis for the legal authority to act is the Federal Food, Drug and Cosmetic Act, as Amended January 1980 (U.S. Congress, 1980). Various sections of the act are applicable: Section 301, Prohibited Acts; Section 401, Standards; Section 402, Adulteration; Section 403, Misbranding; and Section 801, Imports and Exports.

Specific objectives of the act related to food include provisions to:

1. prohibit adulteration of food—Section 301 (b);
2. prevent food from containing any filthy, putrid, or decomposed substances—Section 402 (a) (3);
3. prohibit preparation, packing, or storage under unsanitary conditions whereby it may become contaminated or be rendered injurious to health—Section 402 (a) (4);
4. prohibit misbranding of foods—Section 301 (b);
5. set reasonable definitions and standards of identity and reasonable standards of quality—to promote honesty and fair dealing in the interests of consumers—Section 401;
6. prohibit the importation of any adulterated or mishandled food—Section 801 (a).

The operational program of FDA may specify microbiological criteria. In addition to the presence of foodborne pathogens and/or their toxins, these criteria may include indicator organisms that reflect contamination at harvest, poor manufacturing practices, and/or inadequate storage conditions. (For a discussion of criteria for foodborne pathogens, see Chapter 1, page 52, note 3.)

Compliance Policy Guides

Compliance Policy Guides (FDA, 1982a), where established, describe FDA's official policy on compliance matters and set forth specific criteria that must be met before the agency initiates legal actions. FDA has established microbiological criteria for certain foods susceptible to microbiological contamination. These criteria may be used as the bases for legal actions. Compliance Policy Guides containing microbiological criteria applicable to foods and feeds are listed in Table 8-2. Contaminants covered by these guides include foodborne pathogens, bacterial toxins, mycotoxins, and bacterial indicators such as aerobic plate counts (APC), *Escherichia coli,* coliform, and coagulase-positive staphylococci.

The testing of imported shrimp and frog legs for the presence of salmonellae and the development of block lists involving compulsory testing for such commodities after finding repeated violations are carried out under the authority of Section 801 of the act.

Food Defect Action Levels

Criteria used in food ingredient and finished food product evaluations are identified in the Food Defect Action Levels first published in 1972 by the FDA (see FDA, 1982b). These levels for natural or unavoidable

TABLE 8-2 FDA Compliance Policy Guides Related to Microbiological Problems in Foods and Feeds

Chapter—Title	Guide No.	Food Item(s)	Criteria	Sampling Plan
6—Dairy Industry	7106.08	Cheese & cheese products	Positive test for staphylococcal enterotoxin	Any sample
	7106.10	Fluid milk products	Original and check analyses indicate sample contains aflatoxin M_1 above permitted conc. and identity of aflatoxin M_1 is confirmed	10 pounds composited from not less than 10 units or taken from bulk fluid storage
8—Fish & Seafood Industry	7108.02	Crabmeat, fresh, frozen	*E. coli* by MPN (confirmed) plus APC, coliform group, and coagulase-positive staphylococci	Objective sample consisting of a minimum of 6 subsamples
	7108.09	Langostinos, frozen, cooked	Coliforms or *E. coli* or coag.-pos. staphylococci based on MPN in 20% of subsamples or APC geom. mean of all subsamples	10 subsamples of lot
	7108.16	Chubs, hot processed, smoked	Process controls: $NaNO_2$ or NaCl conc., or time-temp. of cook or time-temp. of cooling and storage, or factory inspection—insanitary conditions. Inhibit *Cl. botulinum*, Type E.	Any sample
	7108.17	Fish, hot processed, smoked	Process controls: NaCl conc. or time-temp. of cook or time-temp. of cooling and storage or insanitary conditions in factory inspection. Inhibit *Cl. botulinum*, Type E.	Any sample
	7108.20	Clams, mussels, oysters, fresh, frozen, or canned	Positive test by bioanalysis for paralytic shellfish poison	Any sample
12—Nuts	7112.02	Peanuts and peanut products	Original and check analyses show aflatoxin above permitted conc. and identity of B_1 is confirmed	Any sample
	7112.05	Tree nuts—nut meats	*E. coli* MPN (confirmed)	In 2 or more subsamples if less than 10 taken. Otherwise, in 20%

12—Nuts	7112.07	Brazil nuts	Original and check analyses show aflatoxin above maximum concentration permitted and identity of aflatoxin B_1 is confirmed	Any sample
	7112.08	Pistachio nuts	Original and check analyses show aflatoxin above max. conc. permitted and identity of aflatoxin B_1 is confirmed	Any sample
	7112.09	Tree nuts—reconditioning	Killing of *E. coli* not permitted during reconditioning. Filth must be removed	
	7112.11	Tree nuts—nut meats	*E. coli* MPN (confirmed)	Without inspectional evidence, in 2 or more subsamples if less than 10 taken. Otherwise, in 20%
19—Import Foods	7119.12	Clams, mussels, oysters, fresh and frozen	*E. coli* or coliforms or APC (35°C)	Average of subsamples or 3 or more of 5 subs. equal or exeed max. number permitted
20—Food—General	7120.20[a]	Foods	Positive tests in one or more composite units for *Salmonella* or *Arizona*	Sampling and testing done based on product category
	7120.26	"	Original and check analyses show aflatoxin above max. conc. permitted and identity of aflatoxin B_1 is confirmed by chemical derivatives and chick Embryo Bio-Assay	Any sample
25—Animal Feeds	7126.13	Animal by-products	Positive test for *Salmonella* plus factory evidence of continuing cross contamination	Action where 30% of subdivisions are positive

TABLE 8-2 (Continued)

Chapter—Title	Guide No.	Food Item(s)	Criteria	Sampling Plan
26—Animal Feed	7126.17	Dry dog food	Positive test for *Salmonella* in at least one of subsamples tested	10 subsamples of 25 grams each per sample
	7126.33	Finished feeds & feed ingredients	Original and check analyses are above max. conc. permitted *and* identity of aflatoxin B$_1$ is confirmed by chemical derivatives *and* by mass spectrometry.	Any sample
Import Alert	45-03	Dried yeast	Positive test for *Salmonella*	Any sample
Import Alert	28-04	Spices and condiments	Positive test for *Salmonella*	Any sample

[a]Includes criteria for *Salmonella* in shrimp and frog legs at import.

SOURCE: FDA, 1982a.

defects in foods are not based on any relationship to a health hazard. The levels are the limits at or above which FDA can take regulatory action to remove the violative food from the market. Specification of levels other than zero is necessary because it is not possible to grow, harvest, and process crops that are totally free of natural defects. The alternative would be increased pesticide utilization to control rodents, insects, and other natural contaminants, which might result in a more serious potential hazard from chemical residuals.

Action levels are specified for 55 of the 76 individual foods and/or classes of foods. Twenty-eight are concerned with visible mold in foods. Twenty-five have limits dealing with direct microscopic mold counts and one has a limit dealing with a direct microscopic count of bacterial cells in dried egg products. In addition, tuna and related fish products have a limit for histamine, a decomposition indicator of microbial activity (FDA, 1982b).

Products that might be harmful to consumers will be acted against regardless of whether the level of contamination exceeds an established level. Also, compliance with defect levels does not prevent action against a manufacturer who does not observe Good Manufacturing Practices, e.g., insanitary plant conditions are a violation.

Efforts for Microbiological Standards

Efforts have been made to establish microbiological quality standards for certain foods for which there are no standards of identity. These have included frozen, ready-to-eat cream-type pies (banana, chocolate, coconut, and lemon) and food-grade gelatin. Aerobic plate counts and coliform counts were the bases for the proposed microbiological standards, which were derived from the results of an FDA survey of all manufacturers known to be shipping these products in interstate commerce at the time of the study (FDA, 1972). After comments on the microbiological standards were received, amendments were made (FDA, 1973) and further objections permitted. Because of questions about the legal status of these regulations, further amendments were proposed and additional time for comment was again provided (FDA, 1976a). These microbiological standards were withdrawn to provide future opportunity to establish consistent domestic and international standards for these food products (FDA, 1978a).

Later, recommended microbiological quality standards were issued for frozen fish sticks, frozen fish cakes, and frozen crab cakes. These were the result of an extensive survey of 47 products performed on samples collected from retail stores in 32 standard U.S. metropolitan statistical areas (FDA, 1980). Various segments of the microbial population were determined, including aerobic plate counts (APCs), coliform and *E. coli* levels, *Staphylococcus aureus*, and yeast and mold counts.

Another survey was carried out on 28 plants in the shrimp-breading industry. The plants' inspection days, sampling intervals, and locations were evaluated using APC at 30° and 35°C (86° and 95°F), coliform, *E. coli*, and *S. aureus* in an attempt to establish GMP guidelines (Duran et al., 1983). These data have been used to develop proposed microbiological defect action levels on raw breaded shrimp (FDA, 1983a).

A fish-breading survey was carried out in a similar fashion in 22 plants to establish in-line microbiological criteria for that industry (R. B. Read, Jr., FDA. 1983. Personal communication). Statistical evaluation of the data obtained in comparisons of frozen versus refrigerated fresh products, batters and mixes, breading procedures, and steps and time in the processing cycle will provide the basis for establishing microbiological criteria for regulating finished fish prior to freezing.

Nineteen plants that produce frozen cream/nondairy substitute pies and that had a history of incompliance were also surveyed to obtain data to establish in-line microbiological criteria (R. B. Read, Jr., FDA. 1983. Personal communication). Samples were collected to determine relative levels of the organisms indicated above at specific points in the production line. At this time, there is no indication of whether, how, or when these data bases will be used to generate recommendations for establishment of microbiological criteria.

In connection with efforts to develop microbiological quality standards for certain foods for which there are no standards of identity, proposals to establish a quality standard and good manufacturing practices for bottled water have been adopted into final regulations (FDA, 1977). The regulations include coliform standards as determined by the multiple fermentation tube and membrane filter methods with appropriate sampling plans on the final packaged products as well as on the original source water.

Cooperative Programs

Recent FDA attempts to establish cooperative programs with food industries have been reported by Majorack (1982). The earlier Cooperative Quality Assurance Program (CQAP) embraced a formal commitment to cooperate; the newer Industry Quality Assurance Assistance Program (IQAAP) is a voluntary program conducted through trade associations that does not require reporting of nonconformance with provisions of the quality assurance plans submitted.

The basic FDA authority to exercise punitive measures against food processors in violation is conferred by the Federal Food, Drug and Cosmetic Act. Other programs in the agency that provide assurance of safety and quality are basically cooperative and/or voluntary in nature and are implemented by the states. Various operational programs were inherited from the former Public Health Service Milk and Food Sanitation programs. Sections of Public Law 410, the Public Health Service Act (U.S. Congress, 1944), provide for the following:

42 USC 241, Section 301	— provides for cooperation in research and investigations
42 USC 243, Section 311	— provides the basis for cooperation with the States
42 USC 246, Section 314(C)—	provides for training of state and local personnel
42 USC 264, Section 361	— provides for control of communicable diseases
	— gives authority for promulgating regulations

One cooperative federal/state activity, the USPHS/FDA Grade A milk program, was discussed from a historical viewpoint in the introductory section of this chapter. The 1978 Grade A Pasteurized Milk Ordinance (PMO) (USPHS/FDA, 1978) documents and translates the newest production, processing, and sanitation technologies into effective public health practices. The PMO is the basic standard used in the voluntary Cooperative State-PHS Program for Certification of Interstate Milk Shippers. The PMO with its Appendices is recommended by FDA for adoption by states and local regulatory agencies to encourage a greater uniformity of milk sanitation practice in the United States and to facilitate shipment and acceptance of milk and milk products in interstate and intrastate commerce. All 50 states participate in the program. It is incorporated by reference in federal specifications for procurement of milk and milk products; it is used as the sanitary regulation for milk and milk products served on interstate carriers; and it is recognized by the public health agencies, the milk industry, and many others as a national standard for milk sanitation.

The National Shellfish Sanitation Program (NSSP) (USDHEW, 1965) is a voluntary cooperative FDA, state, and shellfish industry program in which the states are encouraged to adopt shellfish sanitation regulations based on federal agency recommendations. The heavy import traffic in raw shellfish has led to the involvement of other nations in the program, namely, Canada, Mexico, Republic of Korea, Iceland, Japan, England, and New Zealand. These countries have inspected and approved those shippers on the Interstate Certified Shellfish Shippers List (FDA, 1983b).

Each shellfish-shipping state adopts laws and regulations adequate for sanitary control of the shellfish industry. The federal agency periodically reviews each state's control program. Because growing and processing of shellfish are two distinct phases of the industrial operation, the present NSSP manual (USDHEW, 1965) has been prepared in two parts: I—Sanitation of Shellfish Growing Areas, and II—Sanitation of the Harvesting and Processing of Shellfish. The manual serves as a guide to the states in the certification of interstate shellfish shippers and is used by the FDA in evaluating state shellfish sanitation programs. Microbiological criteria are suggested for the growing waters (coliforms and fecal coliforms by MPN) and for shucked oysters at the wholesale market level (plate count at 35°C (95°F) and fecal coliforms by MPN).

The NSSP was reorganized in September 1982 and is now titled the Interstate Shellfish Sanitation Conference (ISSC). The stated objectives of the conference are to foster and improve the sanitation of shellfish. The role of the states in the ISSC appears to be broadened and FDA will assume a more advisory and consultative position. The overall program is structured along the lines of the National Conference on Interstate Milk Shippers (NCIMS).

A Memorandum of Understanding (MOU) between ISSC and FDA is under consideration for the purpose of establishing a formal basis upon which to foster and improve sanitation and quality of shellfish. It states the responsibilities of FDA and the ISSC in the establishment of the Interstate Shellfish Sanitation Program (ISSP) and the ISSC Procedures.

Another cooperative federal/state program, this one concerned with the safety of food at the retail level, is the Retail Food Protection Program, administered by FDA. This program covers food service, food store, and food-vending industries. Uniform model food codes are available:

1. Food Service Sanitation Manual (FDA, 1976b)
2. The Vending of Food and Beverages (FDA, 1978b)
3. Retail Food Store Sanitation Code (FDA, 1982c)

The statutory authority for providing assistance to state and local government is from the Public Health Service Act, Section 311 (U.S. Congress, 1944). FDA supports state and local regulatory agencies by developing uniform requirements, developing training aids, providing training, giving technical assistance, and evaluating programs.

United States Department of Agriculture (USDA)

The USDA has the specific mission to promote the orderly marketing of wholesome, high-quality agricultural products. These principally advisory functions are carried out under the following legislative actions:

1. Agricultural Marketing Act as Amended (U.S. Congress, 1946);
2. Egg Products Inspection Act (U.S. Congress, 1970);
3. Wholesome Meat Act (U.S. Congress, 1968a) (Currently titled the Federal Meat Inspection Act);
4. Wholesome Poultry Products Act (U.S. Congress, 1968b) (Currently titled the Poultry Products Inspection Act).

The USDA Agricultural Marketing Service (AMS) and Food Safety and Inspection Service (FSIS) programs are applied to dairy products, eggs and egg products, and meat and poultry products. The USDA Seal is placed on products that meet the appropriate plant inspection and product criteria. Industry standards and grades may be designated by participation in the program.

Mandatory inspection is government-funded except for overtime needs. Monitoring of production may be on a continuous resident inspection arrangement or on a continuous supervision schedule. Microbiological criteria provide some bases for evaluating product quality and furnish some indication about conformance to acceptable processing, sanitation, and storage practices. Depending on product and program, finished foods may be evaluated for presence of common foodborne pathogens in addition to indicator organisms, e.g., dried milk. The need for resident and continuous inspection programs in all plants as presently operated has recently been questioned.

Dairy Products

The dairy product program, other than the Grade A milk and milk products program, is located in the Agricultural Marketing Service (AMS) and carried out under the Agricultural Marketing Act (U.S. Congress, 1946). Qualification for the USDA inspection and grading service is contingent upon approval of the dairy plant facilities, processing equipment and procedures, as well as finished product standards for grades, including microbiological criteria. Approval permits the use of official identification on as well as grade assignment for products packed under the USDA inspection program. Microbiological criteria applied in the AMS dairy products program are summarized in Tables 8-3 and 8-4.

Dry Milk Products

A *Salmonella* Surveillance Program (USDA, 1980) is conducted in approved plants manufacturing dry milk products. The program is carried out in accordance with a Memorandum of Understanding with FDA (FDA, 1975). For further detail and discussion, see Chapter 9, Part A.

TABLE 8-3   Microbiological Standards for Raw Milk: USDA-AMS Standards for Grades of Dairy Products

Bacterial Estimate Classification	Direct Microscopic Count, Standard Plate Count, or Plate Loop Count	Resazurin Reduction Time to Munsell Color Standard 5 P 7/4
No. 1		
Can	Not over 500,000 per millimeter	Not less than 2¼ hours
Bulk	"	Not less than 3¼ hours
No. 2		
Can	Not over 3,000,000	Not less than 1½ hours
Bulk	"	Not less than 2½ hours
Undergrade		
Can	Over 3,000,000	Less than 1½ hours
Bulk	"	Less than 2½ hours

SOURCE: USDA, 1975, p. 47919.

Egg Products

The Egg Products Inspection Act (EPIA) (U.S. Congress, 1970) provides for protection against the movement or sale for human food of products that are adulterated, misbranded, or otherwise in violation of the act. The EPIA requires the use of wholesome raw materials and processing procedures, e.g., pasteurization, that will assure the production of wholesome products that are free of *Salmonella*.

Under the present organizational structure, the egg and egg product and the dairy product regulatory activities are in the same division of AMS. Their mechanisms and administrative procedures are very similar. But, whereas the dairy products program has a variety of microbiological criteria that apply to raw milk and to finished products, the USDA egg program relies on a single microbiological criterion: a negative result for *Salmonella* in samples tested. However, as indicated earlier in the discussion of the FDA Defect Action Level program, there are some bacterial standards based on direct microscopic count (DMC) that are applicable to frozen and dried egg products. For further details and discussion, see Chapter 9, Part F.

Meat and Poultry Products

The meat and poultry products programs in USDA are carried out under the Federal Meat Inspection Act and the Poultry Products Inspection Act,

TABLE 8-4 Microbial Standards for Processed Milk Products: USDA-Agricultural Marketing Service Standards for Grades of Dairy Products

Product	Standard		Reference
Nonfat dry milk (spray and roller process)			USDA, 1982a,b
U.S. Extra Grade	50,000/g	SPC	
U.S. Standard Grade	100,000/g	SPC	
U.S. grade not assigned	300×10^6/g	DMC	
Instant nonfat dry milk			USDA, 1982c
U.S. Extra Grade	30,000/g	SPC	
	10/g	Coliform	
U.S. grade not assigned	75×10^6/g	DMC	
Dry whole milk			USDA, 1982d
U.S. Premium	30,000/g	SPC	
	90/g	Coliform	
U.S. Extra	50,000/g	SPC	
U.S. Standard	100,000/g	SPC	
Dry buttermilk			USDA, 1982e
U.S. Extra	50,000/g	SPC	
U.S. Standard	200,000/g	SPC	
Dry whey			USDA, 1982f
U.S. Extra	50,000/g	SPC	
	10/g	Coliform	
Butter and whipped butter	100/g	Proteolytic	USDA, 1975
	20/g	Yeasts and molds	
	10/g	Coliform	
	10/g	Enterococci[a]	
Plastic and frozen cream	30,000/ml	SPC	USDA, 1975
	20/ml	Yeasts and molds	
	10/ml	Coliform	
Cottage cheese	10/g	Coliform	USDA, 1975
	100/g	Psychrotrophic	
	10/g	Yeasts and molds	
Ice cream	50,000/g	SPC	USDA, 1975
plain	10/g	Coliform	
flavored	20/g	Coliform	
Sherbet	50,000/g	SPC	USDA, 1975
	10/g	Coliform	
Sweetened condensed milk	1,000/g	SPC	USDA, 1975
	10/g	Coliform	
	5/g	Yeasts	
	5/g	Molds	
Edible dry casein			USDA, 1982g
U.S. Extra Grade	30,000/g	SPC	
	0/0.1 g	Coliform	
U.S. Standard Grade	100,000/g	SPC	
	2/0.1 g	Coliform	
	0/100 g	Salmonella[b]	
	0/g	Staphylococci[b]	
	5,000/g	Thermophiles[b]	
	5/0.1 g	Yeasts and molds[b]	

[a]Optional except when required or requested.
[b]Optional.

established as the Wholesome Meat Act (U.S. Congress, 1968a) and the Wholesome Poultry Products Act (U.S. Congress, 1968b), respectively. The meat and poultry inspections are designed in part to minimize microbial contamination during slaughter and processing, to prevent the production of products harmful to human health, and to prevent the production and sale of food that is unwholesome or spoiled. Even though animals, carcasses, and products may be rejected in whole or in part to safeguard food quality and safety, the thrust of these program activities is through industry-managed quality assurance programs.

As presently organized, the Food Safety and Inspection Service (FSIS) of the USDA has responsibility for the wholesomeness of meat and poultry products. The microbiological programs have been summarized by Johnston (1982). Of primary concern are organisms that cause human illness and next of concern are problems related to spoilage. Samples are sent to FSIS laboratories under a variety of programs:

1. samples collected by inspectors to evaluate unusual conditions or product abnormalities brought about by process deviation;

2. samples collected as a result of complaints originating from a national (federal/state) epidemiology communications network;

3. samples collected as part of routine monitoring, outbreak, or complaint investigation, and exploratory investigations for development of a data base. This information may lead to subsequent regulatory actions.

An update on the USDA-FSIS approaches to and policies on microbiological criteria for meat and poultry products has been provided (T. B. Murtishaw, USDA-FSIS. 1982. Personal communication):

1. FSIS does not now have nor has it ever had formal regulations for microbiological standards or guidelines. These have not been adopted because wide variations in products and processing procedures exist in inspected products and because production procedures in the food industry are constantly changing.

2. Both acts referred to above (U.S. Congress, 1968a,b) contain language that prevents the sale of food that is unwholesome, spoiled, or deleterious to health. FSIS has consistently maintained that foods containing preformed microbial toxins are considered adulterated, as are ready-to-eat foods containing viable salmonellae. In some instances voluntary recalls have been effected where staphylococcal or clostridial levels of 10^5 or more per gram have been observed without the presence of detectable toxin. Such recalls are considered good examples of an informal policy on microbiological matters that recognizes potential health hazards. Favorable responses from processors have been obtained with regard to product recall and correction of responsible procedural conditions.

3. Informal microbiological criteria are now in use. Examples of these criteria currently being used for advisory purposes are shown in Table 8-5. These are advisory criteria action levels for resubmission of samples in the USDA Meat and Poultry Inspection Programs. When advisory microbiological limits are exceeded in samples taken under a monitoring or surveillance program, supervisory inspection staff initiate additional inspection and retesting. The objective is to locate the problem and get the product and the plant back within limits.

A relatively new development is the Microbiological Monitoring and Surveillance Programs (MMSP) being conducted in regional laboratories at San Francisco; Athens, Georgia; and St. Louis. Methods development and special investigations are carried out in the USDA laboratory at Beltsville, Maryland.

Some greater detail on MMSP activities has been provided by Johnston (1981). There are two categories of programs: microbiological monitoring and microbiological surveillance.

Microbiological monitoring has as its principal purpose the collection of data on new products, on products being processed with new and different procedures, or on products for which there are insufficient data.

Microbiological monitoring programs may be carried out on:

1. raw red meats and their uncooked products;
2. raw poultry and its uncooked products;
3. cooked red meats;
4. cooked poultry products;
5. nonmeat products used as ingredients in meat and poultry products such as spices, plant proteins, and dairy proteins;
6. nonmeat products included in prepared dinners;
7. environmental samples.

Microbiological surveillance programs are directed at plants in which hazardous situations have been detected. Sampling is continued to determine if perceived corrective measures have been effective and that the hazardous situation does not recur. Also, plants operating at the fringes of Good Manufacturing Practices may be studied to provide data to initiate changes in regulations.

Surveillance programs operate with biased sample selection of plant and/or product with defect and with sampling tailored to the process and the problem. The ultimate goals are compliance or change in regulations. A draft describing microbiological criteria for domestically processed meat and poultry products has been under consideration within USDA for some time. The criteria were to be applied to the evaluation of finished products

TABLE 8-5 USDA Meat/Poultry Advisory Criteria: Action Levels for Resubmission of Samples (counts per gram)

Product	APC 35°C	APC 20°C	Coliforms	E. coli	Staphylococci	Salmonella	Gas-Forming Anaerobe (Clostridia)	pH
Beef hearts	Not more than 1 of 5 over 5 million	No action level For information only	Not more than 1 of 5 at 10,000 or more	Not more than 2 of 5 at 1,000 or more	Not more than 2 of 5 at 1,000 or more	No action level For information only	No action level For information only	No action level For information only
Pork hearts	Not more than 1 of 5 over 5 million	No action level For information only	Not more than 1 of 5 at 10,000 or more	Not more than 2 of 5 at 1,000 or more	Not more than 2 of 5 at 1,000 or more	No action level For information only	No action level For information only	No action level For information only
Beef cheek meat	Not more than 1 of 5 over 10 million	No action level For information only	Not more than 2 of 5 at 10,000 or more	Not more than 2 of 5 at 1,000 or more	Not more than 2 of 5 at 1,000 or more	No action level For information only	No action level For information only	No action level For information only
Pork cheek meat	Not more than 1 of 5 over 10 million	No action level For information only	Not more than 2 of 5 at 10,000 or more	Not more than 2 of 5 at 1,000 or more	Not more than 2 of 5 at 1,000 or more	No action level For information only	No action level For information only	No action level For information only
Cooked meat entrees	Not more than 1 of 5 over 50,000	Not done	Not more than 1 of 5 over 10	Not more than 1 of 5 positive	Not more than 1 of 5 positive	None of 5 positive	Not more than 1 of 5 at 1,000 or more	No action level For information only
Cooked poultry entrees	Not more than 1 of 5 over 50,000	Not done	Not more than 1 of 5 over 10	Not more than 1 of 5 positive	Not more than 1 of 5 positive	None of 5 positive	Not more than 1 of 5 at 1,000 or more	No action level For information only
Meat pot-pies	Not more than 1 of 5 over 50,000	Not done	Not more than 1 of 5 over 10	Not more than 1 of 5 positive	Not more than 1 of 5 positive	None of 5 positive	Not more than 1 of 5 at 1,000 or more	No action level For information only

Poultry potpies	Not more than 1 of 5 over 50,000	Not done	Not more than 1 of 5 over 10	Not more than 1 of 5 positive	Not more than 1 of 5 positive	None of 5 positive	Not more than 1 of 5 at 1,000 or more	No action level For information only
Cooked poultry rolls	Not more than 1 of 5 over 50,000	No action level For information only	Not more than 1 of 5 over 10	Not more than 1 of 5 positive	Not more than 1 of 5 positive	None of 5 positive	Not more than 1 of 5 at 1,000 or more	No action level For information only
Chili	Not more than 1 of 5 over 50,000	No action level For information only	Not more than 1 of 5 over 10	Not more than 1 of 5 positive	Not more than 1 of 5 positive	None of 5 positive	Not more than 1 of 5 at 1,000 or more	No action level For information only
Beef barbecue	Not more than 1 of 5 over 50,000	No action level For information only	Not more than 1 of 5 over 10	Not more than 1 of 5 positive	Not more than 1 of 5 positive	None of 5 positive	Not more than 1 of 5 at 1,000 or more	No action level For information only
Pork barbecue	Not more than 1 of 5 over 50,000	No action level For information only	Not more than 1 of 5 over 10	Not more than 1 of 5 positive	Not more than 1 of 5 positive	None of 5 positive	Not more than 1 of 5 at 1,000 or more	No action level For information only

SOURCE: T. R. Murtishaw and R. W. Johnston. USDA, 1983.

at the processing level. Its publication in the *Federal Register*, however, has been indefinitely postponed.

National Marine Fisheries Service (NMFS)

The U.S. Department of Commerce-National Marine Fisheries Service (USDC-NMFS) fishery products inspection program is a voluntary, fee-for-service program involving inspection and grading of fisheries products. A principal objective is to provide certification that fisheries products have passed federal inspection, which in this case consists mainly of physical examination of facilities and organoleptic evaluation of products.

A recent update has been provided on the USDC-NMFS involvement with microbiological criteria (E.S. Garrett, USDC-NMFS. 1983. Personal communication). The NMFS does not establish microbiological criteria for foods, but rather examines fishery products or causes them to be examined for conformance with the microbiological criteria of other organizations including the Food and Drug Administration, the Department of Defense, private manufacturing firms, and/or institutional purchasers of seafoods. The USDC-NMFS inspection program recognizes and determines conformance to microbiological standards, specifications, and guidelines where such are either mandatory through codification in the Federal Regulations or included in a purchasing specification on product destined for either domestic or international trade. Microbiological food examination is used primarily to evaluate a product's safety status as opposed to its quality factors. Determinations of microbiological food safety are generally focused toward fully cooked, ready-to-eat items or the identification of process-induced hazards.

History

The NMFS had its origin in the Agricultural Marketing Act, as Amended (U.S. Congress, 1946), which provided for establishment of a system for distributing and marketing agricultural products based on the authority to inspect, certify, and identify agricultural products moving in interstate commerce. Fish and shellfish as well as processed products thereof were included as agricultural products. Some of the present commodity programs in the USDA are based in this program; however, early efforts did not include fish and shellfish.

The Fish and Wildlife Act (U.S. Congress, 1956) transferred all of the commercial fisheries activities from the USDA to the Bureau of Commercial Fisheries in the newly established Fish and Wildlife Service of the U.S. Department of the Interior. It was here in 1958 that the Fish and

Fisheries Products Inspection Program originated with a commitment to promote better health standards and sanitation. This program and some other commercial fishery activities were transferred in 1970 to the newly established National Marine Fisheries Service of the National Oceanic and Atmospheric Administration (NOAA) of the U.S. Department of Commerce (USDC). The NMFS unit with the greatest involvement in the establishment and use of microbiological criteria is the Division of Seafood Research, Inspection and Consumer Services, which houses the USDC quality-inspection activities (Sackett, 1982).

Current Cooperative Agreements

In addition to the above basic legislative authorities, the USDC fisheries inspection service through NMFS is a participant in six Memorandums of Understanding with other federal agencies to ensure cooperation and co-ordination in seafood inspective activities (E. S. Garrett, USDC-NMFS. 1983. Personal communication). The four Memorandums of Understanding concerned with microbiological criteria are listed in Table 8-6.

The agency also participates in 11 formal federal/state agreements dealing with fishery product inspective activities. The agreements are with Alabama, Alaska, Arkansas, Florida, Hawaii, Louisiana, Maine, Mississippi, New Jersey, Oregon, and Tennessee.

TABLE 8-6   U.S. Department of Commerce Memorandums of Understanding with Other Federal Agencies Concerned with Microbiological Criteria

Participating Agencies	Date	Purpose
FDA/USDC	January 17, 1975	To define respective roles in food inspection activities.
FDA/USDA/USDC	April 2, 1975	To transfer USDA's fish-meal salmonella control program to NMFS.
DOD/USDC	May 14, 1980	To transfer from DOD to USDC logistics agency origin inspection responsibility for DOD procurement.
USDC/FDA	May 22, 1981	To improve research coordination and cooperation and minimize duplication of research effort.

SOURCE: E. S. Garrett, National Marine Fisheries Service, 1983.

Activities Under Memorandums of Understanding.   The FDA has established several microbiological standards that are enforced in the USDC inspection program. These microbiological standards are the "commercially sterile" requirement contained in the Code of Federal Regulations for Low-Acid Canned Food GMP (FDA, 1983c) and the microbiological criteria for whole fish protein concentrate (FDA, 1983d). Additionally, FDA may enforce a requirement for imported fishery products such as shrimp from Asia to be free of *Salmonella*; NMFS then examines the product for this pathogen. FDA also has Compliance Policy Guidelines for crabmeat and cooked langostinos (FDA, 1982a).

The Department of Defense (DOD) purchases fresh and frozen oysters under a Federal Purchasing Document (DOD, 1976) that contains microbiological specifications. The USDC inspection program routinely employs the microbiological specifications when inspecting oysters for military procurement.

Activities With Industry.   The USDC seafood inspection program also determines conformance with a limited number of corporate quality assurance or quality control microbiological standards, specifications, or guidelines. Each firm has its own set of specifications and contracts with NMFS to do the inspection and analyses. Firms using microbiological criteria specified in these programs are either large, sophisticated fishery product processors or institutional purchasers.

Research

The USDC inspection program routinely uses microbiological evaluations to determine safe and suitable processing operations for use in producing fully cooked, ready-to-eat product. In addition, applied research is conducted to assess potential process-induced hazards, such as controlled atmosphere packaging of fishery products. Raw materials entering USDC-inspected plants are surveyed when there is concern, for instance, that polluted glaze water may have been used on a frozen product. When deemed appropriate, a product safety analysis is carried out by actions such as toxin assays of product suspected of contamination with *Clostridium botulinum*.

U.S. Army Natick Research and Development Center

One of the objectives of this center is to provide safe and nutritionally adequate food products in support of existing and future service concepts.

The problems of food procurement for military purposes are somewhat different from those for civilian purposes. While garrison (base) feeding may resemble civilian food service in terms of the degree of misuse and abuse to which foods may be subjected, field rations may be subject to additional abuse. The rations may be stored for extended periods of time and considerable delays may be encountered between preparation and consumption.

The legislative base for activities relative to microbiological criteria is the Defense Cataloging and Standardization Act, P.L. 10 USC, 2451-56 (U.S. Congress, 1976), implemented by Department of Defense (DOD) directive 4120.3, "Defense Standardization and Specification Program (DSSP)" (DOD, 1978). The DSSP includes approximately 400 Military and Federal Food Specifications. Of these, about 35 contain microbiological criteria, most of which apply to finished foods.

Microbiological criteria used for monitoring foods for the military as described in military and federal specifications were listed by Powers (1976). A summary of the current status of these microbiological criteria for foods purchased for the military (including pertinent Military and Federal Specification Numbers and Sampling Plans) prepared specifically for this subcommittee report (G. Silverman, U.S. Army Natick Research and Development Center. 1984. Personal communication.) is presented in Appendix E.

An increasing number of items are now purchased under a Commercial Item Description (CID) to save on inspection and analytical costs. A CID document is applied only to commercially available products for which there is already a civilian market. The company's sales to the government must be less than 50% of its total sales and the company must certify that the product meets certain requirements. Microbiological criteria are included in CIDs only if problems had been encountered with similar products already being procured.

Agencies other than DOD may carry out some of the inspection activities associated with military food purchases. The USDA inspects food plants except where USDA specifications are in disagreement with those of DOD. The NMFS is responsible for assuring that the microbiological criteria are being met in the case of shucked oysters. The military has no specifications on other fresh products.

The input of the Natick Microbiology Branch into specifications is made during the ration developmental stages and modified, if necessary, after initial procurement from commercial processors. The microbiology branch is presently concentrating on updating their criteria to make them uniform for given classes of foods and to benefit from current analytical techniques and concepts. For this reason the microbiological requirements listed in Table 1 of Appendix E are illustrative of those proposed for this class of rations. The criteria are derived from data obtained from analyzing actual production samples. Those listed in other Appendix E tables are current criteria. Critical processing parameters for achieving commercially sterilized or microbiologically stabilized foods are also established but are not listed in the tables in Appendix E. These parameters include minimal Fo values as well as water activity (prefried, canned bacon; cakes) and pH (rice).

Federal and Regional Level Cooperation

State Level

Grade A Milk Products.   The cooperation between FDA and the states relative to grading of milk products is discussed in the section above on cooperative programs and in Chapter 9, Part A. The chemical, bacteriological, and temperature standards of this program are listed in Table 8-1.

Changes have been introduced since the adoption of the Pasteurized Milk Ordinance (PMO), 1978 Recommendations (Table 8-1). Some material has been added on standards for ultrapasteurized and aseptically processed milk and milk products. Testing for antibiotic residuals in milk and milk products using a *Bacillus stearothermophilus* disc assay method has also been approved.

Manufactured Milk Products.   Grade B raw milk or raw milk for manufacturing purposes may be regulated by USDA recommended requirements (USDA, 1972) if they are adopted by the states or by requirements established by the individual states. The products may be subject to the microbiological criteria established in the Standards for Grades of Dairy Products (USDA, 1975) or to criteria established by the individual state. For further comments, see Tables 8-3 and 8-4 and Chapter 9, Part A.

Shellfish and Seafood Sanitation Programs.   The federal and state microbiological criteria for shellfish and other seafoods are listed in the National Fisheries Institute Handbook (Martin and Pitts, 1982). Standards and/or guidelines, advisory and mandatory, as in use in 48 states are included. The states with criteria for shellfish use NSSP regulations for harvest, processing, and distribution of shellfish and also use NSSP procedures for growing area surveys and plant inspections. (See discussion above of the National Shellfish Sanitation Program and the Interstate Shellfish Sanitation Program.) Additional monitoring and laboratory testing may also be applied by state authorities.

Other Foods.   A number of guidelines have been promulgated by the states (Wehr, 1982). Twenty-nine agencies had microbiological guidelines or standards in effect as of November 1981. The number of criteria for a single agency varied from 1 to as many as 40. There is little agreement on foods singled out and the criteria proposed.

The major portion of the criteria are applicable to shellfish, meat and meat products, and delicatessen items. However, criteria are applied narrowly to single items such as pecans or gelatin by some agencies and broadly to "products and levels unspecified" or "non-packaged foods, general" by other agencies. Sampling plans are random or unstated. The bases for the criteria developed by each agency may be existing criteria from another agency, internally generated data, externally generated data, some combination of the three, experience, or opinion. Criteria for a single food, hamburger or ground meat for example, may be implemented at the retail level by one agency, at the distribution and retail levels by another, at the processing and retail levels by a third, and at all three levels by a fourth.

City-County (Local) Level

The objective of local agencies in regard to food surveillance generally is to respond to and solve local problems relating to public health and nuisance abatement. The agencies have a broad interface with small operators involved in food processing or preparation of often very sensitive foods as well as with some aspects of food service.

The local agency may monitor the safety and quality of locally produced and/or consumed food products, principally delicatessen and other specialty food-processing operations and food service establishments. The agency may follow up on local reports of alleged foodborne disease incidents, poor quality products showing evidence of spoilage, insanitary and unsightly facilities, and similar complaints. The scope and depth of food surveillance, the qualifications of the field and laboratory personnel involved, and the adequacy of laboratory facilities and procedures are influenced by the population and area served by the local unit. Some city-county units where food safety and quality are perceived to be a problem may be very well structured and equipped to engage in food surveillance. In addition, the personnel in these units may be adequately trained and experienced to make appropriate interpretations of data. The nature of local food-processing surveillance may be quite formal and well organized. Frequently, however, local units have neither criteria of record nor experience in evaluating the results of microbiological analyses carried out during routine inspection or in the course of an investigation of alleged foodborne disease. These conditions could lead to inappropriate setting of criteria or regulatory actions by the local authority and could result in unnecessary financial burden to industry with no reduction of risk to the public.

The legislative bases for activities of local agencies are local ordinances. The data bases may be meager or nonexistent. The basic information often comes from other agencies or laboratories, and the criteria may have been intended for other uses with other foods. At times there may be little critical evaluation of the pertinence or validity of the application, e.g., applying criteria developed for highly processed foods to unprocessed or fermented foods.

INDUSTRY

Microbiological guidelines and specifications are used by industry in the sale and purchase of raw materials and ingredients for further processing. They are used by industry to:

1. assure safety and wholesomeness of raw material and ingredients and determine their suitability for further processing;
2. establish evidence of adequate processing and assess sanitation;
3. identify and monitor critical control points;
4. determine conformance to finished product microbial limits;
5. assure safety and wholesomeness of finished products;
6. assure compliance with regulatory requirements.

The use of microbiological criteria by food processors varies greatly. Sophisticated companies establish microbiological specifications over a wide variety of critical raw materials and in many cases not only monitor incoming raw materials, but also inspect the facilities in which these products are produced. Such companies, in addition, have established Hazard Analysis Critical Control Point programs (see Chapter 10) to monitor critical control points and where appropriate to utilize microbiological criteria in such monitoring. In addition, finished product testing through microbiological analysis and guidelines is common in the food industry.

At the other end of the spectrum there are processors who make no use of microbiological criteria. Hazards presented by their products are identified as a result of regulatory inspections, consumer complaints, rejection by other processors using their products, or as a result of an outbreak of foodborne disease.

Unfortunately, purchase specifications are frequently written by a purchasing agent whose knowledge of the relevance of such specifications to the microbiological acceptability of the finished product concerned is insufficient for selection of appropriate specifications.

REFERENCES

Clark, D. S.
    1978   The International Commission on Microbiological Specifications for Foods. Food Technol. 32(1):51-54, 67.
DOD (Department of Defense)
    1976   Oysters, fresh (chilled) and frozen: Shucked. Federal Specification PP-O-956G. Dec. 27 (Amendment).
DOD (Department of Defense; Office of Undersecretary of Defense for Research and Engineering)
    1978   Defense standardization and specifications program: Policies, procedures and instructions. Manual DOD 4120. 3M. Philadelphia: U.S. Naval Publ. and Forms Center.
Duran, A. P., B. A. Wentz, J. M. Lanier, F. D. McClure, A. H. Schwab, A. Swartzentruber, R. J. Barnard, and R. B. Read, Jr.
    1983   Microbiological quality of breaded shrimp during processing. J. Food Prot. 46:974-977.
FAO/WHO (Food and Agriculture Organization/World Health Organization)
    1975   Consultation, 1975. Microbiological specifications for foods. Report of Joint FAO/WHO Consultation. Geneva.
    1977   Consultation, 1977. Microbiological specifications for foods. Report of Second Joint FAO/WHO Consultation. Geneva. February 21-March 2.
FDA (Food and Drug Administration)
    1972   Certain foods for which there are no standards of identity. Proposed microbiological quality standards. Federal Register 37(186):20038-20040.
    1973   Part 11—Standards of quality for foods for which there are no standards of identity. Federal Register 38(148):20726-20730.
    1975   Memorandum of Understanding Between AMS/USDA and FDA. No. FDA 225-75-4002.
    1976a   Standards of quality for foods for which there are no standards of identity. Federal Register 41(154):33249-33253.
    1976b   Food Service Sanitation Manual. DHEW Publ. No. (FDA) 78-2081. Washington, D.C.: U.S. Department of Health, Education and Welfare.
    1977   Standards of quality for foods for which there are no standards of identity. Federal Register 42(50):14326.
    1978a   Quality standards for foods with no identity standards. Federal Register 43(45):9272.
    1978b   The vending of foods and beverages. DHEW Publ. No. (FDA) 78-2091. Washington, D.C.: U.S. Department of Health, Education and Welfare.
    1980   Frozen fish sticks, frozen fish cakes, and frozen crab cakes; Recommended microbiological quality standards. Federal Register 45(108):37524-37526.
    1982a   Compliance Policy Guides Manual. #PB-271176. Springfield, Va.: National Technical Information Service.
    1982b   The Food Defect Action Levels. Publ. No. (FDA) 82-2161.
    1982c   Retail Food Store Sanitation Code. 1982. Recommendation of the Association of Food and Drug Officials of the U.S. Department of Health and Human Services. Washington, D.C.: Public Health Services (Food and Drug Administration).
    1983a   Raw breaded shrimp, microbiological defect action levels. Federal Register 48 (175): 40563-40564.

1983b   Interstate Certified Shellfish Shippers List. March 1, 1983.

1983c   Thermally processed low-acid foods packaged in hermetically sealed containers. General provisions. Current good manufacturing practice. Code of Federal Regulations 21 CFR 113.5.

1983d   Food additives permitted for direct addition to foods for human consumption. Special dietary and nutritional additives. Whole fish protein concentrate. Code of Federal Regulations. 21 CFR 172.385.

1983e   1983 NCIMS Actions. Transmittal 83-9. IMS-a-21, 10-3-83 of National Conference of Interstate Milk Shippers to DHHS/FDA/MSD.

ICMSF (International Commission on Microbiological Specifications for Foods)

1974   Microorganisms in Foods. 2. Sampling for microbiological analysis: Principles and specific applications. Toronto: University of Toronto Press.

1985   Microorganisms in Foods. 2. Sampling for microbiological analysis: Principles and specific applications, 2nd Ed. In preparation.

Johnston, R. W.

1981   Microbiological monitoring and surveillance programs. Paper presented at Science Division Directors Seminar, March. Washington, D.C.: U.S. Department of Agriculture.

1982   Microbiology programs of Food Safety and Inspection Service. Paper presented at 7th Annual Eastern Research Highlights Conference, National Food Processors Association, November 8. Washington, D.C.: U.S. Department of Agriculture.

Kimbrell, E. F.

1982   Codex Alimentarius food standards and their relevance to U.S. standards. Food Technol. 36(6):93-95.

Majorack, F. C.

1982   FDA's industry quality assurance assistance program. Food Technol. 36(6):87-88, 95.

Martin, R. E., and G. T. Pitts

1982   Handbook of State and Federal Microbiological Standards and Guidelines. Washington, D.C.: National Fisheries Institute.

Olson, J. C., Jr.

1978   Microbiological specifications for foods: International activities. Food Technol. 32(1):55-57, 62.

Pivnick, H.

1978   Canadian microbiological standards for foods. Food Technol. 32(1):58-60, 62.

Powers, E. M.

1976   Microbiological criteria for food in military and federal specifications. J. Milk Food Technol. 39(1):55-58.

Sackett, I. D., Jr.

1982   Quality inspection activities of the National Marine Fisheries Service. Food Technol. 36(6):91-92.

U.S. Congress

1944   Public Law 410. Public Health Service Act, 58th Stat., 683. Washington, D.C.: Superintendent of Documents.

1946   Agricultural Marketing Act, as Amended. Washington, D.C.: Superintendent of Documents.

1956   Fish and Wildlife Act. Washington, D.C.: Superintendent of Documents.

1968a   Wholesome Meat Act. Washington, D.C.: Superintendent of Documents.

1968b   Wholesome Poultry Products Act. Washington, D.C.: Superintendent of Documents.

1970   Egg Products Inspection Act. Washington, D.C.: Superintendent of Documents.

1976   Defense Cataloging and Standardization Act. PL 10 USC 2451-56. Washington, D.C.: Superintendent of Documents.

1980   Federal Food, Drug and Cosmetic Act, as Amended. Washington, D.C.: Superintendent of Documents.

USDA (U.S. Department of Agriculture)

1972   Milk for manufacturing purposes and its production and processing. (Agricultural Marketing Service). Federal Register 37(68):7046-7066.

1975   General specifications for approved dairy plants and standards for grades of dairy products. (Agricultural Marketing Service). Federal Register 40(198):47910-47940.

1980   Salmonella Surveillance Program, DA Instruction No. 918-72. January 28, 1980. USDA, FSQS/PDQD. Washington, D.C.: U.S. Department of Agriculture.

1982a   United States standards for grades of nonfat dry milk (Spray process). Code of Federal Regulations 7 CFR, Subpart L. 58.2528.

1982b   United States standards for grades of nonfat dry milk (Roller process). Code of Federal Regulations 7 CFR, Subpart M. 58.2553.

1982c   United States standards for instant nonfat dry milk. Code of Federal Regulations 7 CFR, Subpart U. 58.2753, 58.2754.

1982d   United States standards for grades of dry whole milk. Code of Federal Regulations 7 CFR, Subpart S. 58.2704, 58.2705, 58.2706.

1982e   United States standards for grades of dry buttermilk. Code of Federal Regulations 7 CFR, Subpart Q. 58.2655.

1982f   United States standards for dry whey. Code of Federal Regulations 7 CFR, Subpart O. 58.2605.

1982g   United States standards for grades of edible dry casein. Code of Federal Regulations 7 CFR, Subpart V. 58.2803, 58.2804.

USDHEW (U.S. Department of Health, Education and Welfare)

1965   National Shellfish Sanitation Program. (Revised 1965) Part I—Sanitation of Shellfish Growing Areas. Part II—Sanitation of the Harvesting and Processing of Shellfish. Washington, D.C.: U.S. Government Printing Office.

USPHS (U.S. Public Health Service)

1924   Standard Milk Ordinance. Reprint 971, Public Health Reports, November 7.

1925   Report of Committee on Sanitary Control of the Shellfish Industry in the United States. Supplement 53 to Public Health Reports. November 6.

1927   Standard Milk Ordinance and Code. Mimeographed tentative draft. November.

USPHS/FDA (U.S. Public Health Service/Food and Drug Administration)

1978   Grade A Pasteurized Milk Ordinance. 1978 Recommendations. PHS/FDA Publ. No. 229. Washington, D.C.: U.S. Government Printing Office.

Wehr, H. M.

1982   Attitudes and policies of governmental agencies on microbial criteria for foods—an update. Food Technol. 36(9):45-54, 92.

9

Application of Microbiological Criteria to Foods and Food Ingredients

INTRODUCTION

In preceding chapters, conditions necessary for establishing meaningful microbiological criteria were presented. In this chapter recommendations are given regarding the need or lack thereof for microbiological criteria for each of 22 food products or groups of products. The subcommittee elected not to give specific recommendations relative to microbiological limits but chose instead to emphasize that any criteria that are developed should be realistic and should be based on relevant background information. Although the organization of the individual sections of this chapter may vary for each of the foods or groups of foods, the subcommittee has attempted to address the following basic issues in each section: (1) the sensitivity of the food product(s) relative to safety and quality, (2) the needs for a microbiological standard(s) and/or guideline(s), (3) assessment of information necessary for establishment of a criterion if one seems to be indicated, and (4) where the criterion should be applied.

The following foods and food groups are included in this chapter in the order in which they are listed below:

A. Dairy Products
B. Raw Meats
C. Processed Meats
D. Raw (Eviscerated, Ready-To-Cook) Poultry
E. Processed Poultry Products

F. Eggs and Egg Products
G. Fish, Molluscs, and Crustaceans
H. Fruits and Vegetables
I. Fruit Beverages
J. Low-Acid Canned Foods

K. Acid Canned Foods
L. Water Activity-Controlled
   Canned Foods
M. Cereals and Cereal Products
N. Fats and Oils
O. Sugar, Cocoa, Chocolate,
   and Confectioneries
P. Spices

Q. Yeasts
R. Formulated Foods
S. Nuts
T. Miscellaneous Additives
U. Bottled Water, Processing
   Water, and Ice
V. Pet Foods

A. DAIRY PRODUCTS

Introduction

Microbial growth in the more perishable dairy products, i.e., pasteurized milks, condensed milks, ice cream mixes, creams, cottage cheese, and fermented milks, often results in development of objectionable flavors and textural changes. Even under conditions of good production, processing, distribution, and storage (including care in the home) such changes are inevitable and may be expected to occur within two to three weeks or less. However, the high acidity of cottage cheese and fermented milks and the high heat treatment given to ultrapasteurized milk permits somewhat longer shelf-life. Recognition of the perishability of these products has led to the common practice of "sell by date" labelling as a means of alerting distributors and consumers to the products' limited shelf-life. On the other hand, the relatively stable dairy products, i.e., dried milks, evaporated milk, sterilized milk, ice cream, ripened cheese, butter, and sweetened condensed milk, may remain free of microbiologically induced deterioration for several months or years.

In the early part of this century, health of dairy animals and production, processing, and distribution practices were often poor. At that time, unpasteurized milk was a major vehicle for transmission to humans of diseases such as typhoid, diphtheria, septic sore throat, tuberculosis, and brucellosis (Bryan, 1983). Recognition of these problems by government and industry led to a series of recommendations embodied in the Milk Ordinance of 1924 and an interpretion of these recommendations in the Code in 1927. This model milk ordinance, now titled the "Grade A Milk Ordinance" (see below), is an example of the application of the HACCP system to a major food industry.

Maintenance of the quality and safety of dairy products, which includes optimum shelf-life, is now a well-accepted industry responsibility and is a necessity for economic survival in this highly competitive industry. Furthermore, it has become traditional for the public to expect, if not demand, high-quality products that are safe and esthetically acceptable. Therein lies the basis for current safety and quality assurance programs of regulatory agencies and of industry. As a component of such programs, microbiological criteria play an important role.

Sensitivity of Products Relative to Quality

Currently, most state and local regulatory agencies utilize almost exclusively the Grade A Pasteurized Milk Ordinance (USPHS/FDA, 1978) and USDA Standards for Grades of Dairy Products (USDA, 1975) as the bases for their regulatory programs for dairy products. As an integral part of these two documents, microbiological criteria are specified for most products (see Chapter 8, Table 8-4). Furthermore, the testing of dried milk products for *Salmonella* is provided for in accordance with a Memorandum of Understanding (FDA, 1975) (see Chapter 8).

There can be little doubt that application of microbiological criteria has contributed significantly to the provision of high-quality, safe dairy products. With the exception noted below and as needs are uncovered by future investigations and research, there appears to be no basis for imposing more severe standards or additional criteria. Industry imposes on itself criteria far more stringent than those that must be met to avoid the likelihood of noncompliance. This has the salutary effect of providing reasonable assurance that products are esthetically acceptable and that aerobic plate count levels are maintained well below those likely to cause deteriorative changes within a reasonable shelf-life period.

One of the exceptions referred to above is the bacterial count limit for Grade 2 raw milk for manufacturing purposes as specified in the USDA "Standards for Grades" (USDA, 1975). Recent research has revealed the potential for heat-resistant enzymes of microbial origin to be involved in the deterioration of processed dairy products held for prolonged storage periods. Furthermore, these enzymes have been implicated in lowered cheese yields. Psychrotrophs are among the principal organisms that produce these enzymes and because of modern milk-handling practices, they can comprise a large proportion of the microflora of raw milk. Thus, bacterial count levels as high as the 3 million per ml permitted in Grade 2 milk would appear to be excessive. Consideration might well be given to modifying this standard. Certainly, lower count levels are easily attained through application of modern milk-handling practices.

Sensitivity of Products Relative to Safety

Currently the microbiological safety of dairy products can be assured only through application of three preventive measures. These are:

(1) pasteurization or more severe heat treatments; (2) prevention of post-heat treatment contamination; and, (3) for certain products, end-product testing for microorganisms and toxins for certain products. Microbiological criteria are useful in the application of the preventive measures listed above.

Current standards for coliforms as specified in the Grade A Pasteurized Milk Ordinance and the USDA Standards for Grades are useful in detecting post-heat treatment contamination. However, failure to find these organisms in finished products or at critical control points does not necessarily indicate the absence of post-heat treatment contaminants.

Dried Milk

There is ample justification for continued finished-product testing and surveillance of dried milk products for the presence of *Salmonella*. These products are susceptible to *Salmonella* contamination and are often used without further heat treatment for fluid consumption as recombined milk or as ingredients in formulated foods. Furthermore, these recombined or formulated products are often consumed by high-risk populations. Monthly reports of the USDA's *Salmonella* surveillance program (USDA, 1980) administered in accordance with the USDA/FDA Memorandum of Understanding (FDA, 1975) reveal a continuing low level of *Salmonella*-positive environmental samples and finished products from dried milk plants. Concurrent with the USDA/FDA programs, industry conducts extensive testing. Subsequent routine follow-up procedures undoubtedly have prevented contaminated product from reaching the market.

The above-mentioned program as well as FDA surveillance of products offered for import should be continued, strengthened when indicated, and reviewed periodically to ascertain that sampling plans, including methods used, are consistent with the hazards presented and in accord with current developments in methodology and with appropriate statistical concepts. Reference is here made to the USDA document entitled "*Salmonella* Surveillance Program" (USDA, 1980). This document refers to the National Academy of Sciences publication *An Evaluation of the* Salmonella *Problem* (NRC, 1969) and states that the report classifies dried milk and dried milk product in Food Category II and proposes acceptance of a lot on the basis of all negative results on twenty-nine 25-g samples (n = 29). The USDA document states "Instead of analyzing 25-g samples this Instruction provides a procedure whereby each test shall comprise a composite of four 100-g samples." It further states that, "based on low incidence of contamination, this procedure provides comparable sensitivity and permits greater coverage at a reduced cost." In this case n = 16. The sampling plan applies to finished products analyzed quarterly in accordance with the surveillance program. This subcommittee does not agree that a sampling plan of n = 16 provides "comparable sensitivity" to the recommended plan where n = 29, though obviously it must agree that the cost is reduced. In essence the USDA Quarterly Surveillance Program should require the analysis of 2 rather than 1 composite sample. In this case the sampling plan would be n = 32, which would be only slightly more stringent than the plan recommended by the *Salmonella* committee. In practice, on a quarterly basis, the USDA collects samples from 3 days' production (preferably consecutive days). Four samples of product from each day are drawn, for a total of 12 samples. The four samples for each day are composited to yield a 400-g analytical unit that is analyzed for *Salmonella*. Thus, the quarterly finished-product surveillance consists of the analysis of three 400-g samples for a given plant. If the plant produces products other than a nonfat dried milk, i.e., buttermilk and whey, a separate set of 12 samples is taken from the dryer(s) that is (are) used for each product. If the plant has several dry-milk dryers, each with its own bagging head, the product from only one dryer is sampled. The "Instruction" directs that alternately a different dryer be sampled on each successive quarterly survey. This subcommittee believes that samples should be drawn from each dryer since each is an integral unit of production equipment. At the time of the quarterly survey three environmental samples are also collected, these being waste material from the vacuum cleaner, air filters, and tailings. When the surveillance on a plant's production shows a positive test, a letter is sent to the plant manager informing him of the single positive test and the three available options by which the positive product can be handled. These options appear to be adequate to provide reasonable assurance that contaminated product will not reach the market. They provide that the day's production having the positive *Salmonella* test shall be either:

1. segregated, reprocessed and the reprocessed product tested for *Salmonella*;
2. segregated and disposed of in a manner that poses no health problem to humans or animals, e.g., USDA certification that the product was discarded in a sanitary landfill; or
3. retested (verification test) at the rate of twelve 100-g samples. For test purposes the laboratory will composite 4 samples for a total of 3 tests (n = 48). If none of the composites shows a positive test, the results are interpreted as meaning that the incidence of *Salmonella* is insignificant, and the day's production may be used for human purposes. If one or more of the composites shows a positive test, the day's production represented by the test is then handled as in

(1) or (2) above, i.e., segregated, reprocessed, and retested or disposed of. In addition, eight 100-g samples are collected from product manufactured on each of two days immediately preceding the day(s) in which the positive product was noted and this rate of sampling and testing is also performed on each day's production made subsequent to the day(s) having a positive product test until the plant effects a complete cleanup of its drying facilities. This procedure would represent a sampling plan of n = 32, a plan comparable in stringency to that recommended by the *Salmonella* committee.

If, in connection with a quarterly survey, more than one of the three finished product samples are positive, then verification testing (as outlined above) is not permitted. Positive lots are reconstituted and repasteurized or disposed of in a manner that poses no threat to human or animal health. The plant manager is requested to furnish a list of production back to at least two days prior to the positive lot and up to the time of special cleanup. The list should show the date of manufacture, lot number, number of containers in each lot, and the present location of the product. "Because of possible serious contamination, the product should be recalled from distribution channels and held for sampling and testing for *Salmonella*." In this connection eight samples are drawn from each day's production held from distribution. If all eight test results on a day's production are negative, that product may be released for use or distribution. If a positive test is obtained on product for any day, all the product for that day shall be disposed of in such a manner so as to pose no health problem to humans or animals. This subcommittee believes that the actions taken subsequent to the detection of positive lots at time of quarterly surveillance sampling are adequate for the purposes intended.

The effectiveness of cleanup (required as part of one of the three options indicated above) is determined on the basis of tests made on product manufactured subsequent to cleanup. Sampling involves the collection of eight 100-g samples on each of three production days immediately following the cleanup (n = 32). In this instance, if a lot is declared positive, there is no option for verification testing; management must dispose of the product "in such a manner as to pose no health problem to humans or animals" or reprocess the lot and again test it for *Salmonella*. Furthermore, three environmental samples are taken presumably on each post-cleanup production day.

The environmental sampling program is an integral part of the USDA *Salmonella* Surveillance Program. Concomitant collection of environmental samples at the time quarterly finished-product samples are taken materially strengthens the program. Experience has taught that if a *Sal-*

monella problem exists within a milk-drying plant, one is far more apt to detect this problem through the analysis of environmental samples than through finished product analysis. Thus, given an adequate finished product sampling plan (n = 29-30) combined with the testing of environmental samples, there is reasonable assurance that if all samples are negative, a serious *Salmonella* problem did not exist at the time of the quarterly inspection. Furthermore, the sampling programs followed in verification tests have a stringency comparable to that recommended by the *Salmonella* committee (NRC, 1969). The overall weakness of the program lies in the fact that (1) samples are collected only on a quarterly basis; (2) sampling plans used at time of quarterly sampling are not sufficiently stringent, i.e., consistent with recommendations of the NAS/NRC *Salmonella* report (NRC, 1969); and (3) in plants having more than one dryer for a given product, the product from only one of the dryers is sampled. Thus, the USDA surveillance program cannot substitute for in-house surveillance by the processor. As with the USDA program on eggs and egg products, the control of the *Salmonella* hazard in dry milk requires continuous testing of finished product and environmental samples by the processor. The present USDA program is to be commended and should be strengthened as indicated above and continued, with the realization that it is not a substitute for microbiological control by the manufacturer. Accordingly, the dry milk industry should be encouraged to test finished products regularly and in accordance with sampling plans recommended in the NAS/ NRC *Salmonella* report.

Cheese

Cheese is the second dairy product for which finished product testing for presence of a pathogen or its toxins may be indicated. The organism of primary concern is *Staphylococcus aureus*; although pathogenic *Escherichia coli* have caused some concern. Also, the recent series of outbreaks of brucellosis due to unripened raw goat milk queso blanco cheese sold primarily from roadside vendors in the Houston, Texas area has emphasized the hazard of cheese made from unpasteurized milk (Perkins et al., 1983). As in the case of the hazard of raw milk consumption, pasteurization of milk used in the manufacture of this cheese is the only rational means of control. Routine microbiological testing would not serve as an effective control measure.

Certain cheese varieties have served as the vehicle involved in outbreaks of staphylococcal food poisoning. Others, although not involved in outbreaks, have been shown to permit the buildup of potentially hazardous levels of *S. aureus* under certain conditions of manufacture. Although few outbreaks have been reported in the United States in recent years, the problem does persist. The nature and control of the problem, including application of microbiological criteria, has been reviewed recently (ICMSF, 1980, 1985). The following is a brief summary of these considerations.

The hazard of staphylococcal food poisoning presented by cheese is limited largely to hard varieties, i.e., Cheddar and similar types and Swiss or Emmenthaler. Although *S. aureus* has been demonstrated to grow in certain other varieties, i.e., Gouda, Brick, Roquefort, Blue, and Mozzarella, their involvement in outbreaks has been rare or unreported (ICMSF, 1980). At some point during manufacture and subsequent handling, the first group of cheeses undergoes a sufficiently long period at moderate temperatures, which permits growth of lactic starter cultures. Impairment of such growth during these periods permits relatively unrestricted growth of various other organisms that may be present, including *S. aureus*. If the initial population and period of time of favorable growth conditions are sufficient, the number of *S. aureus* may reach several million per gram of product, at which point hazardous levels of enterotoxin may be present. Adequate heat treatment of cheese milk, good sanitary practices to avoid post-heat treatment contamination, and unimpaired starter culture activity are essential elements of good manufacturing practices for control of *S. aureus* in cheese.

Appropriate analytical methods are available for the testing of cheese and the monitoring of critical control points in cheese manufacture. Adequate and relatively simple methods for detection and enumeration of *S. aureus* in cheese are available. *S. aureus* enterotoxins may be detected with specificity, although the procedures are somewhat complicated. Furthermore, a rapid test for staphylococcal thermonuclease is sufficiently reliable for determining whether a particular lot of cheese may contain enterotoxin or whether it may be safely released for distribution (see Chapter 15 of ICMSF, 1985).

At present the incidence of staphylococcal food poisoning by domestically produced cheese does not justify routine testing by regulatory agencies. However, industry should be encouraged to (1) routinely monitor critical control points for presence or indication of staphylococcal growth and to (2) test all cheese for *S. aureus* and/or thermonuclease if abnormal lactic culture activity occurred during manufacture or if other conditions that might lead to extensive staphylococcal growth were encountered. FDA should routinely test all susceptible cheese varieties offered for import for presence of thermonuclease. This routine testing is advisable as regulatory agencies generally do not have knowledge of the cheese production conditions. Lots positive for thermonuclease should be further tested for presence of enterotoxins.

Outbreaks of foodborne illness due to certain pathogenic strains of *E. coli* in imported Camembert cheese occurred in the United States in 1971. These were the first documented foodborne outbreaks due to *E. coli* to be reported in the United States. Nevertheless, they caused considerable concern about cheese as a vehicle for transmission of pathogenic *E. coli* to humans. No further outbreaks of cheeseborne illness due to *E. coli* were reported until 1983. In 1983 several outbreaks occurred again, resulting from consuming imported soft cheese (Brie and Camembert) of French origin. Investigations were not completed at time of this writing, but they seem to indicate that a certain strain of *E. coli* (027:H20) producing a heat-stable toxin was the causative organism (Francis and Davis, 1984).

Following the first episode in 1971 certain control measures were introduced by the French government and the industry. Apparently these measures were effective in view of the 12-year interval between the two series of outbreaks. However, now it would appear prudent for FDA to initiate appropriate research relative to the *E. coli* problem in soft cheese as well as the routine testing of soft cheese offered at import, i.e., Camembert, Brie, and similar varieties, for the presence and quantitative level of *E. coli*. Such studies would serve to further delineate the problem and assist in development of an appropriate control program.

Fluid Milk

Milkborne disease outbreaks caused by consuming legally purchased contaminated raw milk as well as raw milk cheese (see preceding discussion of queso blanco cheese) continue with regularity. Even certified raw milk, which is produced under the most exacting sanitary conditions, continues to cause outbreaks (Werner et al., 1984).

Recently, Bryan (1983) reviewed the epidemiology of milkborne diseases and concluded, as many others have done previously, that pasteurization is an essential process in providing milk that is free of disease-producing microorganisms. Application of microbiological criteria, although useful, cannot assure that contaminated raw milk will be detected.

The problems of preventing the sale and consumption of raw milk have been emphasized in a recent editorial by Chin (1982) (see Appendix F). The sale of raw milk is still legal in some 20 states in spite of the fact that infectious disease professionals consider the scientific case against raw milk to be irrefutable. Nevertheless, the legal aspects involved in preventing the sale of raw milk are complex and provide impediments toward that end. Unfortunately, the small segment of the dairy industry that engages in public sale of raw milk for fluid consumption, deliberately or through ignorance of the consequences, continues to make available to consumers a product that sometimes is hazardous. The subcommittee agrees with Dr. Chin's conclusion that, "It is the responsibility of all health professionals to see that the public and the policymakers are adequately informed about the scientific findings so that public policy on raw milk may be compatible with scientific knowledge and protective of the public's health."

References

Bryan, F. L.
    1983   Epidemiology of milk-borne diseases. J. Food Prot. 46:637-649.

Chin, J.
    1982   Raw milk: A continuing vehicle for the transmission of infectious disease agents in the United States. J. Infect. Dis. 46: 440-441.

FDA (Food and Drug Administration)
    1975   Memorandum of Understanding USDA/FDA on *Salmonella* Inspection of Dry Milk Plants. No. FDA 225-75-4002. Washington, D.C.: U.S. Department of Agriculture.

Francis, B. J., and J. P. Davis
    1984   Update: gastrointestinal illness associated with imported semi-soft cheese. Morb. Mort. Weekly Rpt. 33:16, 22.

ICMSF (International Commission on Microbiological Specifications for Foods)
    1980   Milk and milk products. Pp. 470-520 in Microbial Ecology of Foods. Vol. 2. Food Commodities. New York: Academic Press.
    1985   Microorganisms in Foods. 2. Sampling for microbiological analysis: Principles and specific applications. 2nd Ed. In preparation.

NRC (National Research Council)
    1969   An Evaluation of the *Salmonella* Problem. Committee on *Salmonella*. Washington, D.C.: National Academy of Sciences.

Perkins, P., A. Rogers, M. Key, V. Pappas, R. Wende, J. Epstein, M. Thapar, F. Jensen, T. L. Gustafson, and E. Young
    1983   Brucellosis—Texas. Morb. Mort. Weekly Rpt. 32:548-553.

USDA (U.S. Department of Agriculture)
    1975   General specifications for approved dairy plants and standards for grades of dairy products. Federal Register 40(198):47910-47940.
    1980   *Salmonella* Surveillance Program. DA Instruction No. 918-72. Washington, D.C.: U.S. Department of Agriculture.

USPHS/FDA (U.S. Public Health Service/Food and Drug Administration)
    1978   Grade A Pasteurized Milk Ordinance. 1978 Recommendations. PHS/FDA Publ. No. 229. Washington, D.C.: U.S. Government Printing Office.

Werner, S. B., F. R. Morrison, G. L. Humphrey, R. A. Murray, and J. Chin
    1984   *Salmonella dublin* and raw milk consumption—California. Morb. Mort. Weekly Rpt. 33:196-198.

B. RAW MEATS

Sensitivity of Products Relative to Safety and Quality

The microbiological condition of retail cuts of red meat (beef, pork, and lamb) is the result of a series of conditions and events including:

1. the health and condition of the live animal;
2. slaughtering-dressing practices;
3. conditions of chilling of the carcass such as rate of cooling, temperature, and humidity;
4. sanitary conditions and practices during fabrication of a carcass into primal, subprimal, and retail cuts;
5. packaging conditions such as air versus vacuum-packaging;
6. conditions of distribution and storage (time-temperature profiles);
7. handling of cuts in food service establishments and in the home (proper refrigerated storage, adequate heat treatment, avoiding cross-contamination).

Following is a brief summary of these conditions and events as they relate to shelf-life and wholesomeness of meat and the potential need for microbiological criteria. For more detailed information, the reader is referred to the following reports (APHA, 1984; Ayres, 1955, 1960; ICMSF, 1980; Ingram and Roberts, 1976; and Roberts, 1974).

Conditions prior to slaughter can have an impact on the microbiological condition of meat. Muscle tissue from carcasses of animals that have undergone prolonged muscular activity or long-term stress (lack of feed, temperature changes) before slaughter is often dark, firm, and dry (DFD meat), contains little or no glucose and has a higher pH (≥ 6.0) than that of unstressed animals (approximately 5.5). Under aerobic storage conditions, normal meat spoils when glucose is exhausted and amino acids are attacked. In DFD meat, however, amino acids are attacked without delay. The high pH of vacuum-packaged DFD meat allows the development of *Serratia liquefaciens* and *Alteromonas putrefaciens*, which produce off-odors. For these reasons DFD meat spoils more rapidly than normal meat (Gill and Newton, 1981). Stress also may increase the prevalence of *Salmonella* in pigs as they are transported from production units to slaughtering facilities (Ingram, 1972; Williams and Newell, 1970).

Microorganisms associated with the live animal are located primarily on the surface of the animal (hide, hair, hooves) and in the gastrointestinal tract. The number of microorganisms in the muscle tissue (intrinsic bacteria) of healthy animals is small (Gill, 1979). Carcasses of normal, healthy animals appear to have considerable residual ability to maintain tissue sterility. It is often reported that muscle tissue from stressed animals is more likely to contain "intrinsic" bacteria. It is possible that certain forms of stress depress the immune defense mechanisms and therefore allow the survival of bacteria that otherwise would have been destroyed.

Sources of microbial contamination of a carcass include: the animal (surface and gastro-intestinal tract), workers, clothing of workers, utensils, equipment, air, and water. Hence, the level of microbial contamination of a carcass at this stage depends upon the degree of sanitation practiced during the slaughter-dressing procedures. Aerobic plate counts (APCs) of freshly dressed beef, pork, and lamb carcasses in the United States usually range from 10^2-10^4 per cm^2, most of which are not psychrotrophic. Microbial types reflect the various sources of contamination and include *Micrococcus, Staphylococcus, Bacillus, Enterobacteriaceae, Pseudomonas*, yeasts and molds, and others. Because of location and handling practices certain areas of a carcass are more likely to be contaminated or to remain contaminated than are others. For these reasons, microorganisms are not uniformly distributed over the surface.

Under conditions of rapid chilling, low storage temperature (-1 to $+1°C/$ 30.2 to 33.8°F), proper air movement, and relative low humidity, the number of microorganisms on a carcass may increase little or in some cases actually decrease during the first 24 to 48 hours. During further refrigerated storage, psychrotrophic bacteria will become a more prominent part of the microbial flora.

Fabrication of carcasses into primal, subprimal, and retail cuts involves extensive handling of the meat, markedly increases the surface area, and increases the a_w as newly cut surfaces are made. Because these operations are carried out at refrigeration temperature, contamination at this stage is likely to include a high proportion of psychrotrophic bacteria.

In recent years, approximately 60-70% of the beef leaving meat-packing plants in the United States is vacuum-packaged. Storage of cuts in vacuum packages results in a predominance of lactic acid bacteria, whereas gram-negative, aerobic, psychrotrophic rods such as *Pseudomonas* spp. predominate on aerobically stored cuts. The latter are more active spoilage producers than the lactic acid bacteria. Thus, vacuum-packaged cuts with 10^6-10^7 bacteria per cm^2 may be organoleptically acceptable whereas comparable cuts stored in air-permeable films with similar numbers of gram-negative, aerobic psychrotrophic rods may exhibit off-odors. In vacuum-packaged red meat, high levels of lactic acid bacteria (10^7-10^8 per cm^2) frequently contribute to odors characterized as sour, acid, buttermilk-like, cheesy and less frequently "sulphur-like" or "H_2S-like" (Hanna et al., 1983). When vacuum-packaged cuts are fabricated into steaks or chops and then repackaged in oxygen-permeable films, gram-negative aerobic rods will soon become predominant on the cuts in the display cases.

Conditions of refrigerated storage in the distribution chain (plant, wholesale, retail, food service establishment, home) can have a profound effect on the microbial condition and therefore shelf-life of the product. Cuts with initial low numbers of psychrotrophic bacteria held at proper refrigeration temperature (-1 to $+1°C/30.2$ to 33.8°F) will have a greater shelf-life than will meats produced under less sanitary conditions. Even meats produced under good sanitary conditions will have reduced shelf-life when stored at marginal refrigeration temperatures.

Improper cooking and handling of raw meats in homes and food service establishments is one of the main reasons for foodborne illness caused by consumption of "cooked" meats. It is not yet commercially feasible to produce red meat free from pathogenic bacteria. Small numbers of a variety of pathogenic organisms such as *Salmonella, Clostridium perfringens, Yersinia enterocolitica, Campylobacter jejuni*, and *Staphylococcus aureus* can be present on raw red meats. (See Chapter 4 for more detailed information on these bacteria.) In pork *Trichinella spiralis* can be present. Adequate heat treatment of the meat will destroy most of these pathogens. Spores of *C. perfringens,* however, may survive in cooked meats. If such meats are held at temperatures between 20 to 50°C/68 to 122°F, growth of *C. perfringens* may occur, during either serving operations or subsequent storage, thus creating a health hazard.

To produce red meats with optimum shelf-life and safety requires the monitoring of a series of critical control points pertinent to each of the conditions or events listed above. Most of these critical control points can be monitored by careful inspection of the animals, evaluating the procedures and practices used, and by checking temperatures during chilling operations.

Microbiological guidelines can be applied to monitor some of the critical control points. For example, several relatively simple procedures (APHA, 1984) are available to check the sanitary condition of equipment and utensils. They are useful to evaluate the effectiveness of cleaning and sanitizing procedures. Microbiological count data on freshly dressed carcasses need to be interpreted cautiously (Ingram and Roberts, 1976) because (1) microorganisms are not distributed evenly over the carcass, (2) there is considerable variation in contamination between carcasses, (3) there are differences in contamination due to processing on different days in the same plant and (4) there are differences between plants. In addition, the tests that can be applied to examine carcasses under commercial conditions recover only a fraction (often a variable fraction) of the organisms present, usually from a rather small surface area of the total carcass. Nevertheless, APCs on freshly dressed carcasses may provide data that indicate a trend in the handling of animals during the slaughter-dressing operations.

Several other methods have been tried to monitor microbial activity in red meats such as pH, dye reduction, titratable acidity, volatile nitrogen compounds, volatile acids, extract-release-volume, and others (see Chapter 5). None of these has proved to be a sensitive and reproducible indicator of incipient spoilage applicable to various raw meats.

Critical control points associated with handling in retail outlets, food service establishments, and in the home are beyond the control of the meat processor. To obtain optimum shelf-life and wholesomeness, the HACCP concept has to be applied along the entire production, processing, distribution, and food preparation chain.

Need for Microbiological Criteria

Microorganisms of public health significance such as *Salmonella, C. perfringens, S. aureus, Y. enterocolitica,* and *C. jejuni* often are present in small numbers as part of the natural microbial flora of live animals. Even the best production and processing practices do not eliminate these organisms from raw meats. Therefore, limits for pathogenic microorganisms in microbiological criteria for raw meats are impractical. The same is true for indicator organisms such as the coliform group (coliforms, fecal coliforms, and *Escherichia coli*) because there is no direct relationship between the presence of these types and the presence or absence of pathogens. The courts have held that *Salmonella* is an inherent defect in raw meats (*APHA* v. *Butz*, 1974). This decision was based upon the fact that even with the use of the best manufacturing practices consistent with present technology, *Salmonella* cannot be eliminated from raw meat.

The APC of refrigerated red meats in distribution channels reflects microorganisms acquired from a series of events: slaughter-dressing procedures, chilling, fabrication into primals, subprimals, and retail samples, and growth during refrigerated storage. At points remote from the processing line the APC does not distinguish between microorganisms from the carcass, those acquired during processing, and those resulting from growth during normal refrigerated storage. Although the APCs may be similar, vacuum-packaged cuts on which lactic acid bacteria frequently predominate can be organoleptically acceptable, whereas comparable cuts under aerobic storage, with gram-negative aerobic rods predominating, may be unacceptable. The APC may be of some value to a meat processor to evaluate processing conditions and perhaps shelf-life of a product under well-defined conditions of refrigerated storage. However, the APC of perishable red meats in distribution channels is of little value in the evaluation of the microbial quality of the carcass and processing practices and has no relevance to health.

The history of the Oregon Meat Standard is directly related to the above discussion. In 1973, the state of Oregon adopted a microbiological standard for fresh or frozen red meat at the retail level with limits of APC 5×10^6 and 50 *E. coli* per gram. The standard was revoked in 1977 (State of Oregon, 1977) for the following reasons:

1. There was no evidence that application of the standard improved sanitary conditions in the retail market.

2. There was no evidence of a significant change in the numbers of microorganisms in ground meat and probably no change in quality characteristics of the meat.

3. There was no evidence of a reduction of foodborne illness.

4. The promulgation of the standard may have created the impression on the part of the public that ground meat produced under the standard would have lower microbial counts, improved quality, and fewer health hazards. There was no clear evidence that the expectations were materialized.

5. The additional costs of the program were not justified because the expected benefits, namely lower microbial counts, improved organoleptic quality, and reduced risk to public health, were not clearly demonstrated.

The working group of the Codex Committee on Food Hygiene (FAO/WHO, 1979) also concluded that no benefits would result for either public health or quality through the application of microbiological criteria for raw meats.

In summary:

1. Carcasses, primal, subprimal, and retail cuts of meat from normal, healthy animals contain a variety of microorganisms including low levels of some pathogens.

2. Refrigerated raw meats will spoil eventually even if they are produced from the carcasses of normal, healthy animals, fabricated under good manufacturing conditions, and properly refrigerated.

3. If red meats are not properly cooked, held, cooled, and stored, they can cause foodborne illness.

4. Microbiological standards for raw meats will prevent neither spoilage nor foodborne illness and thus do not appear warranted. Instead, application of the HACCP system to the entire processing and distribution chain including the meat-packing plant, retail units, food service establishment, and home should be used to produce a product with satisfactory shelf-life and public health safety.

5. Microbiological guidelines are applicable to monitor certain critical control points in the processing of raw meats such as the sanitary condition of equipment and utensils and the condition of freshly dressed carcasses.

References

APHA v. *Butz*
   1974   American Public Health Association et al., Appellants vs. Earl Butz, Secretary of Agriculture et al. D.C. Civil Court. Suit to enjoin the Secretary of Agriculture against

alleged violations of the Wholesome Meat Act. Pp. 331-338. 511 F. 2d 331 (D.C. Civ. 1974).

APHA (American Public Health Association)

1984 Compendium of Methods for the Microbiological Examination of Foods. 2nd Ed., M. L. Speck, ed. Washington, D.C.: APHA.

Ayres, J. C.

1955 Microbiological implications in handling, slaughtering, and dressing meat animals. Adv. Food Res. 6:109-161.

1960 Temperature relationships and some other characteristics of the microbial flora developing on refrigerated beef. Food Res. 25:1-18.

FAO/WHO (Food and Agriculture Organization/World Health Organization)

1979 Report of a FAO/WHO working group on microbiological criteria for foods. Geneva: FAO/WHO.

Gill, C. O.

1979 A review. Intrinsic bacteria in meat. J. Appl. Bacteriol. 47:367-378.

Gill, C. O., and K. G. Newton

1981 Microbiology of DFD beef. Pp. 305-327 in The Problem of Dark-cutting in Beef, D. E. Hood and P. V. Tarrant, eds. The Hague: Martines Nijhoff.

Hanna, M. O., J. W. Savell, G. C. Smith, D. E. Purser, F. A. Gardner, and C. Vanderzant

1983 Effect of growth of individual meat bacteria on pH, color and odor of aseptically prepared vacuum-packaged round steaks. J. Food Prot. 46:216-221, 225.

ICMSF (International Commission on Microbiological Specifications for Foods)

1980 Microbial Ecology of Foods. 2. Food Commodities. New York: Academic Press.

Ingram, M.

1972 Meat processing past, present and future. R. Soc. Health J. 92:121-131.

Ingram, M., and T. A. Roberts

1976 The microbiology of the red meat carcass and the slaughterhouse. R. Soc. Health J. 96:270-276.

Roberts, T. A.

1974 Hygiene in the production of meat. Meat Research Institute Memoir No. 696. Langford, Bristol.

State of Oregon

1977 Report of the meat bacterial standards review committee. Salem, Oregon: Department of Agriculture.

Williams, L. P., and K. W. Newell

1970 *Salmonella* excretion in joy-riding pigs. Am. J. Publ. Health 60:926-929.

C. PROCESSED MEATS

Introduction

After the animal carcass is chilled, it is generally broken down into primal, subprimal, and ultimately retail cuts. Unlike poultry, where the various separated parts of the carcass are classified as "processed," the various cuts derived from carcass meat are still classified as "red meat," i.e., unprocessed.

Sensitivity of Products Relative to Safety and Quality

Raw Ground Beef

Ground beef (hamburger) is an important by-product of the retail butcher shop. Trimmings from in-store cutting operations, as well as various "held-over" retail cuts, are ground at the store level. The product may be sold in bulk or may be packaged in oxygen-permeable films.

A substantial quantity of raw ground beef is now being processed in central locations for distribution to retail outlets. The raw materials consist of trimmings from cutting operations, but in addition, substantial quantities of various cuts such as chucks and rounds are also utilized. Such ground meat is generally packaged in an oxygen-impermeable film. In some cases the product is frozen before distribution to retail outlets; in other cases it is shipped under refrigeration.

Generally, the shelf-life of in-store produced ground beef is relatively short, due in part to high microbial numbers in the raw materials, but also due to lax practices with respect to equipment sanitation and temperature control. The initial flora reflects that of the raw materials and thus is comprised chiefly of gram-negative aerobic psychrotrophic bacteria. During storage these organisms are responsible for surface spoilage; in the interior of the meat microaerophilic bacteria (*Lactobacillaceae* and *Brochothrix thermosphacta*) develop (Gardner, 1981).

Packaged ground beef produced at central locations generally has substantially greater shelf-life than in-store produced product. The oxygen-impermeable packaging material creates an environment that inhibits the growth of gram-negative psychrotrophic bacteria. Ultimately spoilage is brought about by the growth of lactic acid bacteria and *B. thermosphacta*. Successful producers of the product must exercise considerable control over the microbiological condition of raw materials, equipment sanitation and temperature control. Though the sensory changes caused by the developing flora in this product are not nearly as disagreeable as those brought about by the gram-negative psychrotrophs, gas production—generally brought about by heterofermentative lactic acid bacteria—is often a serious problem.

Raw ground beef, as such, has not constituted a serious foodborne disease problem. Obviously, those who consume the product without cooking (as in steak tartar) may contract salmonellosis and, at least in theory, this practice could lead to infection with *Yersinia* and *Campylobacter*. The consumption of raw ground meat packaged at a single meat-processing plant, was the cause of a multistate outbreak of *Salmonella newport* disease (Fontaine et al., 1978). Raw ground beef can constitute a trichinellosis hazard if the meat is ground in equipment that has previously been used to grind pork. This is far more apt to happen with raw ground beef produced at the store level than with that manufactured in centralized locations where regulatory control is exercised. Pathogenic *E. coli* (0157:H7) in hamburger has been responsible for outbreaks of hemorrhagic colitis (CDC, 1982). Adequate cooking of the meat should minimize or eliminate the risk of contracting this disease from eating hamburgers. Cooked ground beef as an ingredient in a variety of foods can be associated with foodborne illness (Bryan, 1980).

The critical control points in the production of raw ground beef are the raw meats, equipment sanitation, and temperature control. At centralized locations, the raw materials may be entirely generated ''in-house.'' More often, at least a portion of the raw meats are purchased from outside sources. Outside purchased trimmings are generally inspected upon receipt, and if sensory evaluation indicates off-condition the trimmings should be rejected. The prudent manufacturer will conduct microbiological analyses on the trimmings from various suppliers and eliminate those suppliers shipping raw meats of poor microbiological quality. Proper cleanup of equipment used to convey raw meats, grinders, and packaging machinery is essential to the production of a product with satisfactory shelf-life. Temperature control is of paramount importance. Most manufacturers attempt to grind and package product as near to the freezing point as possible. This is often accomplished through the use of dry ice. If proper steps are not taken, however, the product may be packaged before the ice has sublimed. If this occurs, the packaged product may become ''gassy'' due to evolution of gaseous CO_2 after packaging. Microbiological monitoring of the finished product is only of retrospective value, because results become available after the product has entered merchandising channels. The prudent manufacturer will regularly monitor critical control points to determine whether he has been successful in controlling the microbiological quality of raw meat, the sanitation of processing equipment, and storage temperature.

Perishable Raw Salted and Salted Cured Meats

Examples of these products are fresh pork sausage, Polish and Italian sausage, and uncooked ham, bacon (see also Cooked Cured Meats), and corned beef.

Fresh pork sausage, Polish sausage, and Italian sausage are essentially ground meat to which spices and salt are added. The addition of salt may be somewhat inhibitory to the gram-negative psychrotrophic aerobic bacteria that normally spoil red meats. However, these are highly perishable products that when packaged in oxygen-permeable films support the growth of a heterogeneous microbial flora similar to that of ground beef, though the rate of spoilage is somewhat slower due to the addition of salt. When packaged in oxygen-impermeable films, the spoilage flora is comprised of lactic acid bacteria and *B. thermosphacta* (Gardner, 1981; Johnston and Tompkin, 1984). These products may be merchandised refrigerated. Alternatively, they may be frozen at the processing level and merchandised in the frozen state, or frozen at the processing level and merchandised as refrigerated products. The addition of salt makes these products susceptible to oxidative rancidity. If merchandised in the frozen state, oxidative rancidity is the usual cause of spoilage. If merchandised as refrigerated products, microbial spoilage precedes oxidative rancidity. As with ground beef, the critical control points are the raw materials, temperature and equipment sanitation. Again, finished product analysis is useful but of retrospective value. If properly cooked and promptly served, these products do not constitute an important foodborne disease problem. If not adequately cooked, products containing pork may pose a hazard of trichinellosis (see Chapter 4), e.g., the incorporation of fresh pork sausage in turkey dressing that is not adequately heat treated during roasting.

Uncooked ham, bacon, and corned beef are raw salted cured meats. Uncooked ham is no longer an important commodity in the United States; bacon and corned beef are of considerable importance. In the production of bacon and corned beef, pork bellies and beef briskets respectively are injected with a ''pickle'' containing salt and nitrite and/or nitrate. The pork bellies are then subjected to a mild heat treatment (53.3 to 54.4°C/ 128 to 130°F), a temperature sufficient to ''fix'' the cured meat color but not sufficient to destroy trichinellae. A substantial volume of corned beef is distributed as a raw cured product to which no heat treatment is applied. Currently, most bacon is merchandised as a sliced product packaged in oxygen-impermeable films. Spoilage is due primarily to the growth of lactic acid bacteria. Likewise, uncooked corned beef is merchandised in oxygen-impermeable films and the spoilage flora is also comprised primarily of lactic acid bacteria. If bacon is packaged in oxygen-permeable films, its shelf-life is significantly shorter and the spoilage flora consists primarily of yeasts and micrococci. The critical control points in the production of these products include the microbiological status of the raw materials (beef briskets and pork bellies), the microbiological status of the pickle, and the environment of the packaging area. Generally, the pickle is recirculated and, if adequate control is not exercised, this recirculated pickle can be a significant source of spoilage organisms, including those that cause spoilage due to oxidation of the cured meat pigment. In the past, when it was common to merchandize bacon in oxygen-permeable films, the air in the packaging area was a critical control point as mold growth commonly terminated the shelf-life of sliced bacon. Currently, most bacon is merchandized in oxygen-impermeable films, and mold development is no longer a significant problem.

The perishable raw salted and salted cured meat products do not constitute a significant foodborne illness problem, although, in common with other meat products, misuse by the ultimate consumer can lead to foodborne illness. On occasion, bacon may be consumed by certain ethnic groups without cooking, and outbreaks of trichinellosis have resulted.

Cooked Polish and Italian sausages, as well as heat-processed corned beef, also are merchandised. The spoilage and foodborne disease problems of these products are analogous to those presented by other cooked cured meats (see below).

Shelf-Stable Raw Salted and Salted Cured Meats

Included in this category are salt pork, dry cured bacon, and dry cured ham (country cured ham). These products were extremely important in the early history of the United States and continued to be so until home refrigeration procedures became common. Currently, salt pork, dry cured bacon, and country hams continue to be produced in agricultural regions.

Salted pork, bacon, and hams are prepared by coating the meat with dry salt and storing it at low temperatures (below 10°C/50°F). At intervals, the meat is recoated with dry salt. The product contains high levels of salt and is racked and held at ambient temperatures until the surface of the meat dries. It may then be rubbed with a thin coating of salt and spices, netted, and sold. With bacon and some ham, nitrite and/or nitrate is added to the dry salt used for curing. The product may be hung to dry at ambient temperature for 35 to 140 days before offering it for sale as a shelf-stable meat product. During the initial phases of processing, salt and/or curing agents penetrate and equilibrate in the tissues. Non-spore-forming bacteria of public health concern are subjected to stress or are rendered nonviable. During the subsequent drying period, salt-tolerant micrococci and enterococci grow and appear to render the products even more refractile to the microorganisms of public health concern. The nitrite-and/or nitrate-cured products are required to be held in the dry room for a specified period to destroy trichinellae. Although most U.S. consumers cook these products before eating, dry cured hams have historically been eaten raw in Europe (Johnston and Tompkin, 1984).

Although these products are produced by major meat packers as dry cured hams, a substantial volume is produced by small processors, i.e., as a cottage industry (country cured hams). These operators generally initiate production during the late fall and winter months; the curing process is continued into the early spring of the year. Processors depend upon cool weather to protect the product from spoilage during the curing period. They provide no mechanical refrigeration and, if climatic conditions are unfavorable, internal spoilage of the product may occur before salt and nitrite penetrate by diffusion to protect the product from spoilage. If unseasonably cold weather occurs, freezing of the meat may prevent penetration of salt and nitrite, this leading to spoilage when warm weather appears. Bone taint—deep tissue spoilage near the bone—occurs when improper salt equilibration occurs (Mundt and Kitchen, 1951).

These products have an excellent public health history in the United States. They are merchandised at ambient temperatures, and if properly processed, microorganisms of public health concern constitute no problem. Spoilage problems, as indicated above, relate to improper control of temperature during the curing process. Molds may develop on the finished product during merchandising but to date have constituted no known foodborne disease hazard.

The critical control points in the manufacture of these products are the control of temperature during the curing period and, closely related to this, the proper penetration and equilibration of the curing ingredients. Improper control of humidity during the drying process can lead to the development of surface spoilage microorganisms. Microbiological criteria for either quality control or regulatory purposes are not applicable.

Cooked Uncured Meats

Products in this category include cooked versions of the perishable raw salted items discussed above (pork sausage, and Polish and Italian sausage). In addition, cooked uncured meats are components in a variety of frozen entrees such as "TV dinners," potpies, and sliced cooked meat with gravy. Still other cooked uncured meats are produced for bulk distribution to food service establishments, e.g., cooked ground beef with chili, thinly sliced cooked beef for use in Mexican or other ethnic dishes. These products may be frozen, but more often are distributed under refrigeration. A substantial volume of cooked "roast beef" is distributed to food service establishments. These products are not necessarily prepared from primal cuts. Sometimes they are fabricated from meat trimmings in such a manner that when sliced they have the appearance of cooked roast beef.

Generally, the heat treatment used in the preparation of these products is sufficient to destroy most vegetative microorganisms. A notable exception is precooked roast beef. Post-cooking handling by the manufacturer, the food service worker, and the consumer frequently results in contamination of these products with microorganisms, including those capable of producing spoilage and those of public health concern. If temperature abuse follows, the hazards of spoilage and foodborne disease increase.

In recent years precooked "roast beef" has been a significant vehicle of human salmonellosis in the United States (CDC, 1976a,b; 1977a,b; 1981; and Bryan, 1980). Initially, the multistate outbreaks traced to this product were thought to be due to consumer desire for roast beef presenting a rare appearance and the necessity, therefore, for mild heat processing. Accordingly, research was conducted to determine time-temperature parameters necessary to the destruction of salmonellae in "roast beef" (Goodfellow and Brown, 1978). Despite the promulgation of regulations consistent with the parameters of these studies, outbreaks of salmonellosis traced to cooked beef persist (CDC, 1978). Outbreaks can be attributed either to failure of the processor to comply with the established regulations or to post-heat treatment contamination. In the outbreak cited above, the USDA determined that the processor had not complied with USDA regulations. However, cross-contamination between raw and adequately cooked products is the more usual problem (R. W. Johnston, USDA. 1983. Personal communication). The last outbreak occurred in 1980 (R. W. Johnston, 1984, personal communication). Through a combination of regulation, education of processors, and microbiological monitoring by both industry and the USDA the problem of salmonellae in precooked roast beef appears to have been brought under control. The sampling of products that are rebagged after cooking is more intense than that of products cooked as rolls and not rebagged. However, the USDA requires industry monitoring of both types of product (R. W. Johnston, 1984, personal communication).

The hazard potential for precooked uncured meats produced in commercial establishments is high (NRC, 1964). Yet the incidence of outbreaks traced to cooked meat produced in meat-processing plants has been low, except for the aforementioned important role of precooked roast beef in human salmonellosis. Four cases of botulism have been traced to frozen potpies (CDC, 1960; State of California, 1975; State of California, 1976; and CDC, 1983); in each instance, gross mishandling in homes was the direct cause of illness. Thus, despite the high potential of precooked uncured meats processed in meat-processing plants as a foodborne disease hazard, few outbreaks have been uncovered. However, cooked meat, mishandled in food service establishments and homes, has been an important vehicle of foodborne disease (Bryan, 1980).

The critical control points in the manufacture of these products include, aside from the microbiological quality of raw materials, the heat process and post-heat process handling, proper refrigeration, and adequate re-heating. Assuming adequate heat processing, proper chilling of the heated product is a critical control point. In recognition of this, the USDA (1983) requires that the maximum chill time after cooking of cooked beef, roast beef and cooked corned beef be restricted to no more than six hours during which the product may be in the optimum growth zone for pathogens, defined as 48.9-12.8°C (120-55°F). It further stipulates the chill of the product must continue until the product reaches 4.4°C (40°F) and that the product not be packed until this occurs. Other post-heat treatment handling procedures constitute critical control points, e.g., the slicing of cooked products, boning, packaging, etc. As indicated previously, these procedures may add microorganisms of spoilage and/or foodborne illness significance. Subsequently, improper handling by persons in food service establishments and in homes may lead to spoilage or the potential for foodborne disease. In the commercial production of these products the processor has assumed many of the responsibilities met by the consumer who prepares such foods from raw meat and other ingredients. When the expanding market for these products first developed (in the 1950s and 1960s) there was concern over their high foodborne disease hazard potential (NRC, 1964), but the low incidence of foodborne disease outbreaks traced to them suggests that the processor is more able to circumvent the hazards attendant to their production than is the individual consumer.

Cooked Cured Meats

Cooked cured meats include domestic sausage, (e.g., frankfurters, bologna), luncheon meats (e.g., pepper and pimiento loaf), ham, bacon, and corned beef. The common shared property is that the products are cured, i.e., treated with nitrite and salt, and are subject to heat treatment. Some are ready to eat (bologna, luncheon meats, and fully cooked hams); others are cooked before eating to improve texture and flavor (smoked ham and frankfurters); still others must be cooked before eating to ensure safety, e.g., bacon that does not receive a heat process sufficiently severe to destroy trichinellae.

The physical nature of the raw materials varies from primal cuts of red meats (ham, pork bellies, and beef briskets) to red meat trimmings that are the basic raw materials for domestic sausage and luncheon meats. This necessitates different methods for introducing the curing ingredients (nitrite and salt, with or without nitrate). With ham, bacon, and beef briskets, the curing ingredients are introduced in a solution (pickle). Historically, the primal cuts were submerged in the pickle, which, over a period of time, diffused into the meat. Pork bellies were rubbed with dry salt containing nitrite, with or without nitrate; the curing ingredients dissolved in the moisture phase and, as with ham and beef briskets, penetrated by diffusion. At the present time the curing ingredients are introduced by "pumping" pickle into the primal cuts of meat. This has greatly changed the microbiological problems presented by these products. In former times internal microbial spoilage occurred before complete diffusion of the curing ingredients (see section above on raw salted and salted cured meats). The modern process of injecting the pickle results in rapid distribution of the curing salts within the meats and largely obviates the problem of bone taint. On the other hand, microorganisms contained in the pumping pickle may be instantaneously distributed throughout the meat mass. At times this can result in interior spoilage problems.

With domestic sausage and luncheon meats, the trimmings are ground and the curing ingredients in the form of a dry powder are mixed with the trimmings, generally with the concomitant introduction of various spices, sweeteners, and a curing accelerator.

After the spices and curing ingredients are mixed with ground trimmings, the emulsion is "stuffed" into casings. In the past, natural casings, which were sections of animal intestines, were utilized. Natural casings are still used with some products, but the bulk of domestic sausage products are now processed in synthetic casings. Luncheon meat emulsions are generally introduced into metal containers that are fitted with watertight lids.

Whether the product being manufactured is a primal cut or an emulsion prepared from ground trimmings, development of the stable cured meat color requires heat treatment. For this purpose hams and similar products are wrapped in nets. The netted hams are hung in smokehouses; bacon bellies are attached to metal hangers and hung on "trees." The trees are placed in smokehouses. Domestic sausage products, such as frankfurters and bologna, are generally hung in smokehouses, whereas luncheon meats are usually cooked by submersion in water. Historically, hams, bacon, and briskets were "held in cure" under refrigeration for many days, even weeks, before heat processing. This process has gradually died out in the meat industry. In most plants these products are heat treated soon after the cure is introduced, though some packers may hold the pumped product overnight before heat processing. Domestic sausage and meat emulsions are generally heat processed very soon after the emulsion has been pumped into casings or introduced into metal forms.

The heat process applied to cooked cured meats depends upon the product (for temperatures required in meat processing, see Bailey, 1974). For example, bacon is cooked to a final internal temperature of 48.9 to

54.4°C (120 to 130°F). The heat is applied for the sole purpose of "fixing" the cured color. This requires denaturation of the myoglobin, which takes place at temperatures between 48.9 and 54.4°C (120 and 130°F). Smoked hams, on the other hand, must achieve a temperature of 58.3°C (137°F). This minimum internal temperature is required for the destruction of trichinellae. Fully cooked hams must achieve a minimum internal temperature of 70°C (158°F). Domestic sausage and luncheon meats containing pork must achieve a minimum internal temperature of 58.3°C (137°F) to achieve freedom from trichinellae. From a practical point of view, however, luncheon meats and domestic sausage are processed to much higher temperatures in order to ensure satisfactory shelf-life. The temperatures employed vary with the processor, but generally they range from approximately 68.3 to 76.7°C (155 to 170°F). The maximum temperature, as with the minimum, is self-limiting, since the higher the final temperature the greater the shrinkage loss during heat processing. The processes normally applied are sufficient to destroy non-sporeforming bacteria of public health concern, namely, staphylococci and salmonellae, though the spores of *Clostridium perfringens, Clostridium botulinum*, and *Bacillus cereus* survive. Thermoduric non-sporeforming bacteria, such as Group D streptococci and some lactobacilli, may survive the heat process. The number of survivors is directly related to the level of microorganisms in the unheated product as well as to the degree of heat treatment applied. There is some evidence that surviving non-sporeforming bacteria may be heat injured and thus initiate growth only slowly in properly refrigerated finished product, the degree of heat injury being related to the severity of the process (Greenberg and Silliker, 1961). Various natural spices, e.g., black pepper, may contribute large numbers of aerobic sporeforming bacteria to the sausage or luncheon meat emulsion. These organisms survive the heat process and at times are the predominant surviving microorganisms. They constitute neither a spoilage nor a public health hazard in properly refrigerated cooked cured meats; however, occasionally they may cause product spoilage during the heat process, particularly with large pieces of sausage such as bologna, which must be subjected to a long heat process.

After heat processing, domestic sausage and luncheon meats are generally showered with cold water and placed under refrigeration. The chilled meats are then further treated. The products cooked in molds are removed from the molds as loaves. The luncheon meats are then sliced and packaged. Similarly, domestic sausage products such as bologna are sliced and packaged. With products such as frankfurters that have been heat processed in artificial casings, it is the practice to mechanically remove (peel) the casings. Following this, they are packaged. Natural casings are generally not removed.

It is in the handling of cooked sausage products prior to packaging that the greatest opportunities for contamination with microorganisms occur. For example, a contaminated slicer blade can inoculate the surface of every piece of meat it touches. The equipment used to peel frankfurters can similarly be a source of contamination to every product unit passing through it. Conveyors that transfer sliced or peeled products to packaging equipment can likewise contaminate finished products with spoilage organisms. Most packaging areas are maintained at temperatures that select for the growth of psychrotrophic organisms, 1.1 to 4.4°C (34 to 40°F). This only serves to magnify post-heat treatment handling problems. Cooked cured meats are perishable commodities. In general their shelf-life under refrigerated storage conditions is directly related to the number of microorganisms present upon them at the time of packaging. Most important in this regard is the contamination that occurs after heat processing. These microorganisms are specifically adapted to growth at low temperatures, and if the environment of the processing area is not properly controlled, the organisms are metabolically active. These microorganisms are more capable of initiating growth on the packaged product than are the survivors of the heat process, which may suffer from the effect of heat injury.

Hams may be packaged as whole hams or may be cut to yield half hams or slices. Due to the smoking process, the surfaces of hams tend to be somewhat dry, and some of the components of smoke that are deposited on these surfaces have mild antimicrobial properties. Thus, hams receive less post-heat treatment handling and their surfaces are somewhat more resistant to microbial attack than is the case with domestic sausage and luncheon meats. Bacon, though occasionally sold unsliced, is generally sliced and packaged. As with domestic sausage, if the slicing equipment is not satisfactorily maintained, each sliced piece may become contaminated with spoilage organisms.

The spoilage flora of cooked cured meats depends upon the packaging system employed. In the past, packaging was in oxygen-permeable films, and the spoilage flora was comprised primarily of micrococci and yeasts. In recent years, oxygen-impermeable films have been used and the spoilage flora has consisted primarily of lactic acid bacteria. Formerly, these products had a relatively short shelf-life. Packaging in oxygen-impermeable films has significantly increased shelf-life since the lactic acid bacteria normally developing during refrigerated storage may reach very high levels without significant organoleptic changes. Characteristically, the growth of these lactic acid bacteria is manifested by a milky appearance in the free moisture within the package. This is due to the production of lactic acid, which precipitates protein in the free moisture surrounding the meat.

The public health history of sliced cured meats, domestic sausage, and luncheon meats in this country has been good even though these products are commonly subjected to temperature abuse in the hands of the consumer. Although salmonellae are quite capable of growing on cooked, cured meats, they have rarely been associated with foodborne illness from this source. Though staphylococci are capable of growth on sliced luncheon meats and domestic sausage, it appears likely that the relative freedom from foodborne disease may be attributed to competing microorganisms. The situation with ham is quite different. This cooked cured meat is perhaps the most important source of staphylococcal food poisoning. In general the food poisoning is not related to problems created by the food processor. Rather, most outbreaks of staphylococcal food poisoning are caused by contamination of the ham by food service personnel and persons in their homes after cooking. Such contamination, followed by temperature abuse, is the major cause of foodborne disease traced to this product.

Many critical control points are associated with the production of cooked cured meats. Among these are the raw materials themselves. If, for example, raw materials of poor microbiological quality are utilized, the shelf-life of the finished product will be correspondingly compromised. It is common practice in the meat industry to use "rework" product as a raw ingredient in cooked products. Such product may be generated "in plant." On the other hand, the USDA permits the use of over-age product returned from retail stores if it is not organoleptically spoiled. At least in part, rework consists of over-age product returned from retail sources. Such raw materials may have extremely high loads of microorganisms. A specific problem may relate to microorganisms that cause cured meat discoloration. Such organisms are generally lactic acid bacteria, which under aerobic conditions produce hydrogen peroxide. Some of these are extremely heat-resistant (Niven et al., 1954). A processor experiencing a problem with short shelf-life in his products will have an increasing amount of them returned from the trade and thus increasing amounts that he is tempted, for economic reasons, to rework. If heat-resistant, peroxide-producing lactic acid bacteria are present in the returned product, the use of rework may cause an increasing problem of spoilage that can only be solved through terminating rework as a raw material.

As mentioned previously, spices may on occasion constitute a critical raw material if they contain excessive numbers of aerobic sporeforming bacteria that survive normal heat processing. The heat process itself is a critical control point for these products. The number of survivors is directly related to the severity of the heat process except of course with respect to heat-resistant spores. These spores introduced by spices may lead to spoilage during heat processing of certain products such as large pieces of bologna. The number of survivors of a given heat process is also related to the initial number of organisms in the emulsion or other product being treated.

The sanitation of equipment for handling the cooked product (slicers, peelers, and conveyors) is also a critical control point. If such equipment, through insanitary practices, becomes a site of microbial growth, each product unit may become contaminated with spoilage organisms that reduce shelf-life. The processor must be certain that the processing environment is so controlled that this does not happen. Control is accomplished by microbiological analyses of equipment during the course of the operating day. Cleaning schedules are established upon the basis of such studies to break the cycle of microbiological development. Indeed, the USDA requires a processor to establish that a mid-shift cleanup is unnecessary in the plant. Proof is based upon data indicating that the processing equipment in the plant does not become a site of active microbial growth during the course of an operating shift. Critical control points in the manufacture of cooked cured meats include proper temperature control at all stages of processing, including the handling of raw material, the proper chilling of cooked product, the environment of the packaging operations, and the storage of packaged products. Prevention of cross-contamination and proper cold storage practices are also essential in retail stores, food service establishments, and homes.

Fermented Sausages

The initial steps in the production of domestic sausage are followed in the production of fermented sausage: the raw materials (meat trimmings that are ground, appropriate spices, sugar, and curing agents) are mixed and the emulsion is "stuffed" into natural or artificial casings. At this point, the processes diverge. Fermented sausages are held at a temperature of about 21 to 32°C (70 to 90°F) for 24 to 96 hours. During this period, under proper conditions, lactic acid bacteria develop and their growth results in fermentation of the sugar in the initial emulsion, the development of lactic acid, and a drop in pH to 5.3 or lower. Processors may depend upon the selective nature of the cured meat environment for lactic acid bacteria (natural fermentation) or may inoculate the product with commercially available cultures of lactic acid bacteria to ensure that fermentation occurs. Alternatively, glucono-delta-lactone may be added to the meat emulsion, the hydrolysis of which yields gluconic acid and a rapid decrease in pH. As an alternative to commercial cultures, many processors practice "back slopping," the addition of naturally fermented meat from a previous batch to the new emulsion to provide fermentative organisms. In all procedures the 24- to 96-hour hold in the "green room" at temperatures around 21 to 32°C (70 to 90°F) should, under proper conditions, produce a fermented meat emulsion with a pH of 5.3 or lower. If the product is then subjected to a mild heat process, usually including smoke, a semidry product results. If the emulsion contains pork, the product must be processed to a minimum of 58.3°C (137°F). If it does not contain pork, the degree of processing is then selected by the manufacturer. The finished semidry sausage, e.g., Lebanon bologna, Thuringer, Summer sausage, has a relatively long shelf-life due to the increased acidity produced by fermentation. Experience teaches that these products can be safely merchandised at ambient temperatures, though most of them are merchandised under refrigerated conditions as either sliced or unsliced products.

If, after fermentation in the "green room" the product is held in a "dry room," a room maintained at low humidity with proper air flow, a dry sausage is produced. The product is held in the dry room for an extended period of time varying from several weeks to months, depending upon the volume of the sausage pieces. During this period, the low humidity and air movement in the room result in loss of moisture from the product. Secondary fermentations occur and nuances of flavor develop. Moisture loss results in concentration of salt in the moisture phase of the product. If the product contains pork, the length of time in the dry room is closely regulated by the USDA in order to assure that any trichinellae present in pork ingredients will be destroyed by low water activity. The resulting dry sausage, e.g., dry salami, Genoa, is stable at ambient temperatures and may be merchandized without refrigeration.

Both semidry and dry sausage products are relatively resistant to microbial spoilage. The exteriors of unsliced products may support the growth of mold, but such mold growth has generally been accepted by the consumer as a characteristic of the product. Its occurrence has not been associated with foodborne illness.

The health hazard presented by fermented sausages relates primarily to improper fermentation, in which case the growth of staphylococci with attendant enterotoxin formation may pose a health hazard (Barber and Deibel, 1972). The American Meat Institute has recently formulated Good Manufacturing Procedures in connection with the production of fermented sausages (AMI, 1982). The key factor is rapid acid production, which prevents the development of enterotoxigenic staphylococci. The survival and/or growth of salmonellae in these products is likewise a potential problem. Salmonellae are relatively salt-tolerant.

As indicated above, fermented sausages are resistant to microbial spoilage, except for the surface growth of molds. The foodborne disease hazard relates primarily to the growth of enterotoxin-producing staphylococci where prompt fermentation and pH reduction do not occur. The critical control point is the fermentation itself, and the American Meat Institute has provided leadership by indicating methods for monitoring. Proper control of humidity and air movement in the drying room is likewise a critical control point, as this relates to proper drying, which in turn is directly related to control of the hazard of trichinellosis. This is under control of the USDA, and trichinellosis traced to these products is not a serious problem in the United States.

Canned Uncured Meat

Products in this category include low-acid canned foods (roast beef and gravy, beef stew, chili con carne, and tamales) and acid canned foods (Sloppy Joe and spaghetti with meat sauce). The classification of a given canned meat depends upon the equilibrated pH at the time of retorting. If the pH is 4.6 or below, the food is classified as an acid canned product and need only be processed to an extent assuring stability. If the final pH of the product is above 4.6, it is classified as a low-acid canned food and must be heat processed to assure freedom from *C. botulinum* (see parts J and K in this chapter). In this regard, canned meat products are no different from other canned foods and require no additional discussion in this section.

Shelf-Stable Canned Cured Meats

Shelf-stable canned cured meats include (1) canned viennas, corned beef, frankfurters, and meat spreads—all of which receive a botulinal cook or greater; (2) canned luncheon meat and canned hams that are given less than a botulinal cook; (3) canned sausages with hot oil in the final container and a water activity of <0.92, and sliced dried beef in vacuum-sealed jars and canned prefried bacon that rely upon a water activity of <0.86 for stability; and (4) vinegar pickled meats such as sausages and pig's feet (Johnston and Tompkin, 1984).

Products in category (1) are treated as low-acid canned foods (see canned foods sections of this chapter). Those in category (2) are limited to 3 lbs or less. They receive significantly less than a botulinal cook. Empirically a heat process equivalent to $F_o = 0.1$ to 0.7 has been found to produce a shelf-stable product. This stability is dependent upon the presence of nitrite, salt, a low indigenous level of *C. botulinum* in meat, and a thermal process that injures surviving spores such that they are incapable of growth in the cured meat environment.

Canned sausages, sliced dried beef, and prefried bacon (category 3) do not undergo spoilage unless their water activity is higher than prescribed or the vacuum seal is broken. Theoretically, it may be possible for *S. aureus* to grow if the water activity exceeds 0.86, but this has not been observed in commercial practice. The inability of *S. aureus* to compete with other organisms developing in this environment is probably the major factor contributing to the absence of staphylococcal food poisoning.

Pickled pig's feet, pickled sausages, and similar items in category (4) are immersed in vinegar brine. Their stability may be traced to low pH combined with the presence of undissociated acetic acid, little or no fermentable sugar in the tissue, and/or an airtight package (Niven, 1956). None of these products has been a significant source of foodborne disease or microbial spoilage.

For spoilage problems relating to products in category (1) or those common to other low-acid canned foods receiving a botulinal cook, see Part J of this chapter. With respect to category (2), thermophilic spoilage can occur in products receiving a cook equivalent to $F_o = 0.1-0.7$, if the products are stored at an abnormally high temperature for a sufficient length of time. Furthermore, if inordinately high numbers of mesophilic sporeforming bacteria are present, mesophilic spoilage can occur. Faulty curing resulting in insufficient levels of salt or nitrite can also result in an unstable product. As with other low-acid canned foods, poor manufacturing practices can lead to product spoilage. As previously indicated, products in category (3) do not undergo microbial spoilage unless their water activity is higher than recommended.

Products in category (4) may contain moderate numbers of lactic acid bacteria and viable spores. Large numbers of lactic acid bacteria may develop and cause the brine to become cloudy (Niven, 1956). However, foodborne disease organisms do not survive. Hermetically sealed jars of pickled bone-in meat may develop gas and even explode from the action of the vinegar on bone. This spoilage is of nonmicrobial origin but may prove puzzling to microbiologists investigating this cause of spoilage.

Critical control points in the production of these products include: for category (1), those points essential to the production of low-acid canned foods; for category (2), the proper curing of the meat, the control of the level of aerobic and anaerobic sporeforming bacteria, and proper heat processing; for category (3), the proper control of water activity and of container integrity; for category (4), control of brine and acid content, temperature control during storage for prevention of growth of acid-tolerant bacteria with attendant gas production, and proper container integrity to prevent the growth of mold.

Perishable Canned Cured Meats

These products receive a heat process far less than that necessary for commercial sterility. They are merchandised under refrigeration with a label indicating that they are perishable. The major product in this category is perishable canned ham, which must achieve a minimum temperature of 65.6°C (150°F) during processing. A substantial quantity of canned perishable luncheon meat is also manufactured, primarily for distribution to food service establishments.

Thermoduric lactic acid bacteria and aerobic and anaerobic spores are the major survivors of the heat process. Lactic acid bacteria may grow extensively during extended refrigerated storage with or without evidence of spoilage. Sporeforming bacteria, which generally develop only with temperature abuse, present the chief health hazard. Canned cured perishable meats have enjoyed an excellent public health history.

Hams distributed as retail products are subject to the hazards of mishandling in food service establishments and homes. Contamination of the ham with *S. aureus* by persons during slicing or other improper handling followed by prolonged storage at ambient temperatures or storage of large masses in the refrigerator results in staphylococcal growth and enterotoxin formation.

A substantial quantity of these hams is merchandised as sliced and packaged items. In such cases the hams must be removed from the containers, sliced, and packaged. In this process, the cans are opened and the hams are unloaded onto tables that "feed" the slicing machine. Ham juices and gelatin are attached to the meat and unloaded onto the table. If the sanitation is not carefully controlled, substantial numbers of microorganisms, including those capable of spoilage, may develop on the "unloading table" feeding the slicer. Likewise, the slicing machine, if not maintained in a sanitary condition, is a key source of contamination to the sliced meat.

As indicated, perishable canned cured meats mishandled after cooking may be an important source of foodborne disease, particularly staphylococcal food poisoning. If these products are sliced and packaged at the packing plant, spoilage problems may result from inadequate sanitation of plant equipment.

Critical control points in the manufacturing process are analogous to those in the production of cooked cured meats. The table upon which perishable cured meats are unloaded prior to slicing constitutes a unique critical control point in the production of sliced items derived from perishable canned cured meats.

Dried Meats

Preservation of meat by drying predates recorded history. The combination of this application with salting likely evolved from the prehistoric observation that the meat could be protected from spoilage during drying if it were salted. The following discussion is concerned with meat that is dried without the addition of salt, i.e., where microbial growth is inhibited by reduced water activity achieved simply by the removal of water (ICMSF, 1980).

Substantial quantities of meat are dried commercially, primarily for use in formulated foods, e.g., soup mixes and dried pasta with meat. Two approaches to drying are employed. In the first, meat is defatted, and the lean meat is cooked and minced, spread in thin layers, and dried under controlled ventilation in hot air tunnels. The air-dried product consists of granules of 5 to 10 mm in diameter and has a water content of less than 15%. The meat pieces must be small and must be separated to ensure thorough drying in one to two hours. In the second process, cooked or uncooked meat is freeze-dried. Pieces as large as chops or steaks can be dried, and hence this process has a wider range of uses than has the air-dried, cooked, mince process. During freeze-drying, microbiological problems are minimized by subzero temperatures that are maintained until the water content is reduced to a level at which microbial growth is impossible.

The key to stability and safety of dried meat products lies in water relations. If dried meat is stored at high humidity, water uptake may occur and this may permit the growth of xerophilic molds. Growth of these molds alters the appearance of the meat and may cause musty odors and/ or off-flavors.

The following pathogenic microorganisms may be important for dried meats: (1) Clostridia, *Salmonella,* and other *Enterobacteriaceae* may be introduced by contamination associated with meat; and (2) staphylococci and *B. cereus* may be introduced by contamination during preparation and drying. The most dangerous circumstances arise when water is added to rehydrate dried meat. The rehydrated product is an excellent substrate for microbial growth if it is held in a temperature range permitting such development.

The critical control points in the production of dried meat include the use of meat of suitable microbiological quality, control of contamination during preparation and transport to the dryer, strict control of time/temperature relations during drying, the avoidance of wet spots in the drying mass, drying to a sufficiently low moisture content, protection by suitable packaging of the dried product from reabsorption of moisture, and proper time-temperature control after rehydration to minimize possibilities of microbial multiplication.

Need for Microbiological Criteria

Raw Ground Beef

Microbiological criteria can be usefully applied to assess the microbiological quality of the raw materials used, the effectiveness of equipment sanitation, and the microbiological quality of finished product. The results obtained through the use of such criteria at the processing level are retrospective but serve as a useful guide to the processor. The application of microbiological criteria to the product after it has entered trade channels is without value, even though standards and guidelines have been promulgated by a number of states and municipalities.

Perishable Raw Salted and Salted Cured Meats

The considerations discussed in the preceding paragraph apply equally to the perishable meat products in this category.

Shelf-Stable Raw Salted and Salted Cured Meats

Microbiological criteria have little value in connection with the production of these products, except perhaps in the evaluation of the microbiological condition of raw materials. The application of microbiological criteria to the finished product would be without value. Microbiological control during processing is best exercised over critical control points identified previously, particularly the control of temperature during the curing process and the control of humidity during the postcuring, drying period.

Cooked Uncured Meats

As previously indicated, one product in this category (roast beef) has been a significant vehicle of human salmonellosis in recent years. It appears that this problem has now been brought under control. Regulation of processing as well as education of processors have played key roles. In addition, microbiological monitoring by processors and the microbiological surveillance program of the USDA have proven to be essential to assuring the safety of these products before their release for sale. The continued application of microbiological criteria to precooked roast beef and similar products is indicated.

Cooked Cured Meats

Microbiological criteria can appropriately be used to evaluate the microbiological quality of raw materials, though the results are of retrospective value with respect to the lot produced from them. Similarly, microbiological criteria can usefully be applied in the evaluation of equipment sanitation, particularly at critical control points such as slicers, conveyors, and casing peelers. Microbiological criteria can effectively be applied in the determination of the microbiological quality of finished products. The results of such tests should confirm the effectiveness of the control over critical control points. For example, a sliced product with a significantly higher APC than the unsliced product is an indication of failure to adequately clean and sanitize equipment and/or the use of processing equipment for too long a period before cleanup. High counts on the surface of such products as frankfurters have similar implications, since surface counts should be negligible. The application of microbiological criteria, including purchase specifications to nonmeat ingredients (in particular, spices), may be appropriate for some products. Cooked cured meats have not proven to be a *Salmonella* hazard. The application of microbiological criteria to these products after they have entered retail channels is inappropriate, despite the fact that many states and municipalities have promulgated standards and guidelines.

Fermented Sausages

Microbiological criteria may be useful in the qualitative and/or quantitative evaluation of starter culture activity (see Chapter 5). Such a criterion might be a part of a purchase specification. The primary microbiological hazard is growth and enterotoxin formation by *S. aureus* (Barber and Deibel, 1972). To monitor this hazard, the outer 3-mm layer of the individual sausage may be sampled for viable *S. aureus* at the end of the fermentation cycle before the product is heated and/or dried. Since *S. aureus* death may have occurred in products ready for consumption, it may be necessary to test the casing or outer 4-mm of meat for thermonuclease and/or enterotoxin (Johnston and Tompkin, 1984). These microbiological criteria are best applied at the processing plant. Presence of *Staphylococcus* enterotoxin should not be tolerated. The product at any point in the distribution should be recalled if there is evidence of the presence of enterotoxin. Other microbiological criteria are not warranted.

Canned Uncured Meats

Both low-acid and acid products in this category are discussed in parts J and K of this chapter.

Shelf-Stable Canned Cured Meats

Included in this category are products that receive a "botulinal cook," namely, canned viennas, corned beef, etc. Such products are discussed in the section on canned foods as are luncheon meats and small canned hams that receive less than a "botulinal cook." Products whose stability is related to reduced water activity are also included, i.e., canned sausage and sliced beef (a_w < 0.92) and canned prefried bacon (a_w < 0.86). Microbiological control is best accomplished through monitoring water activity rather than through the use of microbiological criteria. Finally, the routine application of microbiological criteria to vinegar pickled meats seems unnecessary, though spoilage problems, both microbial and nonmicrobial, may occasionally occur.

Perishable Canned Cured Meats

Microbiological criteria are not generally applicable to these products. However, if there is reason to believe that a consignment may have been subjected to temperature abuse, investigative sampling may be indicated (see ICMSF, 1974).

Dried Meats

Microbiological criteria may appropriately be applied to the finished product as a means of assessing the adequacy of moisture control during the drying process. The APC with proper baseline data may be effective in this monitoring. Tests for pathogens such as *C. perfringens, B. cereus, S. aureus,* and *Salmonella* may be appropriately applied, depending upon the ultimate use of the product. Such monitoring is best carried out at the processing level, though regulatory authorities may apply criteria at any point in merchandising channels. A *Salmonella* standard is applicable to these products.

Assessment of Information Necessary for Establishment of a Criterion if One Seems To Be Indicated

These considerations have been largely addressed in sections above. With respect to criteria utilized to assess the microbiological status of various raw materials, e.g., meat trimmings or the adequacy of equipment cleanup, baseline information must be established by the processor. Only on the basis of such information can useful limits be established.

Where Criteria Should Be Applied

See sections on sensitivity of products relative to safety and quality and on need for microbiological criteria.

References

AMI (American Meat Institute)
1982 Good Manufacturing Practices. I. Voluntary Guidelines for the Production of Dry Fermented Sausage; II. Voluntary Guidelines for the Production of Semi-dry Fermented Sausage. Washington, D.C.: American Meat Institute.

Bailey, J. W.
1974 Encyclopaedia of labeling meat and poultry products. St. Louis: Meat Plant Magazine.

Barber, J. E., and R. H. Deibel
1972 Effect of pH and oxygen tension on staphylococcal growth and enterotoxin formation in fermented sausage. Appl. Microbiol. 24:891–898.

Bryan, F. L.
1980 Foodborne diseases in the United States associated with meat and poultry. J. Food Prot. 43:140–150.

CDC (Centers for Disease Control)
1960 Botulism. Morb. Mort. Weekly Rpt. 9:2.
1976a *Salmonella Saint-Paul* in precooked roasts of beef—New Jersey. Morb. Mort. Weekly Rpt. 25(5):34, 39.
1976b *Salmonella bovis-morbificans* in precooked roasts of beef. Morb. Mort. Weekly Rpt. 25(42):333–334.
1977a Multistate outbreak of *Salmonella newport* transmitted by precooked roasts of beef. Morb. Mort. Weekly Rpt. 26(34)277–278.
1977b Follow-up on *Salmonella* organisms in precooked roast beef. Morb. Mort. Weekly Rpt. 26(38):310.
1978 Salmonellae in precooked roasts of beef—New York. Morb. Mort. Weekly Rpt. 27(24):315.
1981a Multistate outbreak of salmonellosis caused by precooked roast beef. Morb. Mort. Weekly Rpt. 30:391–392.
1981b Multiple outbreaks of salmonellosis associated with precooked roast beef—Pennsylvania, New York, Vermont. Morb. Mort. Weekly Rpt. 30:569–570.
1982 Isolation of *E. coli* 0157:H7 from sporadic cases of hemorrhagic colitis—United States. Morb. Mort. Weekly Rpt. 31:580, 585.
1983 Botulism and commercial pot pie—California. Morb. Mort. Weekly Rpt. 32:39–40, 45.

Fontaine, R. E., S. Arnon, W. T. Martin, T. M. Vernon, E. J. Gangarosa, J. J. Farmer, A. B. Moran, J. H. Silliker, and D. L. Decker
1978 Raw hamburger: An interstate common source of human salmonellosis. Am. J. Epidemiol. 107:36–45.

Gardner, G. A.
1981 *Brochothrix thermosphacta (Microbacterium thermosphactum)* in the spoilage of meats. A review. Pp. 139–173 in Psychrotrophic Microorganisms in Spoilage and Pathogenicity, T. A. Roberts, G. Hobbs, J.H.B. Christian, and N. Skovgaard, eds. New York: Academic Press.

Goodfellow, S. J., and W. L. Brown
1978 Fate of *Salmonella* inoculated into beef for cooking. J. Food Prot. 41:598–605.

Greenberg, R. A., and J. H. Silliker
1961 Evidence for thermal injury in enterococci. J. Food Sci. 26:622–625.

ICMSF (International Commission on Microbiological Specifications for Foods)
1974 Microorganisms in Foods. 2. Sampling for microbiological analysis: Principles and specific applications. Toronto: University of Toronto Press. Pp. 143–146.

1980   Microbial Ecology of Foods. Volume 2. Food Commodities. New York: Academic Press. Pp. 378–383.

Johnston, R. W., and R. B. Tompkin
1984   Meat and meat products. In Compendium of Methods for the Microbiological Examination of Foods. 2nd Ed. M. L. Speck, ed. Washington, D.C.: American Public Health Association.

Mundt, J. O., and H. M. Kitchen
1951   Taint in southern country-style hams. Food Res. 16:233–238.

Niven, C. F.
1956   Vinegar pickled meats. A discussion of bacterial and curing problems encountered in processing. Bulletin No. 27. Chicago: American Meat Institute Foundation.

Niven, C. F., L. G. Bultner, and J. B. Evans
1954   Thermal tolerance studies on the heterofermentative lactobacilli that cause greening of cured meat products. Appl. Microbiol. 2:26.

NRC (National Research Council)
1964   An Evaluation of Public Health Hazards from Microbiological Contamination of Foods. Publication No. 1195. Washington, D.C.: National Academy of Sciences.

State of California (Department of Health Services)
1975   Botulism—home canned figs and chicken pot pie. Calif. Morbidity No. 46.
1976   Type A botulism associated with commercial pot pie. Calif. Morbidity No. 51.

USDA (U.S. Department of Agriculture)
1983   Production requirements for cooked beef, roast beef and cooked corned beef. Federal Register 48 (106):24314–24318.

D.   RAW (EVISCERATED, READY-TO-COOK) POULTRY

Sensitivity of Products Relative to Safety and Quality

The poultry industry is one of the most integrated food industries in the United States. A single organization may control an entire operation including breeder farm, hatchery, grow-out farm, processing, and retail operations. Fertile eggs from breeder farms are delivered to hatcheries where the eggs are incubated and then placed in hatchers. After hatching, chicks or poults are delivered to grow-out farms, reared until ready for slaughter, and then transported to processing plants.

The microbiological condition of eviscerated, ready-to-cook poultry (chickens, turkeys, ducks, and quail) is the result of a series of conditions and events (ICMSF, 1980) including:

1. conditions at the breeding farm and hatchery
2. health of the live animal
3. feed supply
4. environmental conditions under which the flock was raised (cross-contamination by man, rodents, wild birds, litter, drinking water)
5. transportation
6. scalding

 7. picking (defeathering)
 8. washing
 9. evisceration (opening of body cavity, viscera pull, inspection, viscera removal)
10. chilling
11. packaging
12. sanitary practices and conditions in the processing plant (involving workers, equipment, utensils)
13. storage (time-temperature profile)
14. thawing, storage, and handling practices in retail stores and kitchens

Microbial contamination of the egg can occur in the ovaries during the development of the egg or later as a result of penetration of the egg shell. Fumigation at the breeder farm is generally practiced to control microbial penetration of eggs. Breeding flocks are tested for the presence of *Salmonella* by blood agglutination tests and subsequent culturing of internal organs. The National Poultry Improvement Plan (USDA, 1982) is the most recognized plan charged with the elimination of *Salmonella pullorum* and *Salmonella gallinarum* from breeder flocks. Chicks or poults on hatching contain an extensive microbial flora.

Microorganisms associated with live poultry are located primarily on the surface of the bird (skin, feet, feathers) and in the gastro-intestinal tract. The numbers and types depend largely on the environmental conditions under which the flock was raised. This population nearly always includes a large variety of microbial types such as *Pseudomonas*, *Moraxella*, *Acinetobacter*, *Micrococcus*, *Enterobacteriaceae*, *Staphylococcus*, *Bacillus*, *Clostridium*, *Flavobacterium*, molds, and yeasts. Soil, litter, feed, and drinking water are primary sources of these microbes. Other reservoirs include insects, rodents, wild birds, and farm workers. These sources contribute not only saprophytic species but may infect or contaminate birds with pathogens such as *Salmonella*, *Yersinia*, and *Campylobacter*. During transportation to processing plants, the incidence of contamination increases because of further distribution of microorganisms from bird to bird primarily through contact with fecal material.

During the overall processing operation in modern broiler or turkey processing plants a significant reduction (90-95%) in total bacterial numbers can be achieved by the scalding, washing, and chilling operations (Gardner and Golan, 1976). In the first, microbial destruction is effected by heat; in the latter two operations, reduction is achieved by the rinsing effect (mechanical removal) of the spray or wash. Bacterial numbers on the carcass may increase during evisceration because of extensive manual handling. This is particularly so for turkey carcasses because of handling associated with carcass trussing, draining, and packaging. Post-chill operations in broiler processing, however, are largely automated.

Microbial contamination of carcasses during processing should be kept to a minimum by employing sanitary handling procedures, proper cleaning and sanitation of equipment and utensils that come in contact with carcasses, and use of adequate quantities of rinse and chill waters.

Microorganisms on freshly processed carcasses are located primarily on the surface, normally at a level of 10^3 to 10^4 per cm^2. They constitute a variety of species including psychrotrophic bacteria and originate from various sources such as the incoming bird (feet, feathers, intestinal tract), water, ice, and air, and are spread from carcass to carcass by processing equipment, utensils, and line workers.

The shelf-life of freshly processed carcasses depends on the number and types of microorganisms present, the time and temperature of storage, and the method of packaging. Shelf-life will be short when initial numbers of psychrotrophic spoilage bacteria are high, particularly when the carcasses are stored at marginal (above 1.7°C/35°F) refrigeration temperatures. When counts of psychrotrophic gram-negative bacteria such as *Pseudomonas*, *Moraxella-Acinetobacter*, and *Flavobacterium* on chilled poultry reach 10^7-10^8 per cm^2, off-odors often followed by slime formation occur. When carcasses are stored refrigerated in vacuum-packages or in modified gaseous atmospheres containing CO_2, lactic acid bacteria usually become predominant. Both of these packaging procedures significantly increase the shelf-life of raw poultry compared to that observed when oxygen-permeable films are used. In vacuum packages and in modified atmospheres containing elevated levels of CO_2, gram-negative aerobic psychrotrophic bacteria are inhibited. Although large numbers of psychrotrophic lactic acid bacteria develop during refrigerated storage, sensory degradation of the product is not as rapid as is observed when gram-negative aerobic psychrotrophic bacteria predominate.

Subsequent handling of carcasses in food service establishments or in homes can spread microorganisms, including pathogens, that may be associated with the carcass to the cooked product or to other foods through contact with knives, tables, cutting boards, and cleaning cloths. Thawing frozen turkeys and then leaving them under conditions that allow microbial growth may lead to increases in bacterial count on the carcass. Proper thawing should be done under refrigeration or in cold running water.

Eviscerated, ready-to-cook poultry carcasses often contain small numbers of pathogens such as *Salmonella*, *Staphylococcus aureus*, *Clostridium perfringens*, *Campylobacter fetus* subsp. *jejuni*, and *Yersinia enterocolitica*. These organisms enter processing plants with live birds and are spread to carcass surfaces during processing. At the present time there are no

commercially applicable methods employed in the United States to eliminate pathogens from carcasses, although ionizing radiation could accomplish this. Good sanitary processing practices, however, can reduce the
prevalence and extent of spread of pathogens in a processing plant. The
presence of pathogens on ready-to-cook carcasses can lead to health hazards if the product is mishandled in a plant, food service establishment,
or in the home (Bryan, 1980; Bryan and McKinley, 1974). These faulty
practices include:

1. inadequate cooking of poultry resulting in survival of pathogens such
   as *Salmonella*, *C. fetus* subsp. *jejuni*, *Y. enterocolitica*, and *S. aureus*
   (spores of *C. perfringens* may survive adequate cooking);
2. transfer of pathogens from the raw carcass via hands, cleaning cloths,
   equipment, and utensils to cooked poultry or to foods that will not
   receive further heat treatment;
3. temperature abuse of adequately cooked poultry containing surviving
   spores of *C. perfringens* or of inadequately cooked poultry containing *Salmonella* or other pathogens (this could involve improper cooling, hot-holding, and reheating);
4. time-temperature abuse of cooked poultry subsequently sliced or
   chopped and recontaminated with *S. aureus* or of salads in which
   this recontaminated poultry is used as an ingredient.

Poultry products so abused have been identified as vehicles in outbreaks
of foodborne disease. From 1968-1977, poultry was responsible for 14%
of foodborne disease outbreaks in which a vehicle was ascertained (Bryan,
1980). Salmonellosis accounted for 19% of these outbreaks, staphylococcal intoxication for 16%, *C. perfringens* enteritis for 10%, other foodborne diseases of known etiology for 2%, and diseases of unknown etiology
for 53%. In summary, cooked poultry products may become a hazard
when raw or cooked products are mishandled.

Need for Microbiological Criteria

Salmonella

The proportion of *Salmonella*-contaminated carcasses from a processing
plant is determined mainly by the incidence of infected or contaminated
live birds and by the extent of subsequent spread during processing (Bryan
et al., 1968a; ICMSF, 1980). Unfortunately, even with the best manufacturing practices, cross-contamination occurs during slaughtering, dressing, and further processing (Bryan et al., 1968a,b). Recommendations to
reduce or eradicate *Salmonella* in animals including poultry have been
discussed in various reports (NRC, 1969; Silliker, 1982). These include:

1. use of *Salmonella*-free feed
2. control of *Salmonella* in breeder flocks, hatchery, and production operations
3. application of the Nurmi concept
4. irradiation of packaged raw poultry
5. education of farm workers, processing plant workers, food service personnel, and homemakers

Salmonella-contaminated feeds remain a major source of *Salmonella* in poultry (NRC, 1969; GAO, 1974). Infected breeding stock can spread *Salmonella* to other farms. The spread of *Salmonella agona* and *Salmonella hadar* in the United States and in England is part of the epidemiological evidence for the involvement of these sources (Clark et al., 1973; Rowe, 1980). Until feeds are decontaminated by heating, irradiation, or chemical means they will continue to be a major source of *Salmonella*.

The Nurmi concept (Pivnick et al., 1981; Stersky et al., 1981) involves oral administration of the gastrointestinal flora from adult birds into newly hatched chicks and poults. Newly hatched birds may be infected by a single *Salmonella*; however, immediately after introduction of gastrointestinal flora from adult birds, chicks become resistant to between 1,000 and 1,000,000 infectious doses of *Salmonella*. The term "competitive exclusion" has been used to describe this phenomenon. Colonization of the intestinal tract with normal gut flora apparently discourages colonization with *Salmonella*. Two important factors may be involved: (1) production of volatile fatty acids in the caecum and (2) occupation of sites on the mucosa that *Salmonella* normally invade. Recently, inocula derived from pure cultures isolated from the feces of adult birds have shown the protective effect achieved through the use of fecal material or mixed cultures derived from feces (H. Pivnick, 1983. Personal communication). The use of defined pure cultures, instead of fecal material or mixed cultures, may lead to a more widespread application of the Nurmi concept.

Irradiation of poultry with a dosage of up to 0.7 Mrad is effective in eliminating pathogens, especially *Salmonella* (Kampelmacher, 1983). The World Health Organization (WHO) has cleared irradiation of foods with up to 0.7 Mrad and declared these foods unconditionally safe for human consumption (FAO/IAEA/WHO, 1977). In the Netherlands, Canada, and the USSR, clearance has been given for test marketing of chilled and frozen poultry irradiated with dosages of 0.3, 0.75, and 0.6 Mrad, respectively (Vas, 1977).

Government, industry, and educational institutions have made sporadic attempts to educate the public about foodborne illness including salmonellosis. A Gallup study (Anonymous, 1979) has shown that these efforts have been ineffective. Educational efforts such as those in Denmark and

Canada that are directed to the young homemaker perhaps may be more successful.

Until changes are made to minimize the infection and contamination of birds on the farm and/or until a method of decontamination is routinely applied to packaged carcasses, it is questionable whether practical microbiological criteria can be set for *Salmonella* on raw poultry without risk of eliminating poultry as food. A working group of the Codex Committee on Food Hygiene (FAO/WHO, 1979) concluded that application of microbiological criteria for raw poultry would not improve safety. Nevertheless, concern must be maintained about *Salmonella* being brought into home kitchens, hospitals, and food service establishments on raw poultry, and being spread via hands, equipment utensils, and cleaning cloths back to either the cooked poultry or other foods. Extensive and continuous efforts should be made to educate the food service industry and public about the contamination potential associated with the handling of raw poultry, to inform them of the need to cook poultry to temperatures that kill *Salmonella*, to hold cooked poultry at temperatures that preclude multiplication of these organisms, and to reheat leftovers thoroughly.

Campylobacter fetus subsp. jejuni and Yersinia enterocolitica

Much of what has been said about *Salmonella* on raw poultry is applicable to *C. fetus* subsp. *jejuni* and *Y. enterocolitica* because these organisms also are frequently present on raw poultry products. Poultry-associated outbreaks of *Campylobacter* infection have been reported in recent years (Cunningham, 1982). Prevention depends on thorough cooking and proper storage of cooked products rather than on microbiological criteria for raw poultry products.

Clostridium perfringens

C. perfringens is a part of the intestinal flora of fowl and is shed in their feces. Furthermore, it is found in soil, dust, or feces that get on their skin, feet, and feathers. Thus, it is impractical at this time to eliminate *C. perfringens* from live fowl. Even strict adherence to Good Manufacturing Practices cannot prevent some contamination of poultry carcasses with *C. perfringens*. Microbiological criteria for *C. perfringens* for raw poultry would not accomplish anything because it only becomes a problem when cooked poultry (in which the spores have become heat activated and the redox potential is reduced) is held at sufficiently high temperatures for spores to germinate and the resulting cells to multiply to large numbers.

Staphylococcus aureus

S. aureus is part of the nasopharynx and skin flora of poultry and is sometimes associated with arthritic and bruised tissue. Staphylococci from these sources are readily spread during defeathering. Therefore, some contamination of raw poultry carcasses with *S. aureus* can be expected. These organisms neither compete well with the microbial flora on raw carcasses nor multiply on chilled carcasses. A microbiological criterion for *S. aureus* on raw poultry meat is impractical because the foodborne disease problem arises when cooked poultry (frequently leftovers) is contaminated with *S. aureus* by persons who handle it and then subjected to room-temperature storage or improper refrigeration.

Other Bacteria

Microbiological criteria involving aerobic plate counts (APCs) and indicator organisms have limited application for eviscerated ready-to-cook poultry carcasses. Microbiological guidelines for psychrotrophic aerobic bacteria and indicator bacteria such as coliforms on carcasses immediately post-processing may be useful to indicate that a sanitation problem exists somewhere along the processing line. Counts in excess of those normally found should alert the processor to inspect critical control points more closely to locate and remedy the problem. With proper sanitary practices along the processing line, control of fecal contamination of carcasses and washing of carcasses, coliform contamination on the freshly processed carcasses can be limited (Gardner and Golan, 1976). These guidelines, however, are not applicable to poultry in distribution channels or at the retail level as suggested by some state standards or guidelines. This is so because aerobic, psychrotrophic bacteria responsible for quality loss and ultimate spoilage of refrigerated raw poultry (packaged in oxygen-permeable film) continue to multiply on carcasses even at recommended cold storage temperatures. Microbiological guidelines are, however, applicable to monitor the sanitary condition of equipment and utensils.

Assessment of Information Necessary for Establishment of a Criterion if One Seems To Be Indicated

Adequate data base is available (ICMSF, 1974, 1980, 1985; APHA, 1976, 1984) to guide processors in establishing and interpreting microbiological guidelines that they may wish to apply.

Where Criteria Should Be Applied

A HACCP program should be applied to the entire poultry production, processing, distribution, and food preparation chain. Critical control points at the farm include sanitary condition of feed, drinking water, equipment, and surroundings in which the birds are raised, and control of microbial contamination by farm workers, insects, rodents, and wild birds. Although each of these control measures can affect the general microbial population, the principal focus should be on reducing the incidence of pathogens, primarily *Salmonella* and *Campylobacter*.

Critical control points to be monitored at the processing plant (eviscerated ready-to-cook carcasses only) should include (1) carcass washing, cooling, and storage procedures, which include amount of water, degree of chlorination and temperature of water, and temperature of storage; (2) cleaning and sanitation of equipment; and (3) employee sanitary practices during processing. Microbiological guidelines should be applicable to: (1) periodic evaluation of equipment surfaces to check cleaning and sanitizing procedures and to check on potential buildup of microbial contaminants, and (2) examination [APC at 20-25°C (68-77°F) for 2-3 days and coliforms] of freshly processed carcasses. Excessive counts should alert the processor to check the product at various stages of processing to pinpoint the problem. Reduction of the number of birds infected with *Salmonella* perhaps will be possible sometime in the future by application of several measures such as use of *Salmonella*-free feed, application of the Nurmi concept, and irradiation of packaged raw poultry.

References

Anonymous
  1979   Report on the Scandinavian Salmonella control programs in poultry with added observations from Finland, Germany and Switzerland. Health/Agriculture/Industry Committee on *Salmonella*, Ottawa, Canada.
APHA (American Public Health Association)
  1976   Compendium of Methods for the Microbiological Examination of Foods. M. L. Speck, ed. Washington, D.C.: APHA.
  1984   Compendium of Methods for the Microbiological Examination of Foods. 2nd Ed. M. L. Speck, ed. Washington, D.C.: APHA.
Bryan, F. L.
  1980   Foodborne diseases in the United States associated with meat and poultry. J. Food Prot. 43:140–150.
Bryan, F. L., and T. W. McKinley
  1974   Prevention of foodborne illness by time-temperature control of thawing, cooking, chilling and reheating turkeys in school lunch kitchens. J. Milk Food Technol. 37:420–429.

Bryan, F. L., J. C. Ayres, and A. A. Kraft
  1968a Contributory sources of salmonellae on turkey products. Am. J. Epidemiol. 87:578–591.
  1968b Salmonellae associated with further-processed turkey products. Appl. Microbiol. 16:1–9.
Clark, G. M., A. F. Kaufman, E. J. Gangarosa, and M. A. Thompson
  1973 Epidemiology of an international outbreak of *Salmonella agona*. Lancet ii:490–493.
Cunningham, F. E.
  1982 Microbiological aspects of poultry and poultry products—An update. J. Food Prot. 45:1149–1164.
FAO/IAEA/WHO
  1977 Wholesomeness of irradiated food. Report of a joint FAO/IAEA/WHO Expert Committee. WHO Techn. Rep. Ser. 604.
FAO/WHO (Food and Agriculture Organization/World Health Organization)
  1979 Report of an FAO/WHO working group on Microbiological Criteria for Foods. Geneva: FAO/WHO.
GAO (U.S. General Accounting Office)
  1974 Report to the Congress, *Salmonella* in raw meat and poultry: An assessment of the problem [B-164031 (2), July 22, 1974]. Washington, D.C.: U.S. General Accounting Office.
Gardner, F. A., and F. A. Golan
  1976 Water usage in poultry processing—An effective mechanism for bacterial reduction. Pp. 338–355 in Proc. 7th Natl. Symposium on Food Processing Wastes, Atlanta, GA. Cincinnati: U.S. Envir. Prot. Agency.
ICMSF (International Commission on Microbiological Specifications for Foods)
  1974 Microorganisms in Foods. 2. Sampling for microbiological analysis: Principles and specific applications. Toronto: University of Toronto Press.
  1980 Microbial Ecology of Foods. Vol. 2. Food Commodities. New York: Academic Press.
  1985 Microorganisms in Foods. 2. Sampling for microbiological analysis: Principles and specific applications, 2nd Ed. In preparation.
Kampelmacher, E. H.
  1983 Irradiation for control of *Salmonella* and other pathogens in poultry and fresh meats. Food Technol. 37(4):117–119, 169.
NRC (National Research Council)
  1969 An evaluation of the *Salmonella* problem. Committee on *Salmonella*. Washington, D.C.: National Academy of Sciences.
Pivnick, H., B. Blanchfield, and J.-Y. D'Aoust
  1981 Prevention of *Salmonella* infections in chicks by treatment with fecal cultures from mature chickens (Nurmi Cultures). J. Food Prot. 44:909–916.
Rowe, B.
  1980 *Salmonella hadar*—England and Wales. Morb. Mort. Weekly Rpt. 29:506–508, 513.
Silliker, J. H.
  1982 The *Salmonella* problem: Current status and future direction. J. Food Prot. 45:661–666.
Stersky, A., B. Blanchfield, C. Thacker, and H. Pivnick
  1981 Reduction of *Salmonella* excretion into drinking water following treatment of chicks with Nurmi culture. J. Food Prot. 44:917–920.
USDA (U.S. Department of Agriculture)
  1982 National Poultry Improvement Plan and Auxiliary Provisions. APHIS-Veterinary Services, APHIS 91-40.

Vas, K.
1977   General survey of irradiated food products cleared for human consumption in different countries. Joint FAO/IAEA/ WHO advisory group on international acceptance of irradiated food. GA-143/INF/2-IAEA, Vienna.

E. PROCESSED POULTRY PRODUCTS

Sensitivity of Products Relative to Safety and Quality

The term "further-processed poultry product" refers to any product beyond the ready-to-cook carcass, frozen or nonfrozen. Further-processed poultry products comprise a significant part of poultry marketed in the United States. In 1982, about 60% of the 16.8 billion pounds of broilers produced in the United States were in the form of cut-up parts and other further-processed products, and of the 2.5 billion pounds of turkey consumed, about 90% was in the form of further-processed products (USDA, 1983). Examples of these further-processed products are:

Broilers: Noncooked—tray pack (chilled or frozen)
          Cooked—wieners, bologna

Turkeys: Noncooked—tray-pack, tenderloin, roasts, further-processed whole birds (injected,basted)
          Cooked—boneless breast, cured smoked breast, hams, rolls, roasts, bologna, salami, pastrami, wieners

The microbiological condition of further-processed products and hence shelf-life and safety depends upon a series of conditions and events including:

1. *Microbiological condition of the carcass entering further processing*
          concern: numbers and types of microorganisms, particularly psychrotrophic bacteria and *Salmonella*
2. *Processing procedures*
    a. *parts removal*—removal of drum, wings, tail, and neck
       concern: sanitary handling
    b. *hand deboning*—removal of breast tissue and thigh tissue from carcass
       concern: sanitary handling
    c. *mechanical deboning*—grinding of racks and other bones followed by deboning
       concerns: sanitary condition of equipment, extensive increase in surface area of tissue, temperature increase of tissue at separation, handling of mechanically deboned poultry meat (MDPM): rate of cooling, time-temperature profile during storage

d. *trim operation*—trimming of major muscles, breast, and thigh
concerns: sanitary handling, continuity of product flow

e. *blending*—mixing of different tissues (dark, light, trim meat), seasonings and additives (salt, sugar, phosphates, erythorbate, sodium nitrite)
concerns: sanitary condition of equipment, microbial condition of additives, time-temperature profile of product, use schedule of equipment (continuity of product flow)

f. *emulsification*—emulsification of tissue fractions
concerns: sanitary condition of equipment, time-temperature profile of product (heat generation), increase in tissue surface area, use schedule of equipment (continuity of product flow)

g. *stuffing*—placing product in casing such as for wieners, bologna, salami, pastrami, rolls, roasts
concerns: sanitary condition of equipment, time-temperature profile of product (time between stuffing and cooking)

h. *product formation (forming)*—to provide shape to a product (for example, boneless turkey breast)
concerns: sanitary condition of equipment, sanitary handling, time-temperature profile of product

i. *massaging (tumbling)*—to extract protein to surface to bind product tissues together when cooked (examples turkey breast, rolls)
concerns: sanitary condition of equipment, time-temperature profile of product

j. *curing*—to add or inject curing ingredients to tissue for flavor and preservative action
concerns: microbiological condition of curing ingredients or solution, sanitary condition of equipment

k. *heat treatment (cooking, smoking, canning)*—to provide desirable body and texture characteristics and for destruction of microorganisms
concern: time-temperature profile of product

l. *chilling*
concern: rapid chilling of cooked product

m. *packaging*
concerns: sanitary condition of equipment (slicers for example), sanitary practices (particularly in repacking

and weighing of cooked product), type of packaging film, container integrity, gaseous atmosphere
n. *storage of further-processed products*
concerns: time-temperature profile of product, sanitary condition of coolers and freezers, inventory control and
rotation
(Note: not all processing steps are applicable to each further-
processed product.)
3. *Handling in food service operations and in the home*
a. *storage conditions of frozen and refrigerated products*
concern: time-temperature profile of product
b. *thawing of frozen product*
concern: time-temperature profile of product
c. *cross-contamination*
concern: contamination from raw to cooked product via cutting boards, handling, etc., and from raw product
to food that receives no further heat treatment
d. *cooking of product*
concern: time-temperature profile of product
e. *cooling of cooked product*
concerns: rate of cooling, time-temperature profile of product
f. *storage of cooked product*
concern: time-temperature profile of product
g. *reheating of product*
concern: time-temperature profile of product

Quantitatively, there will be differences in the degree of "concern"
depending upon the type of further-processed product. The significance
of individual concerns associated with various processing, storage, and
preparation practices for individual further-processed products are dealt
with on the following pages. No attempt will be made to evaluate the
sensitivity of all of the above-listed types of further-processed poultry
products relative to safety, shelf-life, and microbiological criteria. Instead,
these issues and the need for microbiological criteria will be discussed for
a few typical further-processed poultry products as examples of the various
factors that should be considered:

1. tray-pack product (chilled or frozen): cut-up broilers (breast, wish-
bone, wings, drum, thigh, back, neck); turkeys (drum, tail, wings,
neck)
2. mechanically deboned poultry meat product: turkey wieners
3. trim meat product: sliced turkey ham
4. muscle product: boneless turkey breast

5. canned product: canned chicken
6. poultry pot pies

To evaluate shelf-life and safety of other types of products, it would be necessary to conduct a hazard analysis and establish and monitor critical control points for these products.

Tray-Pack Product

The shelf-life of a tray-pack product stored at refrigeration temperatures depends upon the extent of microbial activities, primarily those of psychrotrophic spoilage bacteria such as *Pseudomonas* spp. Critical control points include the microbiological condition of the carcasses from which the parts were derived, sanitary handling of the product during the cut-up operation, sanitary condition of equipment, and the time-temperature profile of the product during processing and storage. Chill-packs should be held at the plant at −2.8°C (27°F), a temperature not conducive for rapid growth of psychrotrophic spoilage bacteria. At the retail level somewhat higher storage temperatures (0 to 4.5°C/ 32 to 40°F) can be expected, resulting in more rapid growth of psychrotrophic bacteria. As the aerobic plate count (APC) of raw poultry parts approaches 10^7 to 10^8 viable cells per cm^2, off-odors often become noticeable with subsequent slime formation at somewhat higher APC.

Safety of tray-pack products as well as that of ready-to-cook carcasses (see Raw Poultry section) can best be assured by adhering to the following practices in food service operations and in the home:

1. adequate cooking
2. proper hot and cold storage of cooked product
3. avoidance of cross-contamination of cooked food from raw food and from contaminated equipment and utensils
4. sanitary handling of raw and cooked product
5. proper cooling of cooked product
6. adequate reheating of cooked chilled product

Bryan (1980) and Bryan and McKinley (1974) have shown that failure to observe these practices commonly leads to outbreaks of meat- and poultry-borne diseases. *Clostridium perfringens* enteritis, staphylococcal intoxication, and salmonellosis are the more common foodborne diseases associated with poultry. Low levels of *C. perfringens* are common on raw poultry. When poultry is cooked, some *C. perfringens* spores survive. As the temperature of the hot cooked product reaches 50°C (122°F) during holding at room temperature or on a warming device or during storage in a refrigerator (when product is stored in thick layers), spore germination and multiplication of vegetative cells begin. Multiplication is favored by the absence of competitive bacteria and the low Eh of the cooked product. If there is enough time during warm holding or slow cooling, cells may reach numbers that can cause illness. If such foods are consumed without adequate reheating to kill vegetative cells, illness may occur.

Contamination of cooked poultry with *Staphylococcus aureus* usually occurs through handling by humans. If such product is left without refrigeration for several hours or cools slowly in refrigerators (when stored in containers in thick layers) growth of *S. aureus* and enterotoxin formation may occur. Growth of *S. aureus* in a cooked product is favored by lack of competitive bacteria, which are destroyed by heat.

Small numbers of *Salmonella* may often be present on raw poultry. *Salmonella* on cooked poultry result either from inadequate cooking or from recontamination of adequately cooked poultry by contact with contaminated hands, equipment, and utensils.

Perishable Cooked Further-Processed Products: Wieners, Ham, Boneless Breast

A flow diagram of basic processing procedures utilized in the production of turkey wieners, sliced turkey ham, and turkey boneless breast is given below:

> *Wieners*:   (turkey, water, salt, sugar, phosphates, erythorbate, nitrite and flavoring)
> Mechanically deboned turkey meat→ packaged→ frozen→ flaking→ emulsification→ blending→ emulsification→ stuffing→ cooking→ chilling→ peeling→ packaging→ storage.
>
> *Sliced turkey ham*:   (turkey, water, salt, sugar, phosphates, erythorbate, nitrite, flavoring)
> Hand-deboned thigh meat→ trimming→ blending→ stuffing→ cooking→ chilling→ peeling→ slicing→ packaging→ storage.
>
> *Boneless breast*:   (turkey, salt, sugar, phosphates)
> Hand-deboned breast skin and breast muscles→ trimming→ tumbling→ forming→ cooking→ chilling→ repackaging→ storage.

Factors that influence the microbiological condition of further-processed poultry products listed in the beginning of this section apply to turkey wieners, sliced ham, and boneless breast. The importance of using carcasses with low numbers of spoilage bacteria for further-processed products is obvious. Unless sanitary procedures are used, hand-boning and trimming can contaminate products. Mechanical deboning systems offer opportunities for increases in bacterial counts. This is possibly an effect of increases in product temperature and increased nutrient availability due to increased surface area of tissue.

Many pieces of equipment are used in the manufacture of further-processed products. To keep increases in bacterial numbers to a minimum, it is advisable to design a cleaning and sanitizing program to fit the production operations of a plant. Equipment and utensils should be periodically cleaned and sanitized thoroughly. Product accumulation on equipment coupled with infrequent cleanup operations should be avoided because they result in substantial increases in bacterial count of the product. Extensive interruptions in product flow increase opportunities for microbial growth in the product.

Proper cooking destroys most vegetative cells, including pathogens such as *Salmonella, Yersinia, Campylobacter*, and *S. aureus*. Cooked poultry must reach an internal temperature of at least 71°C (160°F); cured and smoked poultry at least 68°C (155°F) (Bailey, 1974). Surviving bacteria are primarily sporeformers. APCs of these products immediately post-cook usually are low, but recontamination may occur through contact with hands (packaging) and contaminated equipment such as in peeling, slicing, and packaging operations. Presence of pathogens such as *Salmonella, Campylobacter, Yersinia*, and *S. aureus* on a fully cooked perishable product indicates a lack of sanitary processing practices in post-cook operations.

The hazard associated with eating a product recontaminated with *Salmonella* depends upon the method of food preparation. Cooked poultry products such as rolls and roasts are not always reheated before eating. Salmonellosis has been traced to recontaminated precooked turkey roasts and rolls (Bryan, 1980).

Wieners, sliced ham, and luncheon meats such as bologna, salami, and pastrami prepared from poultry meat are perishable cooked cured meats and are subject to shelf-life problems similar to those described for products produced from beef and pork (see Chapter 9, part C). Cooked cured poultry products such as wieners, ham, bologna, and a wide variety of luncheon meats have a relatively long shelf-life [about 30 days at 1.7 to 4.4°C (35 to 40°F)]. Cooking [internal temperature of at least 68°C (155°F)] destroys most microorganisms except for some thermoduric bacteria and spores. Salt and nitrite have an inhibitory effect on some of the survivors and contaminants. During prolonged refrigerated storage in oxygen-permeable films, micrococci, enterococci, lactic acid bacteria, and yeasts may develop. When packaged in oxygen-impermeable films (vacuum-packaged) lactic acid bacteria become dominant and eventually cause shelf-life problems.

Canned Poultry Products

For a discussion on the sensitivity of canned poultry products relative to shelf-life and safety see the sections in this chapter on canned foods.

Poultry Potpies

Commercially prepared and homemade potpies contain poultry meat, vegetables, gravy, and seasoning materials. They are cooked during processing and the contents are protected from subsequent recontamination by the crust or shell. Proper cooking destroys most vegetative cells, including *Salmonella*, *S. aureus*, *Campylobacter*, and *Yersinia*, but some spores can survive. If these products are subjected to temperature abuse, spoilage usually occurs. More serious, however, is that under such conditions spores of *C. botulinum*, which can survive cooking, germinate, and multiply. Mishandled poultry potpies have been implicated as a vehicle in family outbreaks of botulism (CDC, 1976). Temperature abuse of these products also presents a potential risk for *C. perfringens* enteritis.

Need for Microbiological Criteria

Most critical control points related to further-processed poultry products can be monitored by: (1) checks of time-temperature profile of product during processing (checking temperature during cooking, cooling, and storage), (2) evaluation of sanitary condition of processing equipment and facilities, and (3) evaluation of sanitary practices of employees.

Microbiological criteria for pathogens in raw poultry would accomplish little because (1) low numbers of pathogens such as *Salmonella*, *Campylobacter*, *Yersinia*, *C. perfringens*, and *S. aureus* are often present on raw poultry and for the most part are unavoidable under present conditions of handling, and (2) foodborne disease problems arise when cooked products are mishandled in processing plants, food service operations, or in the home. A working group of the Codex Committee on Food Hygiene (FAO/WHO, 1979) concluded that application of microbiological criteria for raw poultry would not improve safety (see Part D, above).

Microbiological guidelines (APC) are useful to check the condition of incoming carcasses to be used for further processing, particularly if they were obtained from other sources. Relatively simple microbiological procedures (rinse, swab, direct agar contact) are available to evaluate the sanitary condition of equipment and utensils after each cleaning and sanitizing schedule and to monitor buildup of microorganisms on equipment during the processing day (APHA, 1984). The results of counts on incoming carcasses as well as those on equipment and utensils are of retrospective value. They are useful because counts on carcasses can identify suppliers that provide products with excessively high counts. High counts on equipment and utensils would alert the processor to intensify cleanup operations or review cleaning procedures. Microbiological guidelines for products after a critical control point or for finished products can be useful (1) to check conditions along the processing line and (2) to meet "guaranteed shelf life" of product or purchaser specifications. In a cooked product the guideline should include APC (to evaluate general condition along the processing line), *S. aureus* (to identify lack of hygienic practices and potential temperature abuse), *Salmonella* (post-heat cross-contamination), and coliforms (post-heat contamination). For raw finished products, microbiological guidelines (APC) may be helpful to evaluate process control. If counts exceed guidelines that can be met when operating under good processing practices, then the processor will be alerted to check critical control points to locate and remedy the problem.

Assessment of Information Necessary for Establishment of a Criterion if One Seems To Be Indicated

Although several studies have reported on the microbiological condition of further-processed poultry products (Bryan et al., 1968a; Mercuri et al., 1970; Zottola and Busta, 1971; Robach et al., 1980), few published reports (Bryan et al., 1968b; Denton and Gardner, 1982) are available that characterize the effect of individual processing practices on the microbial flora of these products. Information in reports by ICMSF (1974, 1980, 1985) and APHA (1976, 1984) should provide useful guidelines in evaluating the microbiological condition of further-processed poultry.

Where Criteria Should Be Applied

A hazard analysis critical control point program should be applied for these products at the plant level. Various procedures including microbiological guidelines to monitor these control points have been discussed earlier in this section. Mishandling of poultry occurs in food service operations and in homes. Control of this problem should be through monitoring of critical control points, which include thawing, cooking, hot-holding, handling after cooking, chilling, and reheating. The HACCP concept described for food service operations should also be applied to the handling of foods in the home. This approach requires education of all persons in food handling procedures with particular emphasis at the grade and high school levels.

References

APHA (American Public Health Association)
1976   Compendium of Methods for the Microbiological Examination of Foods. M. L. Speck, ed. Washington, D.C.: APHA.
1984   Compendium of Methods for the Microbiological Examination of Foods. 2nd Ed., M. L. Speck, ed. Washington, D.C.: APHA.

Bailey, J. W.
1974   Encyclopedia of Labeling Meat and Poultry Products. 2nd Ed. St. Louis: Meat Plant Magazine.

Bryan, F. L.
1980   Foodborne diseases in the United States associated with meat and poultry. J. Food Prot. 43:140–150.

Bryan, F. L., and T. W. McKinley
1974   Prevention of foodborne illness by time-temperature control of thawing, cooking, chilling and reheating turkeys in school lunch kitchens. J. Milk Food Technol. 37:420–429.

Bryan, F. L., J. C. Ayres, and A. A. Kraft
1968a   Destruction of salmonellae and indicator organisms during thermal processing of turkey rolls. Poultry Sci., 47:1966–1978.
1968b   Salmonellae associated with further processed turkey products. Appl. Microbiol. 16:1–9.

CDC (Center for Disease Control)
1976   Foodborne and Waterborne Disease Outbreaks. Annual Summary 1975. Atlanta: Center For Disease Control.

Denton, J. H., and F. A. Gardner
1982   Effect of further processing systems on selected microbiological attributes of turkey meat products. J. Food Sci. 47:214–217.

ICMSF (International Commission on Microbiological Specifications for Foods)
1974   Microorganisms in Foods. 2. Sampling for microbiological analysis: Principles and specific applications. Toronto: University of Toronto Press.
1980   Microbial Ecology of Foods. 2. Food Commodities. New York: Academic Press.
1985   Microorganisms in Foods. 2. Sampling for microbiological analysis: Principles and specific applications. In preparation.

Mercuri, A. J., G. J. Banwart, J. A. Kinner, and A. R. Sessoms
1970   Bacteriological examination of commercial precooked Eastern-type turkey rolls. Appl. Microbiol. 19:768–771.

Robach, M. C., E. C. To, S. Meydav, and C. F. Cook
1980   Effect of sorbates on microbiological growth in cooked turkey products. J. Food Sci. 45:638–640.

USDA (U.S. Department of Agriculture)
1983   Poultry-Production, Disposition & Income 1981–1982. Statistical Reporting Service. Pou-2-3, April 83.

Zottola, E. A., and F. F. Busta
1971   Microbiological quality of further-processed turkey products. J. Food Sci. 36:1001–1004.

F. EGGS AND EGG PRODUCTS

Sensitivity of Products Relative to Safety and Quality

Eggs and egg products are regulated by the USDA, the legislative base being the Egg Products Inspection Act of 1970 (U.S. Congress, 1970). The term "egg" means the shell egg of domesticated chicken, turkey, duck, goose, or guinea. The term "egg product" means any dried, frozen, or liquid eggs with or without added ingredients, excepting products that contain eggs only in a relatively small proportion. Processors of egg products are subject to continual USDA inspection. Though shell eggs are covered under the Egg Products Inspection Act, their processing is not under continual inspection.

Historically, consumption of eggs and egg products has been an important cause of human salmonellosis. Between 1963 and 1975 there were 651 outbreaks of human salmonellosis reported to the Center for Disease Control, and the vehicle of transmission was identified in 463 (71%) of these occurrences. Of these, poultry accounted for 99 (21%), meat for 69 (15%), and eggs for 53 (11%). These data, reviewed by Cohen and Blake (1977), show that poultry, meat, and eggs were vehicles in approximately half of the outbreaks of human salmonellosis during this 13-year period. The percentage of outbreaks caused by eggs decreased dramatically after 1966 (see Figure 9-1). Of 10 egg-related outbreaks occurring between 1968 and 1975, 9 were associated with shell eggs and only 1 with egg products. The vastly improved safety position of eggs and egg products has been maintained since 1975 through to the present time. This may be traced to consumer education and to improvements made by egg producers and processors. Of great importance was enforcement of the Egg Products Inspection Act of 1970, which placed egg products, as well as shell eggs, under supervision by USDA. The Egg Products Inspection Act, as of July 1972, eliminated human consumption of high-risk shell eggs, namely, checks, dirties, incubator rejects, and leakers. Furthermore, the Egg Products Inspection Act required that all egg products be pasteurized to render them free of salmonellae.

Shell Eggs

The interior contents of sound shell eggs are virtually free of microorganisms, e.g., $< 10/g$ (Bergquist et al., 1984). However, shell eggs are subject to spoilage if microbial invasion occurs. This is apt to occur with "leakers," eggs of which the shell and shell membranes are broken.

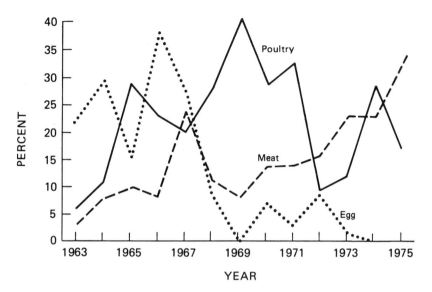

FIGURE 9-1 Percentage of salmonellosis outbreaks (outbreaks caused by unidentified vehicle are eliminated) caused by poultry, meat, or eggs. United States, 1963-1975.

SOURCE: Cohen and Blake, 1977.

The egg contents may become contaminated with microorganisms if improper washing or storage conditions are used. For example, if the wash solution temperature is lower than the temperature of the egg, the wash water may be drawn into the egg through shell pores when the contents contract.

Despite the perishability of shell eggs, microbiological criteria are of little value. Before marketing, shell eggs go through a mechanized process of sorting, washing, drying, candling, weighing, and packaging. The procedures, particularly candling, are depended upon to eliminate shell eggs of poor quality from entering commercial channels. At the present time, egg-associated foodborne disease outbreaks almost always involve consumer misuse of shell eggs, viz. their use as ingredients in foods under conditions where the shell egg contents are not subjected to pasteurizing temperatures—as components of eclairs, meringues, and ice cream. In such circumstances, contamination by bacteria residing on the surface of the shell is carried to the "broken out egg" and thereafter into the food that is prepared without cooking. Compounding the problem is the frequent exposure of broken out shell egg contents to temperatures permitting microbial growth prior to their use as ingredients. To the degree that eggs continue to be a source of human salmonellosis, this is the most significant route of human infection.

Clearly, microbiological criteria can play no significant role in the control of shell egg quality. Both safety and general microbiological quality are dependent upon sorting (elimination of defective eggs from commerce) and candling, as well as proper washing and storage conditions.

Egg Products

Egg products present quite different microbiological problems from those of shell eggs. The contents of shell eggs are subject to contamination during the breaking operation and subsequently during further handling of the broken out egg contents. A single highly contaminated egg can contaminate a large volume of fluid egg with spoilage and/or pathogenic microorganisms. If the liquid egg is to be dried, then it must first be desugared. Microbial growth usually occurs during the desugaring process, even when this is accomplished by enzyme treatment. Whether the liquid eggs are frozen or dried, they must be pasteurized. Egg albumen cannot withstand as high temperatures as can whole eggs and yolks. As a consequence, spray-dried albumen must be held at a temperature of not less than 54.4°C (130°F) for not less than 7 days and until it is negative for *Salmonella*. Pan-dried albumen must be held at a temperature not less than 51.7°C (125°F) continuously for not less than 5 days and until it is negative for *Salmonella* (USDA, 1980).

The risk of postprocessing contamination exists with both liquid and dried egg products. Finally, frozen eggs must be thawed before use, and if this is not done properly, microbial growth may occur. Similarly, dried eggs must be reconstituted. If the thawed frozen eggs or reconstituted dried eggs are not held under proper conditions (time and temperature), microbial growth may lead to spoilage and/or the growth of *Salmonella*. If egg products are contaminated with salmonellae, there is the added hazard of cross-contamination to other products in the food-processing or kitchen environments.

The only pathogen of concern is *Salmonella*. Federal law requires that to assure that adequate pasteurization has occurred, pasteurized egg products and heat-treated dried egg whites shall be sampled and analyzed for the presence of *Salmonella* (USDA, 1980). Thus, a standard requiring that egg products be free of *Salmonella* exists.

Other than a direct microscopic standard, no standards relating to spoilage or indicator organisms exist. Microbiological criteria may be profitably used by the processor and user of egg products. APCs may be used to assess the microbiological quality of raw materials and processing conditions. Pasteurized products may be tested for coliforms to detect post-pasteurization contamination. Many processors of egg products use microbiological criteria to monitor critical control points, and purchase specifications commonly include criteria with limits for aerobic plate count and coliforms, as well as for salmonellae.

The *Salmonella* Standard

As indicated above, federal law has established a standard requiring that egg products, except unpasteurized salted egg products used in acidic dressings, be free of *Salmonella*. The USDA is responsible for administration of this standard. Details of this activity are contained in AMS-PY instruction number 910, Egg Products-1 (USDA, 1975). This document recognizes three different types of sampling and testing, namely certification, surveillance, and confirmation.

Certification means certifying to the quality of a specific lot. Samples are drawn by the USDA inspector and submitted to a USDA laboratory. An attribute sampling plan is prescribed. Samples are randomly drawn from the final shipping containers. The number of containers sampled is determined by the number of containers in the lot. For example, with liquid and frozen egg products, the sampling plan below is used.

No. of shipping containers in the lot	No. of shipping containers to select for sampling	Quantity to be analyzed
1,200 or less	4	1 x 100 g
1,201-3,200	8	2 x 100 g
Over 3,200	16	3 x 100 g

For dried egg products the following sampling plan is prescribed.

No. of shipping containers in the lot	No. of shipping containers to select for sampling	Quantity to be analyzed
50 or less	4	1 x 100 g
51-150	8	2 x 100 g
151-500	12	3 x 100 g
501-1,500	16	4 x 100 g
Over 1,500	20	5 x 100 g

In applying this plan, the units randomly selected for sampling are segregated into groups of four. Two to three ounces of product are withdrawn from each unit in the group, and these samples are combined in a single container, mixed, and a 100-g composite sample is taken and analyzed for *Salmonella*. With reference to dried products, then, a single 100-g sample is analyzed for lots comprised of 50 or fewer containers;

whereas 5 x 100-g composites are analyzed for lots comprised of over 1,500 containers. Thus, the stringency of the sampling plan is related to the number of containers within a lot. If one considers a lot to be comprised of an infinite number of 25-g units, then for dried egg products, the plan applied varies from n = 4 to n = 20. For liquid and frozen egg products, the plan varies from n = 4 to n = 16. As indicated in Chapter 6, lot size has little effect on the probability of acceptance of large lots. Selecting the number of sample units as a percentage of lot size really serves no purpose. In the above case, however, lot size not only influences the number of units sampled but also the amount of sample analyzed. Thus, the USDA approach to certification samples encompasses variation in the stringency of the sampling plan with lot size, and furthermore the plan utilized may vary from one that is extremely loose to one that has a moderate degree of stringency.

Surveillance as applied to the Egg Products Inspection Act means "the sampling of pasteurized products on a statistical basis and analyzing for the presence of *Salmonella* by any laboratory using the USDA method of analysis" (AMS-PY instruction no. 910) (USDA, 1975). Plants without an established history of producing products free of *Salmonella* are required to start sampling 100% of the lots in the order produced. As indicated in Figure 9-2, if 83 consecutive lots are found negative for *Salmonella,* the plan permits inspection of every other lot. If 83 inspected lots at this level are found negative for *Salmonella* then the frequency is shifted to one lot in four (level 2). If 83 inspected lots are found negative, then the sampling rate becomes one in eight lots (level 3). As further indicated in Figure 9-2, the finding of a positive lot "triggers" an increased frequency of sampling. The sampling plan initially applies to each day's production, each category of product, or each product. When a product is found to be positive, that product or category of product has a separate sampling plan until a satisfactory history of analyses is established. Any reduction or tightening of frequency of sampling applies separately to each product or category and not to cumulative results. It is of interest to note that the USDA instruction (AMS-PY instruction no. 910) (USDA, 1975) states that no rigid or set sampling pattern is to be followed. It suggests alternation between frozen and liquid product and between first and last product packed. For surveillance sampling a single 100-g frozen or liquid product is subjected to analysis. For dried samples three separate 25-g samples are analyzed (H. Maguire, 1982. Personal communication). Thus, again considering a lot to be composed of an infinite number of 25-g units, for liquid products n = 4 and for dried products n = 3.

Confirmation is "sampling and analyses, at government expense and direction, to verify the accuracy of the company's surveillance program

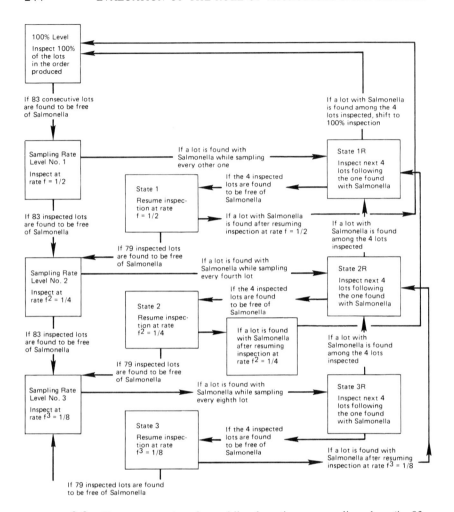

FIGURE 9-2   Flow process chart for multilevel continuous sampling plans ($i = 83$, $f = \frac{1}{2}$, $f^2 = \frac{1}{4}$, $f^3 = \frac{1}{8}$).

SOURCE: USDA, 1975 (From AMS-PY Instruction No. 910 [Egg Products]—1; Exhibit 8.)

and analyses'' (USDA, 1975). The USDA inspector draws confirmation samples from pasteurized liquid, frozen, and dried egg products in the final type of package in which the product is to be shipped. The inspector does not draw confirmation samples when the plant submits all their surveillance samples to a USDA laboratory. A 4-oz. sample is submitted for analysis, and the USDA laboratory analyzes 100 grams ($n = 4$). The confirmation sampling program is a ''spot check'' program for frozen and liquid products; the frequency of sampling is related to the surveillance sampling rate. For example, if a plant is on a 100% or a one in two surveillance sampling program for frozen or liquid products, then one confirmation sample per week is submitted for analysis. For a surveillance sampling program of one in four, two confirmation samples per month are submitted. For a surveillance level of one in eight, one confirmation sample per month is analyzed. For dried products the frequency of confirmation samples is one per week for yellow products (whole egg or yolk), two per month for spray dried egg whites, and one per month for pan-dried egg whites.

The USDA provides for retesting of lots found positive for *Salmonella* (USDA, 1977). Plants with known *Salmonella* problems are not permitted to resample. When permission is granted to resample, product is divided into sublots of not more than 100 containers or not more than 3,000 pounds. The number of containers to be drilled for a sample is the square root of each sublot. A 100-g sample is analyzed from each sublot, and each sublot is analyzed separately. The product may be released when the retest results of all the sublots are negative for *Salmonella*. If the retest result of any one sublot is positive for *Salmonella*, the entire original lot or day's production for the product involved is repasteurized and retested.

Probabilities Associated with the "*Salmonella* Standard"

The National Research Council (NRC) Committee on *Salmonella* categorized foods according to degree of risk to the consumer (NRC, 1969). Egg products, most conservatively, would be placed in Category III as they have historically been considered potential sources of salmonellae in finished products. Furthermore, during their use egg products may be exposed to conditions permitting the growth of salmonellae. Since egg products are subjected to a pasteurizing step capable of destroying salmonellae, they are subject, in theory, to only two of the three hazard potentials delineated in the NRC report. One might argue that pasteurized egg products are subject to post-pasteurization contamination or, on the other hand, that they are consumed by high-risk populations. Accordingly, a case may be made for placing them in a higher hazard category, namely I or II. Thus, these products could be placed in Category I, II, or III, depending upon one's point of view. According to the NRC report, Category III products are to be analyzed by a sampling scheme involving the analysis of thirteen 25-g samples, all of which must be negative. Given these results, there is a 95% probability of one organism or less in 125 g of product. The USDA surveillance sampling plan for dried eggs, based upon the analyses of three 25-g samples per lot, falls far short of NRC recommendations. Indeed, based upon the assumption of random distribution of salmonellae within a particular lot, the probability of accepting a lot with an average *Salmonella* contamination of one organism per 125 grams is 55% (see Figure 9-3). Thus a lot of the quality that should be rejected according to the NRC Category III sampling plan would be accepted by the USDA sampling plan 55% of the time. And this, in fact, is the USDA surveillance sampling plan that is used to determine how frequently a given processor must conduct *Salmonella* tests on his products. The statistics are only slightly more favorable using the sampling plan prescribed for liquid or frozen eggs wherein a single 100-g sample is analyzed (n = 4 instead of n = 3).

With respect to certification samples, the USDA program similarly falls short of the NRC recommendations. Here, the number of samples analyzed (n) is determined by the number of shipping containers within a lot. The virtue of this approach, of course, lies in the fact that the larger the number of units, the more individuals at risk, ignoring the unit weight of the containers themselves. But for the smallest lot (50 containers or less), n = 4, thus employing a consumer's risk far greater than contemplated by the NRC committee. For the largest lot (greater than 1,500 shipping containers of dried eggs), n = 20, the sampling plan is somewhere between a Category II and Category III, according to the NRC report. For liquid and frozen eggs, the sampling plan for the largest lot involves the analyses of three 100-g composite samples (n = 12), which falls short of the stringency recommended by the NRC. In terms of assessing the microbiological safety of individual lots of product, it is difficult to justify the stringency of varying sampling plans depending upon lot size (see Chapter 6).

Likewise, the USDA confirmation sampling program falls far short of NRC recommendations. A single 100-g sample (n = 4) is analyzed.

Since the USDA surveillance sampling program is based upon somewhat unsound statistical premises, it may be argued that the total surveillance program is in question. The credibility of the USDA certification, surveillance and confirmation sampling plans could be significantly improved simply by increasing the weight of the samples analyzed in connection with this program. If one classifies these products as Category III, then the analysis of a single composite 325-g sample (n = 13) would give 95% probability of 1 *Salmonella* or less in 125 g of product. If one were to consider these products in Category II, then the analysis of a total of 725 g of product would give a 95% probability of 1 organism or less in 250 g. The present USDA sampling schemes fall far short of those rec-

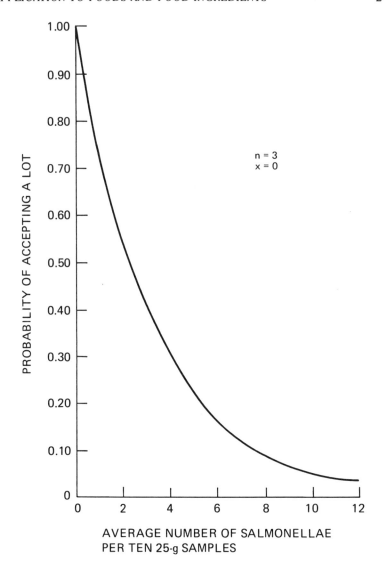

FIGURE 9-3 Operating characteristic curve—homogeneous distribution of salmonellae contamination.

SOURCE: Recommendations by the Subcommittee on Sampling and Methodology for Salmonellae in Eggs, Egg Products and Prepared Mixes, Inter-Industry Committee on Salmonellae in Foods (Anonymous, 1966), p. 124. Reprinted from *Food Technology*. Copyright © 1966 by Institute of Food Technologists.

ommended by the NRC and reliance upon them carries far too great a consumer risk.

Fortunately there has been only one outbreak of human salmonellosis traced to egg products since the Egg Products Inspection Act (CDC, 1977a,b). This outbreak was caused by dried egg albumen, contaminated with *Salmonella infantis*. The product was an ingredient of a "Precision Isotonic Diet," a formula for oral or tube feedings used in hospitalized individuals of all ages. One cannot, however, attribute the good recent public health record of egg products to the effectiveness of the USDA sampling programs. The fact is that producers of these products have employed far more stringent sampling plans than those prescribed by the USDA. Furthermore, users of egg products have, through their purchase specifications, required that products be analyzed according to the sampling plans recommended by the NRC Committee on *Salmonella*.

The dramatic decrease in egg-associated outbreaks attests to the success of mandatory pasteurization of egg products, as well as the Egg Products Inspection Program of USDA. The subcommittee recommends the continuation of the USDA program, with the intensification of the *Salmonella* sampling and testing indicated in this chapter.

References

Anonymous
    1966   Recommendations for sampling and laboratory analysis of eggs, egg products and prepared mixes. A report. Food Technol. 20(4):121–129.
Bergquist, D., A. Kraft, O. Cotterill, and H. Maguire
    1984   Eggs and Egg Products. In Compendium of Methods for the Microbiological Examination of Foods, M. L. Speck, ed. Washington, D.C.: APHA.
CDC (Center for Disease Control)
    1977a   *Salmonella infantis*—California, Colorado. Morb. Mort. Weekly Rpt. 26:41.
    1977b   Follow-up on *Salmonella infantis*—United States. Morb. Mort. Weekly Rpt. 26:84.
Cohen, M. L., and P. A. Blake
    1977   Trends in foodborne salmonellosis outbreaks: 1963-1975. J. Food Protect. 40:798-800.
NRC (National Research Council)
    1969   An Evaluation of the *Salmonella* Problem. Committee on *Salmonella*. Washington, D.C.: National Academy of Sciences.
U.S. Congress
    1970   Eggs Products Inspection Act. P.L. 95-597 (H. R. 19888). Dec. 29.
USDA (U.S. Department of Agriculture)
    1975   Section 8—Sampling for bacteriological, chemical and physical testing. AMS-PY Instruction No. 910 (Egg Products)—1. Implementation of Egg Products Inspection Act. Washington, D.C.: Agricultural Marketing Service, USDA.
    1977   Implementation of Egg Products Inspection Act. Section 9—Handling *Salmonella* Positive Samples. Revised. Washington, D.C.: Agricultural Marketing Service.
    1980   Regulations governing the inspection of eggs and egg products. Code of Federal Regulations 7 CFR Part 2859.

G. FISH, MOLLUSCS, AND CRUSTACEANS

Sensitivity of Products Relative to Safety and Quality

Safety

Fish, molluscs, and crustaceans can acquire pathogenic microorganisms or toxins from the natural aquatic environment, from sewage-contaminated harvesting areas, and from contamination by workers, utensils, and equipment during harvesting, processing, distribution, and food preparation. Even freshly caught fish and shellfish from unpolluted waters may contain pathogens such as *Clostridium botulinum* type E and *Vibrio parahaemolyticus*. For many of the fish-borne and shellfish-borne diseases, faulty harvesting or postharvesting practices are necessary to cause an outbreak of disease. Included in this category are outbreaks caused by *C. botulinum, V. parahaemolyticus, Staphylococcus aureus*, hepatitis A, scombroid poisoning, *Salmonella, Shigella*, and *Clostridium perfringens*. For botulism, staphylococcal intoxication, or *C. perfringens* enteritis time-temperature abuse of a heated seafood usually is involved; for scombroid poisoning time-temperature abuse of the raw fish usually is involved. For *V. parahaemolyticus* infection time-temperature abuse of raw-contaminated or heated-recontaminated seafood is necessary. *Salmonella, Shigella*, and hepatitis A may enter seafood either from contaminated waters, from contamination post-harvesting, or from contamination post-heating and cause disease in humans. Fish and shellfish that have ingested certain types of toxic dinoflagellates can be directly responsible for disease outbreaks. Paralytic shellfish poisoning (PSP) and ciguatera belong to this category.

From 1970-1978 fish, molluscs, and crustaceans were responsible for 7.4, 1.9, and 1.4%, respectively, of the foodborne disease outbreaks in the United States (Bryan, 1980). The more prominent disease outbreaks associated with these products were: for fish: ciguatera, scombroid poisoning, and botulism; for molluscs: paralytic shellfish poisoning, hepatitis A, and *V. parahaemolyticus;* and for crustaceans: *V. parahaemolyticus* and staphylococcal intoxication. The agents responsible for these diseases are discussed in detail in Chapter 4. They are mentioned here relative to the use of and need for microbiological criteria as related to safety of fishery products.

Hepatitis A has been associated with eating raw or undercooked shellfish harvested from estuaries polluted with sewage. In the United States sanitary control of the shellfish industry is primarily based upon classification and control of the harvest areas through comprehensive sanitary survey of the shoreline, microbiological monitoring of growing area waters, and prohibition of harvesting from areas not meeting "approved" growing area criteria. Routine control procedures are based upon guidelines in the National Shellfish Sanitation Program (NSSP) Manual of Operations (US-DHEW, 1965). Shellfish safety has been predicated upon the level of coliforms or fecal coliforms present in the water and the direct relationship of these organisms to known sources of pollution. The only microbiological standard for shellfish meats developed by the NSSP is for APC and fecal coliforms in the product as received at the wholesale market. Fresh or frozen shellfish are considered to be satisfactory if the fecal coliform MPN does not exceed 230 per 100 g and the APC at 35°C (95°F) is not more than 500,000 per g. Historically, it appears that strict adherence to NSSP recommendations for the control of shellfish growing areas generally has resulted in the production of safe shellfish where the hazard has been directly associated with sewage outfalls. Even so, for continued assurance of safety of shellfish, further refinements in the criteria are needed to reflect the impact of quality of growing waters, particularly with reference to the presence of viruses. Since *Escherichia coli* is the best indicator for fecal contamination, testing water and shellfish for this organism by rapid direct plating methods (see Chapter 5) may be more effective than testing for coliforms or fecal coliforms.

Ciguatera is a chemical intoxication resulting from eating fish (usually barracuda, grouper, jack, and red snapper) that have ingested toxic dinoflagellates. In the United States, the illness is usually associated with fish caught in tropical or subtropical waters of areas such as those around Hawaii and Florida. Simple, reliable tests to detect toxic fish are not yet available. An understanding of the ecology and epidemiology of the disease is helpful in predicting to some extent which fish and what areas are likely sources of intoxication.

Scombroid poisoning results from eating scombroid fish such as tuna in which histidine has been converted to histamine by microbial activity. This problem can be controlled best by proper harvesting (control of time in net) and postharvesting practices, i.e., proper cooling of fish. FDA (1982) will take regulatory action against canned albacore, skipjack, or yellowfin tuna that contains 20 mg or more of histamine per 100 g. Tuna with between 10-20 mg of histamine per 100 g that shows a second indicator of decomposition (spoilage odors or honeycomb appearance) is also subject to regulatory action. In view of the adverse reaction of humans to certain levels of histamine, the above criteria (defect action levels) appear useful. Additional information is needed about the toxic substances involved in scombroid poisoning and on the levels of histamine associated with human toxicity. A recently developed rapid screening test for histamine (Lerke et al., 1983) perhaps could be applied to monitor incoming scombroid fish and thus reduce the incidence of scombroid poisoning.

Paralytic shellfish poisoning (PSP) is caused by eating shellfish that have ingested certain dinoflagellates, primarily *Gonyaulax* species. PSP is best controlled by monitoring shellfish for toxins (mouse assay test) during the months of May to October, when this problem occurs most frequently. When the concentration of PSP in representative samples equals or exceeds 80 μg per 100 g of edible portion of raw shellfish, the state shellfish control authority prohibits harvesting in that area (USPHS, 1975). In view of the serious health hazards associated with the ingestion of saxitoxin and other related toxins a microbiological criterion for PSP appears fully justified. With increased interest in and application of shellfish aquaculture, serious consideration should be given to potential PSP problems.

V. parahaemolyticus gastroenteritis is not a serious public health problem in the United States. *V. parahaemolyticus* can become a problem when a seafood, usually crustaceans, is grossly abused in preparation and storage such as by time-temperature abuse of raw or undercooked product or by cross-contamination of a cooked product and subsequent storage within a temperature range at which this organism multiplies. Thorough cooking, prevention of cross-contamination, and proper cold storage will prevent *V. parahaemolyticus* gastroenteritis. A microbiological criterion involving *V. parahaemolyticus* does not appear useful or practical at the present. In addition, there is some uncertainty about the precision and accuracy of present methodologies (see Chapter 4).

Vibrio cholerae has in recent years become a concern in the United States, particularly with reference to the consumption of raw or undercooked shellfish (Blake et al., 1980; Bryan, 1980; CDC, 1981). Accumulating evidence (Colwell et al., 1977, 1981; Kaper et al., 1979; Blake et al., 1980; Hood et al., 1981) suggests that *V. cholerae* (O1 and non-O1) is a component of the autochthonous flora of brackish water and estuarine and salt marshes of coastal areas in temperate regions and poses a potential danger to public health. Measures to minimize this risk include strict adherence to the NSSP regulations for harvesting shellfish, proper refrigerated storage of seafoods, adequate heat treatment, and avoidance of cross-contamination.

Other *Vibrio* species associated with the marine environment, such as *V. vulnificus, V. fluvialis, V. mimicus,* and *V. hollisae* are also associated with human disease (Hickman et al., 1982). Their role as causative agents of foodborne illness is not clear. Studies need to be conducted about their ecology, epidemiology, and role in foodborne illness.

Botulism from ingestion of fishery products such as smoked and canned products can be controlled best by strict adherence to proper processing and storage practices. For example, smoked fish must be properly heated during smoking and then refrigerated so as not to allow growth of *C. botulinum*. Thermal processing of products in hermetically sealed containers must be adequate and container integrity must be maintained (see sections on heated canned foods and Chapter 4).

Conflicting reports have appeared in the literature regarding the botulism hazard of raw fish stored under refrigeration in vacuum packages or in modified gaseous atmospheres (Eyles and Warth, 1981; Eklund, 1982; Lee et al., 1983; Lindsay, 1983; Llobrera, 1983). Some investigators claim that raw fish stored in modified gaseous atmospheres becomes organoleptically unacceptable before toxin can be detected; others have shown that toxicity can occur without overt signs of spoilage. Whether or not the product will have spoiled before toxin is present most likely depends upon a number of conditions such as fish species, film permeability, gaseous atmosphere, time-temperature profile of storage, initial number of *C. botulinum* spores, initial number of bacteria (particularly psychrotrophic spoilage bacteria), and the judgment of the evaluator. Information on the effect of most of these variables on toxin production is inadequate. Thorough studies are needed to evaluate the potential hazard of refrigerated storage of raw fish in vacuum packages and in modified gaseous atmospheres. Until such time that the safety of this storage method for raw fish is validated, this practice is not recommended by this subcommittee because of its potential health risks.

S. aureus, Salmonella, Shigella, and *C. perfringens* have occasionally been responsible for foodborne disease outbreaks from consumption of fishery products. Proper postharvesting practices can greatly reduce the likelihood of such outbreaks. Preventive procedures for illness caused by *S. aureus* and *C. perfringens* include not holding heated fishery products for prolonged periods within a temperature range at which these organisms can grow. For prevention of salmonellosis, avoid harvesting fish and shellfish from polluted waters and heat the seafood thoroughly. To prevent shigellosis, good personal hygiene is an important measure.

The FDA imposed a *Salmonella* standard as an index of failure to apply good manufacturing practices in order to detain contaminated imported shrimp and frog legs from the U.S. market. Frog legs often are contaminated by *Salmonella* because of cross-contamination during handling and processing (Nickelson et al., 1975). Application of the HACCP system including monitoring of processing techniques and cleaning and sanitation of equipment and utensils can effectively reduce *Salmonella* on commercially processed frog legs (Nickelson et al., 1975). APC and *E. coli* are suggested as parts of microbiological guidelines to monitor critical control points in processing frog legs—for example, to monitor exposure of legs to intestinal contents during removal of legs from the frog.

Quality

Faulty harvesting, processing, and distribution methods can result in microbiological activities leading to loss of quality and subsequent spoilage of fish, molluscs, and crustaceans and of products derived from them. The use of meaningful microbiological end-product criteria to assess quality in raw fishery products appears extremely difficult, costly, and hard to enforce. These products are derived from very large numbers of fish and shellfish species, which differ in composition, are harvested from waters differing in temperature, salinity, and degree of pollution, and are subjected to a variety of processing and handling techniques. A more realistic approach to prevent inferior quality (because of microbial activities) products from entering market channels would be to inspect the raw materials at the plant for traits such as odor and appearance (see Chapter 5) and to assure that subsequent processing and handling steps meet Good Manufacturing Practices. A system of self-certification, through a HACCP system designed for a particular industry, should be implemented and enforced. Agencies such as the National Marine Fisheries Service, and the Food and Drug Administration and trade organizations should assist plants in developing a HACCP system. With periodic monitoring, a viable and effective system for insuring quality would be created.

In recent years, FDA has applied organoleptic evaluation and indole content (see Chapter 5) to check imported shrimp for decomposition. This evaluation is not applied to domestically processed shrimp because FDA has access to the plants.

Other tests that are associated with quality of fishery products such as trimethylamine, total volatile nitrogen, indole, and ethanol are discussed in Chapter 5.

Need for Microbiological Criteria

The safety and quality of fish and fishery products can best be assured by application of the HACCP system. For fresh products, monitoring of critical control points should consist primarily of inspection of incoming materials for odor and appearance, proper temperature control (refrigeration and/or freezing), cleaning and sanitizing of equipment and utensils, and handling of product by employees. In addition, for molluscan shellfish it should include analysis of the growing water and the product (at wholesale) for fecal coliforms and of the product for saxitoxin and related toxins. For processed tuna, histamine is the agent of concern (see previous discussion on scombroid poisoning). For cooked ready-to-eat products such as cooked peeled deveined shrimp and crabmeat, microbiological guidelines for the finished products should include APC, *E. coli,* and *S. aureus.* These parameters are useful to evaluate faulty processing and/or handling practices such as inadequate heating, cross-contamination with raw product, contamination from workers, and inadequate refrigeration which may create health hazards. For all processed fish and seafoods, the HACCP system is recommended as the basis for assuring safety and quality and within this system microbiological guidelines should be implemented where needed to monitor critical control points.

An examination of microbiological criteria that exist for fishery products in the various states shows that the most common criterion is that for shellfish as developed by the NSSP, or one closely resembling that criterion (Martin and Pitts, 1981). However, some states and local regulatory agencies have additional microbiological criteria for fish and seafoods (Wehr, 1982). Unfortunately, most of these criteria are not based on sound data or experience and are impractical from the standpoint of compliance or enforcement. If there is a need for additional microbiological criteria these should be based on properly designed and executed studies.

Recently, quality standards have been recommended for frozen crab cakes, frozen fish cakes, and frozen fishsticks (FDA, 1980, 1981). However, these products constitute neither a health hazard nor a serious quality problem. In addition, the methods used to establish "m" and "M" for these microbiological criteria are inconsistent with the principles on which the 3-class plan was established (Clark, 1982; ICMSF, 1974; see Chapter 6). The limit "M" represents the level at which a food is considered defective and unacceptable because (1) the number of organisms is so high that shelf-life is unacceptably short, (2) the microbiology is indicative of unacceptable sanitary conditions during manufacturing or handling, or (3) the microbiological data indicate that the product is unsafe or is a health hazard. "M" for frozen crab cakes, fish cakes, and fishsticks was so selected that it exceeded 99% of the survey population with 99% confidence. In addition, data used for these criteria were based on bacteriological surveys conducted at the retail level. Because of the potential for changes in the microbiological characteristics of the food between manufacture (at the plant level) and the time of purchase, it would be difficult to place the responsibility for an unsatisfactory condition at the retail level on unsatisfactory processing or handling at the manufacturing level. (For further discussion of microbiological quality standards, see Chapter 2.)

Assessment of Information Necessary for Establishment of a Criterion if One Seems To Be Indicated

To implement the recommended HACCP system to assure safety and quality of fishery products, an up-to-date HACCP system should be developed for the various products. For some products such as frozen breaded shrimp (see Chapter 8), breaded fish products (see Chapter 8), and processed blue crab (Phillips and Peeler, 1972; National Blue Crab Industry Association, 1982), extensive information is already available.

GMP recommendations such as those developed by the Tri-State Seafood Committee (National Blue Crab Industry Association, 1982) should be useful to processors.

Where Criteria Should Be Applied

As described above, for certain products, microbiological criteria are applied to the growing water (shellfish); for others, they are applied at the processing plant level. Purchase specifications may be useful to food service operators to monitor incoming products as part of their HACCP program unless the manufacturer can provide data about the quality and safety of the products.

References

Blake, P. A., D. T. Allegra, J. D. Snyder, T. J. Barrett, L. McFarland, C. T. Caraway, J. C. Feeley, J. P. Craig, J. V. Lee, N. D. Puhr, and R. A. Feldman
  1980   Cholera—a possible endemic focus in the United States. New Engl. J. Med. 302:305-309.
Bryan, F. L.
  1980   Epidemiology of foodborne diseases transmitted by fish, shellfish and marine crustaceans in the United States, 1970-1978. J. Food Prot. 43:859-876.
CDC (Centers for Disease Control)
  1981   Cholera—Texas. Morb. Mort. Weekly Rpt. 30:389-390.
Clark, D. S.
  1982   International perspectives for microbiological sampling and testing of foods. J. Food Prot. 45:667-671.
Colwell, R. R., J. Kaper, and S. W. Joseph
  1977   *Vibrio cholerae, Vibrio parahaemolyticus,* and other vibrios: occurrence and distribution in Chesapeake Bay. Science 198:394-396.
Colwell, R. R., R. J. Seidler, J. Kaper, S. W. Joseph, S. Garges, H. Lockman, D. Maneval, H. Bradford, N. Roberts, E. Remmers, I. Huq, and A. Huq
  1981   Occurrence of *Vibrio cholerae* serotype O1 in Maryland and Louisiana estuaries. Appl. Environ. Microbiol. 41:555-558.
Eklund, M. W.
  1982   Significance of *Clostridium botulinum* in fishery products preserved short of sterilization. Food Technol. 36(12):107-112, 115.
Eyles, M. J., and A. D. Warth
  1981   Assessment of the risk of botulism from vacuum-packaged raw fish: A review. Food Technol. Austral. 33(11):574-580.
FDA (Food and Drug Administration)
  1980   Frozen fish sticks, frozen fish cakes, and frozen crab cakes; Recommended microbiological quality standards. Federal Register 45 (108):37524-37526.

1981   Frozen fish sticks, frozen fish cakes, and frozen crab cakes; Recommended microbiological quality standards. Federal Register 46 (113):31067-31068.

1982   Defect action levels for histamine in tuna; availability of guide. Federal Register 47 (178):40487-40488.

Hickman, F. W., J. J. Farmer, III, D. G. Hollis, G. R. Fanning, A. G. Steigerwalt, R. E. Weaver, and D. J. Brenner

1982   Identification of *Vibrio hollisae* sp. nov. from patients with diarrhea. J. Clin. Microbiol. 15:395-401.

Hood, M. A., G. E. Ness, and G. E. Roderich

1981   Isolation of *Vibrio cholerae* serotype O1 from the Eastern oyster, *Crassostrea virginica*. Appl. Environ. Microbiol. 41:559-560.

ICMSF (International Commission on Microbiological Specifications for Foods)

1974   Microorganisms in Foods. 2. Sampling for microbiological analysis: Principles and specific applications. Toronto: University of Toronto Press.

Kaper, J., H. Lockman, R. R. Colwell, and S. W. Joseph

1979   Ecology, serology and enterotoxin production of *Vibrio cholerae* in Chesapeake Bay. Appl. Environ. Microbiol. 37:91-103.

Lee, D. A., M. Solberg, D. Furgang, and J. J. Specchio

1983   Time to toxin detection and organoleptic deterioration in *Clostridium botulinum* inoculated fresh fish fillets during modified atmosphere storage. Paper (No. 483) presented at the 43rd Annual IFT Meeting, New Orleans.

Lerke, P. A., M. N. Porcuna, and H.' B. Chin

1983   Screening test for histamine in fish. J. Food Sci. 48:155-157.

Lindsay, R. C.

1983   Safety and technology of modified-atmosphere packaging of fresh fish. Paper (No. 152) presented at the 43rd Annual IFT Meeting, New Orleans.

Llobrera, A. T.

1983   Bacteriological safety assessment of *Clostridium botulinum* in fresh fish and shellfish packaged in modified atmosphere containing CO_2. Ph.D. dissertation, Texas A&M University, College Station. August.

Martin, R. E., and G. T. Pitts

1981   Handbook of State and Federal Microbiological Standards and Guidelines. Washington, D.C.: National Fisheries Institute.

National Blue Crab Industry Association

1982   Tri-State Seafood Committee GMP Recommendations. Washington, D. C.: National Blue Crab Industry Association.

Nickelson, R., L. E. Wyatt, and C. Vanderzant

1975   Reduction of *Salmonella* contamination in commercially processed frog legs. J. Food Sci. 40:1239-1241.

Phillips, F. A., and J. T. Peeler

1972   Bacteriological survey of the blue crab industry. Appl. Microbiol. 24:958-966.

USDHEW (U.S. Department of Health, Education and Welfare)

1965   National Shellfish Sanitation Program. Manual of Operations. Part 1—Sanitation of Shellfish Growing Areas. PHS Pub. 33 (Revised 1965). Washington, D.C.: U.S. Government Printing Office.

USPHS (U.S. Public Health Service)

1975   National Shellfish Safety Program. Federal Register 40 (119):25916-25935.

Wehr, H. M.

1982   Attitudes and policies of governmental agencies on microbial criteria for foods—an update. Food Technol. 36(9):45-54, 92.

H. FRUITS AND VEGETABLES

Sensitivity of Products Relative to Safety and Quality

Raw fruits and vegetables are not common causes of foodborne illnesses in the United States (CDC, 1971; 1972; 1973; 1974; 1976a,b; 1977; 1979; 1981a,b). The high acidity of many fruits inhibits the growth of bacteria pathogenic for humans and the edible portions often are protected from contamination by a skin or thick rind. Although the vegetables that are eaten raw, such as in salads, may yield APCs of 10^7/g or greater (Fowler and Foster, 1976), they have not presented a serious public health problem in the United States and Canada because the microorganisms are mainly saprophytic species (Splittstoesser, 1970). However, in countries where polluted water or raw sewage are used for irrigation or fertilization of crops, enteric pathogens such as salmonellae and parasites are common contaminants (Ercolani, 1976; Tamminga et al., 1978). Certain imported fruits and vegetables, then, might be potential sources of foodborne illness.

A recently recognized potential problem has been the presence of *Clostridium botulinum* spores on raw potatoes that will be baked in foil. It has been hypothesized that a botulism outbreak occurred because foil-wrapped baked potatoes that were used in a potato salad had been held at room temperature for a number of days. Laboratory studies showed that botulinum spores can survive baking and that vegetative growth and toxin production can occur in the foil-wrapped product (Seals et al., 1981).

Mung bean and other vegetable sprouts that are often consumed raw develop high populations of bacteria during the sprouting process. Although sprouts usually are negative for foodborne pathogens (Patterson and Woodburn, 1980), at least one outbreak has been attributed to *Bacillus cereus* (Portnoy et al., 1976).

Nonsterile processed fruits and vegetables, such as frozen and desiccated products, have rarely been responsible for foodborne illnesses. The few cases that are reported each year have generally been due to contamination or mishandling by persons in food service establishments or home kitchens (see for example CDC, 1981b).

Commercially canned fruits and vegetables have an excellent public health record (see sections on canned foods). Home-canned vegetables, on the other hand, have been a major cause of botulism in the United States with 48 outbreaks occurring during the period 1970 to 1979 (CDC, 1971; 1972; 1973; 1974; 1976a,b; 1977; 1979; 1981a,b). The application of microbiological criteria would not have reduced the incidence of botulism since the outbreaks were due to underprocessing in the home.

Need for Microbiological Criteria

Raw Products

There is little use for microbiological criteria for fresh fruits and vegetables at the present time. However, future changes in irrigation and fertilization practices in this country or changes in the source of imported produce could mandate testing for certain pathogens or indicator organisms.

Nonsterile, Shelf-Stable Products

Because of an excellent public health record, standards are not needed for foods such as frozen or desiccated fruits and vegetables. Guidelines, on the other hand, may aid in the promotion of Good Manufacturing Practices.

These fruits and vegetables commonly receive a treatment at some processing step that destroys most of the epiphytic microflora and field contaminants. High viable counts on the finished product, therefore, usually reflect insanitary equipment, although actual microbial growth on the food also may occur (Splittstoesser, 1973). Most fruits and vegetables are succulent products whose solubles provide an excellent medium for a wide variety of microorganisms. The nutrients may collect in equipment areas difficult to clean (such as the interior of slicers), and significant microbial buildup may occur. Lactic acid bacteria often predominate on vegetable-processing lines although a variety of other mesophilic organisms including coliforms and *Geotrichum* make up a portion of the normal microflora (Splittstoesser and Mundt, 1976). Yeasts, molds, and aciduric bacteria predominate in fruit-processing plants, but other organisms including coliforms may be present in low numbers.

Aerobic plate counts are useful for the assessment of sanitation and manufacturing practices for low-acid vegetables. The enumeration of yeasts and molds and lactic acid bacteria is useful for fruits. Critical control points for sampling would include conveyor belts and unit operations such as size graders, cutters, slicers, and filling machines. Analyzing for diacetyl, a microbial metabolic product, has also served as a useful criterion for citrus products (Hill and Wenzel, 1957). Since coliforms, including fecal coliforms such as *Klebsiella pneumoniae,* are a part of the normal microflora of the raw product and processing lines, there is little reason to include them in microbiological criteria (Splittstoesser et al., 1980a). Testing for *Escherichia coli,* on the other hand, may be informative since this organism usually is not present on these foods.

Because of an excellent public health record, the routine testing of frozen and dried fruits and vegetables for common foodborne pathogens is not justified. Studies indicate that staphylococci are absent or are present only in low numbers and that salmonellae are usually absent (Splittstoesser et al., 1965; Splittstoesser and Segen, 1970).

Commercially Sterile Fruits and Vegetables

As discussed in Chapter 5, Howard mold count and rot fragment count procedures are used mainly to detect the inclusion of moldy materials in canned fruit and tomato products, and the enumeration of *Geotrichum candidum* hyphae has been used to detect insanitary processing machinery in vegetable canneries (AOAC, 1980). These microscopic count criteria are useful because viable counts cannot, of course, be applied to a thermally processed food.

Assessment of Information Necessary for Establishment of a Criterion if One Seems To Be Indicated

The microbiology of frozen vegetables depends upon the vegetable type and the method of processing (Barnard et al., 1982; Duran et al., 1982; Splittstoesser and Corlett, 1980). For example, green beans usually show higher aerobic plate counts than do peas, and French-style green beans are more heavily contaminated than are the cut variety. Presently lacking are modern data that would relate the microbiology of these foods to Good Manufacturing Practices. This information can be generated only through extensive factory surveys. Similar studies would be needed for frozen fruits as well as for nonsterile fruits and vegetables that are preserved by other means.

The Howard mold count and rot fragment standards have been used for many years (FDA, 1978). Although *G. candidum* has long been promulgated by FDA as an indicator of insanitation in tomato processing (Eisenberg and Cichowicz, 1977), more data would be needed (again, developed from extensive factory surveys) before meaningful limits based on filament counts could be established for this and other vegetables (Splittstoesser et al., 1980b).

A number of states have guidelines for horticultural products such as frozen potatoes, frozen onion rings, and pasteurized fruit juices (Wehr, 1982). There is little evidence to justify them.

Where Criteria Should Be Applied

Microbiological guidelines would usually be applied to frozen and dried fruits and vegetables following packaging. The samples can therefore be taken from the processing plant, warehouses, or retail markets. While market samples would show the microbiological condition of a food as purchased by the consumer, they might not permit an interpretation as to the reason for the particular findings.

When the objective of the guideline is to monitor a critical control point in the process line, samples would be collected at or following this point.

References

AOAC (Association of Official Analytical Chemists)
    1980   Official Methods of Analysis, 13th Ed. Washington, D.C.: AOAC.
Barnard, R. J., A. P. Duran, A. Swartzentruber, A. H. Schwab, B. A. Wentz, and R. B. Read, Jr.
    1982   Microbiological quality of frozen cauliflower, corn and peas obtained at retail markets.
            Appl. Environ. Microbiol. 44:54-58.
CDC (Centers for Disease Control)
    1971   Foodborne Outbreaks. Annual Summary 1970. Atlanta: Centers for Disease Control.
    1972   Foodborne Outbreaks. Annual Summary 1971. Atlanta: Centers for Disease Control.
    1973   Foodborne Outbreaks. Annual Summary 1972. Atlanta: Centers for Disease Control.
    1974   Foodborne and Waterborne Disease Outbreaks. Annual Summary 1973. Atlanta: Centers for Disease Control.
    1976a   Foodborne and Waterborne Disease Outbreaks. Annual Summary 1974. Atlanta: Centers for Disease Control.
    1976b   Foodborne and Waterborne Disease Outbreaks. Annual Summary 1975. Atlanta: Centers for Disease Control.
    1977   Foodborne and Waterborne Disease Outbreaks. Annual Summary 1976. Atlanta: Centers for Disease Control.
    1979   Foodborne and Waterborne Disease Outbreaks. Annual Summary 1977. Atlanta: Centers for Disease Control.
    1981a   Foodborne Disease Outbreaks. Annual Summary 1978. Atlanta: Centers for Disease Control.
    1981b   Foodborne Disease Outbreaks. Annual Summary 1979. Atlanta: Centers for Disease Control.
Duran, A. P., A. Swartzentruber, J. M. Lanier, B. A. Wentz, A. H. Schwab, R. J. Barnard, and R. B. Read, Jr.
    1982   Microbiological quality of five potato products obtained at retail markets. Appl. Environ. Microbiol. 44:1076-1080.
Eisenberg, W. V., and S. M. Cichowicz
    1977   Machinery mold—Indicator organism in food. Food Technol. 31(2):52-56.
Ercolani, G. L.
    1976   Bacteriological quality assessment of fresh marketed lettuce and fennel. Appl. Environ. Microbiol. 31:847-852.
FDA (Food and Drug Administration)
    1978   The food defect action levels. Food and Drug Administration, HFF-342, Washington, D.C.
Fowler, J. L., and J. F. Foster
    1976   A microbiological survey of three fresh green salads—Can guidelines be recommended for these foods? J. Milk Food Technol. 39:111-113.

Hill, E. C., and F. W. Wenzel.
  1957   The diacetyl test as an aid for quality control of citrus products. 1. Detection of
          bacterial growth in orange juice during concentration. Food Technol. 11:240-243.
Patterson, J. E., and M. J. Woodburn
  1980   *Klebsiella* and other bacteria on alfalfa and bean sprouts at the retail level. J. Food
          Sci. 45:492-495.
Portnoy, B. L., J. M. Goepfert, and S. M. Harmon
  1976   An outbreak of *Bacillus cereus* food poisoning resulting from contaminated vegetable
          sprouts. Am. J. Epidemiol. 103:589-593.
Seals, J. E., J. D. Snyder, T. A. Edell, C. L. Hatheway, C. J. Johnson, R. C. Swanson, and
J. M. Hughes
  1981   Restaurant-associated type A botulism: Transmission by potato salad. Am. J. Epi-
          demiol. 113:436-444.
Splittstoesser, D. F.
  1970   Predominant microorganisms on raw plant foods. J. Milk Food Technol. 33:500-505.
  1973   The microbiology of frozen vegetables. Food Technol. 27(1):54-56,60.
Splittstoesser, D. F., J. Bowers, L. Kerschner, and M. Wilkison
  1980b   Detection and incidence of *Geotrichum candidum* in frozen blanched vegetables. J.
          Food Sci. 45:511-513.
Splittstoesser, D. F., and D. A. Corlett, Jr.
  1980   Aerobic plate counts of frozen blanched vegetables processed in the United States.
          J. Food Protect. 43:717-719.
Splittstoesser, D. F., and J. O. Mundt
  1976   Fruits and vegetables. In Compendium of Methods for the Microbiological Exami-
          nation of Foods. M. L. Speck, ed. Washington, D.C.: American Public Health
          Association.
Splittstoesser, D. F., and B. Segen
  1970   Examination of frozen vegetables for salmonellae. J. Milk Food Technol. 33:111-
          113.
Splittstoesser, D. F., G. E. R. Hervey II, and W. P. Wettergreen
  1965   Contamination of frozen vegetables by coagulase positive staphylococci. J. Milk Food
          Technol. 28:149-151.
Splittstoesser, D. F., D. T. Queale, J. L. Bowers, and M. Wilkison
  1980a   Coliform content of frozen blanched vegetables packed in the United States. J. Food
          Safety 2:1-11.
Tamminga, S. K., R. R. Beumer, and E. H. Kampelmacher
  1978   The hygienic quality of vegetables grown in or imported into the Netherlands: A
          tentative survey. J. Hyg., Camb. 80:143-154.
Wehr, H. M.
  1982   Attitudes and policies of governmental agencies on microbiological criteria for foods—
          An update. Food Technol. 36(9):45-54, 92.

I. FRUIT BEVERAGES

Fruit beverages include single-strength juices, juice concentrates, and drinks that contain a small percentage of fruit juice plus added sugar, acids, flavors, and colors. They may be preserved as frozen concentrates, by refrigeration, as pasteurized shelf-stable products, or with the addition of benzoate and/or sorbate.

Many of the criteria and principles useful for fruit beverages also apply to sweetened and acidified beverages that contain no fruit juice.

Sensitivity of Products Relative to Safety and Quality

Fruit beverages have had an excellent public health record. Most possess a low pH, which prevents growth of pathogenic bacteria, and many juice products are given a thermal process that kills microorganisms of spoilage and public health significance.

While it is believed that enteric pathogens usually die off rapidly when in a highly acidic environment, *Salmonella typhimurium* has been shown to survive when inoculated into apple juice (Goverd et al., 1979) and nonpasteurized cider was responsible for a large outbreak of salmonellosis (CDC, 1975).

Heat-resistant molds, mainly species of *Byssochlamys, Aspergillus fisheri,* and *Penicillium vermiculatum* may cause spoilage of pasteurized fruit beverages because their ascospores are sufficiently resistant to survive the usual heat treatments that are given to these foods (Splittstoesser and Splittstoesser, 1977; Van der Spuy et al., 1975). The spores are present in orchards and vineyards (Splittstoesser et al., 1971), and thus are introduced into the beverage via the fruit. It is not uncommon to find low numbers of viable ascospores in juice concentrates.

Usually only a limited amount of mold growth occurs in a canned fruit beverage due to the low levels of oxygen present. However, off-flavors may be apparent and some heat-resistant molds may produce mycotoxins such as patulin (Rice et al., 1977).

Need for Microbiological Criteria

Standards are not needed because fruit juice beverages are rarely responsible for foodborne illnesses.

Guidelines are useful for the assessment of good manufacturing practices. Counts of yeasts and lactic acid bacteria in most fruit juices (Luthi, 1959; Murdock, 1976) and levels of diacetyl in citrus juices (Hill and Wenzel, 1957) often can be correlated with conditions of sanitation. Trace levels of patulin in apple juice are indicative of the pressing of fruit rotted by *Penicillium expansum* and other molds (Lindroth and Niskanen, 1978). A criterion for patulin in apple juice might be useful. Testing for coliforms is of limited value because they constitute a part of the normal processing line microflora and their presence does not indicate fecal contamination (Dack, 1955; Patrick, 1953).

Purchase specifications that limit heat-resistant mold spores in juice concentrates are useful. Also, specifications for mesophilic bacteria, yeasts, and molds in sugar to be used in nonpasteurized beverages are applicable (see Chapter 9, Part O).

Assessment of Information Necessary for Establishment of a Criterion if One Seems To Be Indicated

While companies may possess a wealth of data that relate processing conditions to the microbiology of their products, little information is available in the literature. Therefore, extensive surveys of fruit beverage processing lines might be required if a guideline were to be applied.

Where Criteria Should Be Applied

Guidelines can be applied to frozen, nonsterile products such as fruit juice concentrates at all stages of processing including the end product. With thermally processed beverages, on the other hand, analyses are most useful at critical control points prior to pasteurization. Beverages to be treated with preservatives are usually analyzed prior to packaging. Ingredients subjected to specifications should be tested after receipt by the purchaser.

References

CDC (Center for Disease Control)
   1975   *Salmonella typhimurium* outbreak traced to a commercial apple cider. Morb. Mort. Weekly Rpt. 24:87.
Dack, G. M.
   1955   Significance of enteric bacilli in foods. Am. J. Pub. Health 45:1151-1156.
Goverd, K. A., F. W. Beech, R. P. Hobbs, and R. Shannon
   1979   The occurrence and survival of coliforms and salmonellae in apple juice and cider. J. Appl. Bacteriol. 46:521-530.
Hill, E. C., and F. W. Wenzel
   1957   The diacetyl test as an aid for quality control of citrus products. 1. Detection of bacterial growth in orange juice during concentration. Food Technol. 11:240-243.
Lindroth, S., and A. Niskanen
   1978   Comparison of potential patulin hazard in home made and commercial apple products. J. Food Sci. 43:446-448.
Luthi, H.
   1959   Microorganisms in noncitrus juices. Pp. 221-284 in Advances in Food Research. Vol. 9. E. M. Mrak and G. F. Stewart, eds. New York: Academic Press.
Murdock, D. I.
   1976   Fruit drinks, juices, and concentrates. In Compendium of Methods for the Microbiological Examination of Foods. M. L. Speck, ed. Washington, D. C.: American Public Health Association.

Patrick, R.
  1953   Coliform bacteria from orange concentrate and damaged oranges. Food Technol.
          7:157-159.
Rice, S. L., L. R. Beuchat, and R. E. Worthington
  1977   Patulin production by *Byssochlamys* spp. in fruit juices. Appl. Environ. Microbiol.
          34:791-796.
Splittstoesser, D. F., and C. M. Splittstoesser
  1977   Ascospores of *Byssochlamys fulva* compared with those of a heat resistant *Aspergillus*.
          J. Food Sci. 42:685-688.
Splittstoesser, D. F., F. R. Kuss, W. Harrison, and D. B. Prest
  1971   Incidence of heat-resistant molds in eastern orchards and vineyards. Appl. Microbiol.
          21:335-337.
Van der Spuy, J. E., F. N. Matthee, and D. J. A. Crafford
  1975   The heat resistance of moulds *Penicillium vermiculatum* Dangeard and *Penicillium
          brefeldianum* Dodge in apple juice. Phytophylactica 7(3):105-107.

J. LOW-ACID CANNED FOODS

The U.S. Food and Drug Administration defines a low-acid canned food as one with an equilibrium pH >4.6 and a water activity >0.85. There is an exclusion to pH 4.7 for tomatoes and tomato products (FDA, 1983). Low-acid canned foods are packed in hermetically sealed containers. These products must be processed to achieve commercial sterility, i.e., a condition achieved by application of heat that renders such food free of viable forms of microorganisms having public health significance, as well as any microorganisms of non-health significance capable of reproducing in the food under normal nonrefrigerated conditions of storage and distribution (FDA, 1983).

The degree of heat treatment applied varies with the physiochemical nature of the product. For example, canned low-acid vegetables and uncured meats receive a "botulinum cook" (see below). Lesser heat treatments are applied to shelf-stable canned cured meats as well as to foods in which reduced water activity provides a barrier to the growth of spore-forming bacteria. These treatments may also be applied to aseptically processed low-acid canned foods wherein commercially sterilized cooled product is filled into presterilized containers followed by aseptic hermetical sealing with a presterilized closure in a sterile environment.

Sensitivity of Products Relative to Safety and Quality

Safety

Botulism is the prime hazard in low-acid canned foods. If spores of *Clostridium botulinum* survive the thermal process and thereafter grow and produce toxin in the canned product, and if the food is not adequately heated to destroy the toxin before it is eaten, consumption may lead to botulism, an often fatal disease. About 30 billion cans of low-acid food are consumed in the United States each year. From 1940 to 1982 there were 6 botulism outbreaks with 8 deaths caused by low-acid commercially canned foods in the United States. During this period there were an additional 7 instances in which the presence of *C. botulinum* or its toxin was detected in low-acid canned foods but from which no illness resulted. Of the 13 incidents, 5 were attributed to postprocessing contamination (NFPA-CMI, 1984).

The excellent public health history of low-acid canned foods is largely attributable to the application of the 12-D concept. From the classic studies of Esty and Meyer (1922) and Townsend et al. (1938), it was determined that the time required at 121.1°C (250°F) to reduce the survivor population of *C. botulinum* spores in phosphate buffer by a factor of 12 decimal units was 2.45 min (F_o[1] of 2.45). This work was based upon studies using the most heat-resistant strain of *C. botulinum*. Determination of processing schedules for the destruction of *C. botulinum* in other heating menstra, e.g., a canned vegetable, requires inoculated-pack studies in the food under consideration. On the basis of such studies, necessary time/temperature parameters for a 12-D process on the specific food are established.

Shelf-stable canned cured meats receive heat processes far below that dictated by the 12-D process, e.g., expressed as F-values, the heat treatment frequently corresponds to F_o = 0.4 to 0.6, but F_o-values as low as 0.05 are used. These processes alone do not account for the excellent public health record of these low-acid products. Rather the products' safety with respect to botulism is due to the combined effects of heat injury, curing salts, and the low incidence of *C. botulinum* spores in the raw materials (see ICMSF, 1980).

Quality

Though application of the 12-D process has resulted in the production of products with excellent public records, this heat treatment does not assure commercial sterility. There are many nontoxigenic sporeforming bacteria with D values much greater than *C. botulinum*. Among them are thermophilic anaerobes, including the flat-sour group (*Bacillus stearothermophilus*), the gaseous-spoilage group (*Clostridium thermosacchar-*

---

[1]F_o is a term used to denote the number of minutes a product is exposed to 250°F. In practice, the total heat process applied to a product is determined and through mathematical calculations this is equated to equivalent minutes at 250°F.

olyticum), and the sulfide stinkers (*Desulfotomaculum nigrificans*). Also included are mesophilic putrefactive anaerobes, e.g., *Clostridium sporogenes*. To avoid serious economic losses due to spoilage, the severity of heat processes generally applied to low-acid canned foods is greater than that necessary to assure destruction of *C. botulinum*, i.e., the generally acknowledged 12-D process. Even with the application of more severe heat processes, it is necessary to rigidly control the level of these sporeforming bacteria in raw materials, if severe economic losses due to product spoilage are to be avoided (APHA, 1976, 1984; see also parts M and O of this chapter).

Need for Microbiological Criteria

The presence of *C. botulinum* in processed low-acid canned foods is expected to occur so infrequently that no conceivable sampling plan for microbiological testing of finished product or by incubation test is a practical means of assuring safety. The Food and Drug Administration (FDA, 1973a) suggests finished product incubation and evaluation for aseptically processed canned foods, the primary purpose of which is to detect sterility breaks in the aseptic canning system. The U.S. Department of Agriculture requires incubation of approximately 1 container of meat and poultry containing low-acid canned foods per 1,000 processed as a check against gross underprocessing or container failure.

The safety of low-acid canned foods is based upon the establishment of heat processes capable of destroying *C. botulinum*, or in the case of shelf-stable cured meat, the control of the interrelated factors preventing *C. botulinum* outgrowth in the cured meat environment. The control of spoilage depends upon the establishment of heat processes capable of destroying spoilage organisms, some of which are more resistant than *C. botulinum*, and/or controlling the numbers of these organisms through judicious selection of raw materials.

The control of safety and stability is accomplished through the application of the HACCP system. In no phase of food processing is monitoring of critical control points so essential to the safety and stability of finished products as it is in the manufacture of low-acid canned foods. Indeed, monitoring, the extent of which has been reviewed by Ito (1974), is subject to federal regulations (FDA, 1973a,b; FPI, 1975). Physical and chemical tests are performed during production to ensure that all factors necessary to the application of the established safe processes have been adequately controlled. Numerous checks and tests are made at various critical control points, including the adequacy of ingredient blending, determination of consistency, ratio between solids and liquids, weight of product placed in the container, amount of head space, adequacy of double seam, time and temperature during sterilization, quality of cooling water, and post-processing handling of cooled cans. There is no intent above to indicate all the points that are monitored. Rather, the object is to emphasize the importance of checking each critical control point to ensure that the established procedures have been properly carried out. This necessitates specification of the method for measuring each parameter, determination of satisfactory limits for each test, determination of the frequency with which tests and checks should be employed, and recording of the results of these tests. If a defect is observed, remedial action should be taken and documented.

The U.S. Food and Drug Administration requires that operators of retorts, aseptic processing and packaging systems, product-formulating systems, and container closure inspectors be under the supervision of a person who has satisfactorily completed prescribed courses approved by the FDA Commissioner. At the same time, FDA inspectors are trained in the elements of the HACCP system as it relates to low-acid canned foods. The net result is a cost-effective approach to the control of safety and stability based upon both industry and regulatory knowledge of effective control of critical control points.

It is the opinion of this subcommittee that the HACCP system as applied to low-acid canned foods should serve as a model for the rest of the food industry. The identification of critical control points and the establishment of effective monitoring systems for these foods evolved as a result of joint government/industry efforts. Were the same approach to be taken in other phases of the food industry, similar cost-effective solutions to the problems of food safety and stability might be achieved. Training of inspectors in the HACCP approach should likewise be extended to other types of food-processing operations.

Where Criteria Should Be Applied

Microbiological criteria to determine the adequacy of raw materials can and are in most cases incorporated as a part of purchase specifications. The application of National Food Processors Association (formerly the National Canners Association) criteria to such commodities as sugar and starch has a well-established and effective history in the food industry.

Microbiological criteria are also useful for monitoring critical control points such as cooling water and equipment surfaces.

References

APHA (American Public Health Association)
 1976   Compendium of Methods for the Microbiological Examination of Foods. M. L. Speck, ed. Washington, D.C.: APHA.
 1984   Compendium of Methods for the Microbiological Examination of Foods. 2nd Ed., M. L. Speck, ed. Washington, D.C.: APHA.
Esty, J. R., and K. F. Meyer
 1922   The heat resistance of spores of *B. botulinus* and allied anaerobes. XI. J. Infect. Dis. 31:650-663.
FDA (Food and Drug Administration)
 1973a   Thermally processed low-acid foods packaged in hermetically sealed containers. Part 128B (recodified as Part 113). Federal Register 38(16):2398-2410, Jan. 14.
 1973b   Emergency permit control. Part 90 (recodified as Part 109), Federal Register 38(92):12726-12721. May 14.
 1983   Thermally processed low-acid foods packaged in hermetically sealed containers. General provisions. Definitions. Code of Federal Regulations 21 CFR 113.3.
FPI (Food Processors Institute)
 1975   Canned Foods—Principles of thermal process control in container closure evaluation, 2nd Ed. National Canners Association, eds. Berkeley, Calif.: FPI.
ICSMF (International Commission on Microbiological Specifications for Foods)
 1980   Microbial Ecology of Foods. Vol. 1. Factors affecting life and death of organisms. New York: Academic Press.
Ito, K.
 1974   Microbiological critical control points in canned foods. Food Technol. 28(9):46-48.
NFPA-CMI (National Food Processors Association—Can Manufacturers Institute, Container Integrity Task-force)
 1984   Botulism risk from post-processing contamination of commercially canned foods in metal containers. J. Food Prot. 47(10):801-816.
Townsend, C. T., J. R. Esty, and F. C. Baselt
 1938   Heat-resistant studies on spores of putrefactive anaerobes in relation to determination of safe processes for canned foods. Food Res. 3:323-346.

K.   ACID CANNED FOODS

The U.S. Food and Drug Administration defines acid canned foods as those with a natural pH of ≤ 4.6 (below 4.7 for tomatoes and tomato products). An acidified food is a low-acid food to which acid(s) or acid food(s) have been added. It has a water activity > 0.85 and a finished equilibrium pH of ≤ 4.6 (FDA, 1983a).

Acid and acidified canned foods packed in hermetically sealed containers are rendered commercially sterile by the application of heat sufficient to produce a food free from microorganisms capable of growth in the food at normal, nonrefrigerated conditions. The heat treatments are not designed to inactivate spores of *Clostridium botulinum* because this organism cannot grow at pH 4.6 or below. Example treatments are the

"*Bacillus coagulans* cook" for tomato juice of 0.7 min at 121.1°C (250°F) or equivalent and the hot-fill and hold processes for products with greater acidity (pH 3.7 to 4.5) such as tomato paste, puree, and ketchup (90.6°C/ 195°F for 3-5 min). The heat treatment is designed to inactivate vegetative forms and sporeformers capable of multiplication in the product. The acid content of the food is relied upon to act as a barrier to growth of spores such as *C. botulinum* that are not inactivated by the relatively mild thermal treatment.

Sensitivity of Products Relative to Safety and Quality

Safety

Acid and acidified canned foods prepared commercially in the United States have a remarkable record with respect to safety. This record undoubtedly is due to careful control of pH below the limits of growth of most pathogens, including *C. botulinum*.

Quality

Certain acid and acidified canned foods are susceptible to spoilage by flat-sour microorganisms such as *Bacillus coagulans*. Care must be taken to use ingredients with low initial counts of this organism and to destroy them with thermal treatment or limit their ability to reproduce by choice of a suitably low pH and/or high titratable acidity.

Need for Microbiological Criteria

Acid canned foods are considered less critical than low-acid canned foods with respect to control of manufacture. However, the U.S. Food and Drug Administration in 1979 promulgated Good Manufacturing Practices for Acidified Foods (FDA, 1983b). Many of the controls, records, and procedures listed for low-acid canned foods must also be followed for acidified foods.

The critical issues unique to successful processing of acid and acidified canned foods are: (1) destruction of microorganisms capable of reproduction in the food and (2) provision of a pH/acidity barrier to the growth of those microorganisms that survive. This barrier must control not only the acid-generating flat-sour types that would cause spoilage of economic (but not public health) concern but also acid utilizing microorganisms whose reproduction might result in the elevation of pH to the point where a pathogenic sporeformer such as *C. botulinum* could grow. Criteria, usually purchase specifications, should be applied to ingredients such as starch and sugar to prevent the use of raw materials that could lead to these types of spoilage.

Where Criteria Should Be Applied

The critical control points in the manufacture of acid and acidified canned foods are much the same as those already outlined for low-acid canned foods. Selection of ingredients of low spore load is important. The thermal process is of great importance to prevent loss of product due to spoilage. Control of pH and the provision of sound containers are critical. The presence and growth of microorganisms that can elevate the pH of the food and permit reproduction of pathogens must be precluded.

References

FDA (Food and Drug Administration)
1983a Acidified foods. General provisions. Definitions. Code of Federal Regulations. Title 21: part 114.3.
1983b Acidified foods. General provisions. Good manufacturing practices. Code of Federal Regulations 21 CFR 114.5

L. WATER ACTIVITY-CONTROLLED CANNED FOODS

The Code of Federal Regulations requires that a low-acid canned food have a pH greater than 4.6 and a water activity (a_w) greater than 0.85 (FDA, 1983). If a canned food has a pH greater than 4.6 and a_w greater than 0.85, it should receive a *C. botulinum* cook.

There are, however, a number of foods in hermetically sealed containers with pH >4.6 and a_w >0.85 that do not receive a *C. botulinum* cook because the severe heat treatment would jeopardize product acceptability. Examples include cheese spreads and canned cakes and breads, as well as a multitude of syrups and toppings. The reason for this seeming contradiction of the regulation lies in the fact that *C. botulinum* and most other sporeformers are unable to grow at a_w levels below 0.93. Therefore, if enough heat is applied to inactivate all vegetative forms and the a_w is controlled below 0.93, shelf-stable products result. However, manufacturers of these products must register their plants, file their processes, and demonstrate that spores of microorganisms not destroyed by the thermal treatment are incapable of growth in the food under normal nonrefrigerated conditions of storage and distribution.

In fact, parameters such as pH, a_w, heat, and possibly others may interact to result in a stable product. The long safety record of processed cheese spreads attests to the efficacy of multiple inhibitory factors. Research is now under way to identify and quantitate the interaction of pH, a_w, salt and phosphate concentrations, and possibly other factors that contribute to the stability of cheese spreads.

Sensitivity of Products Relative to Safety and Quality

Safety

Canned foods of reduced a_w have had a remarkable safety record in the United States. This record is the result of careful application of the available knowledge on water activity control of microorganisms.

Quality

Canned foods of reduced a_w are susceptible to spoilage by organisms that gain entry as a result of lack of container integrity. Some of the post-process contaminants, such as certain yeasts and molds, can grow in environments of low water activity.

Need for Microbiological Criteria and Assessment of Information Necessary for Establishment of a Criterion if One Seems To Be Indicated

Because reduced water activity is the barrier to growth of those microorganisms surviving the mild thermal treatments given these foods, control of water activity is critical. However, the level of reduced water activity needed for commercial sterility may vary depending on food composition. For example, *C. botulinum* has not been demonstrated to grow under ideal conditions in laboratory media below a water activity of 0.93, the exact level for inhibition depending upon the humectant used to control available water. Therefore, it is reasonable to expect that complex foods of varying ingredient mixtures combined with sublethal heat treatments will prevent the growth of *C. botulinum* at water activities somewhat higher than 0.93. There is a need to destroy vegetative forms, particularly *Staphylococcus aureus*, yeasts, and molds in all thermally processed, water activity-controlled canned foods.

Where Criteria Should Be Applied

Careful control of finished product water activity is essential for the low-acid foods that do not receive the botulinum process. This control must include a thorough procedure to monitor and standardize the accuracy and precision of the instrument used to measure water activity. Checks on each batch of product prepared are indicated. Microbiological criteria are not applicable.

References

FDA (Food and Drug Administration)
    1983   Thermally processed low-acid foods packaged in hermetically sealed containers. General provisions. Definitions. Code of Federal Regulations CFR 21 113.3.

M.   CEREALS AND CEREAL PRODUCTS

Raw cereal grains include wheat, corn, oats, rye, rice, barley, and millet. When processed into flours, meals, flakes, grits, etc., they serve as the basic materials in bakery items, breakfast foods, dry mixes, pastas, and refrigerated doughs. They also are used as ingredients in foods such as canned goods, confectioneries, meat products, and baby foods (APHA, 1976). Soybeans, which are pulses, are included in this section because many soy products are similar to those produced from cereals.

Sensitivity of Products Relative to Safety and Quality

Grains and Milled Grain Products

Under normal growing and harvesting conditions, cereal grains are exposed to a wide variety of microorganisms indigenous to the environment (APHA, 1976; Hesseltine et al., 1978; ICMSF, 1980; Swain et al., 1981). The types and numbers are related to:

1. soil type and species of plant
2. environmental conditions during growth, harvest, transport, and storage
3. grain quality
4. extent of contamination from man, animals, equipment surfaces, and storage facilities
5. abusive handling such as permitting water uptake with subsequent microbial growth

Grains normally contain bacterial populations of about 10^6/g. A wide variety of species are present, including sporeformers, lactic acid bacteria, pseudomonads, and coliforms (Rogers et al., 1915; APHA, 1976; ICMSF, 1980). These microorganisms are usually of little concern because their growth is prevented by the low water activity of the unprocessed grain.

However, many may carry through and survive the milling process and some may be potential spoilers of cereal products. For example, flour may be contaminated with heat-resistant bacterial spores, particularly thermophiles, which may survive the process given canned foods. Flour also may be contaminated with mucoid variants of *Bacillus subtilis* and *Bacillus licheniformis* which can cause "ropy" bread (Pylor, 1973; ICMSF, 1980): When the spores of these species survive baking, their subsequent germination and growth in the bread results in ropiness, which consists of a soft and sticky interior, brown discoloration, and a peculiar odor.

Yeast and mold populations on cereal grains often are as high as 10^4/g. Various molds, mainly species of *Alternaria, Fusarium, Helminthosporium,* and *Cladosporium* have the ability to invade kernels while the plants are growing. When grains have been properly dried to 13% water, these field fungi will slowly die off during storage. When grains contain higher levels of moisture due to inadequate drying or storage under wet conditions, molds are the principal spoilage organisms. Members of the *Aspergillus glaucus* group will grow at water activities as low as 0.73 and thus commonly spoil some of the lower moisture grains.

Cereal grains and their milled products have seldom been implicated as sources of foodborne disease. However, low numbers of pathogenic bacteria including salmonellae, *Bacillus cereus, Clostridium perfringens,* and *Clostridium botulinum* may be introduced from soil, feces, and other environmental sources.

B. cereus, a soil organism commonly found on grains, has been the cause of foodborne disease when cooked rice dishes have been held for extended periods under conditions suitable for spore germination and vegetative growth (ICMSF, 1980; Bryan et al., 1981).

Soybeans and soy products have, at times, been responsible for salmonellosis in animals and humans (Elliott, 1967; ICMSF, 1980). Commercially prepared tofu (soybean curd) was the source of an outbreak of yersiniosis involving 87 cases; two strains of *Yersinia enterocolitica* were isolated (Aulisio et al., 1983).

Mycotoxins are another potential health hazard since they are produced by some of the fungi that are present on cereals and their milled products. Aflatoxins are of particular concern because they are potent carcinogens; *Aspergillus flavus* and *Aspergillus parasiticus* are common contaminants of certain grains (Busby and Wogan, 1979; Labuza, 1983). The prevention of mycotoxins in milled cereal products depends upon the application of HACCP principles (see Chapters 1 and 10), which includes the prevention of mold growth on grains after harvest and the careful inspection of incoming shipments. The observation of fluorescence when kernels are examined under black light indicates mold presence and possible aflatoxin contamination (see Chapter 5), while the finding of pink kernels suggests that vomitoxin (2-deoxydivalenol) may be present (Trenholm et al., 1981).

Pasta Products

There are two basic types of pasta products. The first, noodles, is composed of mainly wheat flour, enrichment nutrients, and eggs or egg yolks, the latter at a level of not less than 5.5% of the total solids content (FDA, 1982). The second, macaroni, spaghetti, vermicelli, and related pastas, is similar but does not contain the eggs.

The ingredients are mixed with water to form a stiff dough of approximately 30% moisture, which then is extruded, shaped, cut, and dried. The dough is not heated during its preparation and, traditionally, the subsequent steps are conducted at temperatures that will support microbial growth. Drying to < 13% moisture for example, may be at 35 to 40°C (95 to 104°F) for a period as long as 18 hours. Since the dough provides an excellent growth medium, high microbial populations can result, particularly if good sanitation is not practiced during the blending and extrusion steps (APHA, 1976; ICMSF, 1980; Swartzentruber et al., 1982). Newer drying procedures, which involve several stages and higher temperatures, have minimized the opportunity for microbial growth. For example, in one process macaroni is dried 40 minutes at 71°C (159.8°F) followed by 4 hours at 74°C (165.2°F).

Staphylococcus aureus and salmonellae can survive the manufacturing process given pasta products (Lee et al., 1975; Walsh et al., 1974; Walsh and Funke, 1975). The heat resistance of *S. aureus* and *Salmonella anatum* has been shown to increase during the drying process, particularly within the intermediate moisture range, thereby increasing the probability that some cells will survive (Hsieh et al., 1976). Market surveys have revealed that pasta products may contain viable staphylococci and *Salmonella* (Walsh and Funke, 1975; Rayman et al., 1981; Swartzentruber et al., 1982.) These pathogens die off relatively rapidly during storage of the dried products (Lee et al., 1975) and will be killed by normal cooking, although staphylococcal enterotoxins would remain (Denny et al., 1966; Lee et al., 1975).

Pastries

Pastry products are baked doughs that are filled or topped with meat-containing gravies, custards, creams, imitation cream fillings, sauces, and/or meringues. These materials are often excellent growth media for spoilage and pathogenic microorganisms (Bryan, 1976; ICMSF, 1980). An exception is the butter cream filling composed of sucrose, water, and shortening that does not support microbial growth due to its low water activity. The different pastry products are distributed and retailed at ambient, refrigerated, or freezer temperatures.

Cream- and custard-filled pastries have been implicated in numerous foodborne disease outbreaks; *S. aureus* usually has been the causative organism although *Salmonella* have been responsible at times (see for example CDC, 1981a,b). In recent years the incidence of foodborne illnesses from pastries has decreased as a result of educational programs; improvements in manufacturing, sanitation, and refrigeration; and changes in formulations. In the 1940s cream-filled pastries were implicated in 15% of the outbreaks, but by the 1970s they accounted for only 2% (Bryan, 1976), and no foodborne disease outbreaks were attributed to them in 1978 and 1979 (CDC, 1981a,b).

Need for Microbiological Criteria

Cereal grains and their milled products have seldom been implicated as vehicles of foodborne disease and thus there does not appear to be a need for bacterial standards. On the other hand, because these foods are susceptible to mold growth, regulatory action levels for aflatoxins exist and are appropriate. Similar criteria for other mycotoxins may also be necessary if future studies show that there is a health hazard. Soy products that do not receive a heat treatment should be free of salmonellae and *Yersinia*.

Because grains, flour, grits, and related items are essentially raw agricultural products, and there is little opportunity for microbial growth during their processing, the microbiology of these foods usually does not correlate well with manufacturing practices. Guidelines for these foods, therefore, have little application.

Specifications may be useful when flour or some other grain product is used as a food ingredient, e.g., limits on thermophilic spores. Ready-to-eat cereal products, such as bakery items, should be free of enteric pathogens and toxins. The application of the HACCP concept is the best means for assuring that these foods will not be vehicles for foodborne illnesses.

Assessment of Information Necessary for Establishment of a Criterion if One Seems To Be Indicated

Information that can be utilized for the development of microbiological criteria is available in the literature (APHA, 1976; ICMSF, 1978, 1980;

Rayman et al., 1981). It is advisable for manufacturers to develop additional data through appropriate microbiological surveillance studies.

Where Criteria Should Be Applied

Criteria for mycotoxins should be applied to grain shipments as received at the mill. Microbiological specifications and guidelines for milled products, and especially for foods that contain them, might best be applied at the factory processing level as a component of an ongoing HACCP program. These criteria should be used for monitoring in-process critical control points as well as finished products for safety, wholesomeness, and stability.

References

APHA (American Public Health Association)
  1976   Compendium of Methods for the Microbiological Examination of Foods. M. L. Speck, ed. Washington, D.C.: APHA.
Aulisio, C.C.G., J. T. Stanfield, S. D. Weagant, and W. E. Hill
  1983   Yersiniosis associated with tofu consumption; serological, biochemical and pathogenicity studies of *Yersinia enterocolitica* isolates. J. Food Prot. 46:226-230,234.
Bryan, F. L.
  1976   Public health aspects of cream-filled pastries. A review. J. Milk Food Technol. 39:289-296.
Bryan, F. L., C. A. Bartleson, and N. Christopherson
  1981   Hazard analysis in reference to *Bacillus cereus* of boiled and fried rice in Cantonese-style restaurants. J. Food Prot. 44:500-512.
Busby, W. F., and G. N. Wogan
  1979   Foodborne Mycotoxins and Alimentary Mycotoxicoses. In Food-borne Infections and Intoxications. 2nd Ed., H. Riemann and F. L. Bryan, eds. New York: Academic Press.
CDC (Centers for Disease Control)
  1981a   Foodborne Disease Outbreaks. Annual Summary 1978. Atlanta: Centers for Disease Control.
  1981b   Foodborne Disease Outbreaks. Annual Summary 1979. Atlanta: Centers for Disease Control.
Denny, C. B., P. L. Tan, and C. W. Bohrer
  1966   Heat inactivation of staphylococcal enterotoxin A. J. Food Sci. 31:762-767.
Elliott, R. P.
  1967   Bacteriological Problems in the Manufacture of Oilseed Proteins. A presentation at the Conference on Engineering of Unconventional Protein Production. Santa Barbara, Calif.: American Institute of Chemical Engineers.
FDA (Food and Drug Administration)
  1982   Macaroni and Noodle Products. Code of Federal Regulations 21 CFR 139.
Hesseltine, C. W., R. F. Rogers, and R. J. Bothast
  1978   Microbiological study of exported soybeans. Cereal Chem. 55(3):332-340.

Hsieh, F., K. Acott, and T. P. Labuza
    1976   Death kinetics of pathogens in a pasta product. J. Food Sci. 41:516-519.
ICMSF (International Commission on Microbiological Specifications for Foods)
    1978   Microorganisms in Foods. 1. Their significance and methods of enumeration. Toronto: University of Toronto Press.
    1980   Microbial Ecology of Foods. Vol. 2: Food Commodities. New York: Academic Press.
Lee, W. H., C. L. Staples, and J. C. Olson, Jr.
    1975   *Staphylococcus aureus* growth and survival in macaroni dough and the persistence of enterotoxins in the dried products. J. Food Sci. 40:119-120.
Pylor, E. J.
    1973   Baking Science and Technology. 2nd Ed., Vol. 1. Chicago: Seibel Publishing.
Rayman, M. K., K. F. Weiss, G. W. Riedel, S. Charbonneau, and G. A. Jarvis
    1981   Microbiological quality of pasta products sold in Canada. J. Food Prot. 44:746-749.
Rogers, L. A., W. M. Clark, and A. C. Evans
    1915   The characteristics of bacteria of the colon type occurring on grains. J. Infect. Dis. 17:137-159.
Swain, E. W., H. L. Wang, and C. W. Hesseltine
    1981   Heat-Resistant Aerobic Bacterial Spores in Soybeans. Peoria, Ill.: Northern Regional Research Center, ARS, USDA.
Swartzentruber, A., W. L. Payne, B. A. Wentz, R. J. Barnard, and R. B. Read, Jr.
    1982   Microbiological quality of macaroni and noodle products obtained at retail markets. Appl. Environ. Microbiol. 44:540-543.
Trenholm, H. L., W. P. Cochrane, H. Cohen, J. I. Elliot, E. R. Farnworth, D. W. Friend, R.M.G. Hamilton, G. A. Neish, and J. F. Standish
    1981   Survey of vomitoxin contamination of the 1980 white winter wheat crop in Ontario, Canada. J. Amer. Oil Chem. Soc. 58(12):992A-994A.
Walsh, D. E., and B. R. Funke
    1975   The influence of spaghetti extruding, drying and storage on survival of *Staphylococcus aureus*. J. Food Sci. 40:714-716.
Walsh, D. E., B. R. Funke, and K. R. Graalum
    1974   Influence of spaghetti extruding conditions, drying and storage on the survival of *Salmonella typhimurium*. J. Food Sci. 39:1105-1106.

N. FATS AND OILS

Sensitivity of Products Relative to Safety and Quality

Fats and oils per se do not support growth of microorganisms. However, when in the presence of moisture and other essential nutrients, these products are subject to degradation by a variety of microorganisms. Such a condition is provided by several processed foods in which fats and oils are the major ingredients. Among such products, mayonnaise, salad dressings, peanut butter, margarine, and butter are of concern. Peanut butter differs from mayonnaise, salad dressing, margarine, and butter in that the water content (a_w) is too low to permit microbial growth and spoilage. If moisture is permitted to deposit on the surface of peanut butter, mold growth might, however, be possible.

Each of these products is an emulsion. Butter, margarine, and peanut butter represent foods that are emulsions comprised of oil (or fat) as the continuous phase and water as the discontinuous phase. Mayonnaise, salad dressing, and related products are emulsions in which water is the continuous phase and fat the discontinuous phase.

The form of emulsion has a profound relationship to microbial stability. With oil-in-water emulsions such as mayonnaise the growth rate of microorganisms is not affected by the water dispersion; only the chemical composition of the water phase plays a role. On the other hand, with water-in-oil emulsions such as butter the water exists as microscopic droplets that are dispersed throughout the oil matrix. If microorganisms are present in these droplets, their growth is restricted by limited water and food supply as well as by inhibitory factors in the aqueous phase, such as salt, preservatives, and organic acids (ICMSF, 1980).

Mayonnaise and Salad Dressings

The microbiology of these products has been reviewed by Smittle (1977) and ICMSF (1980). Mayonnaise and salad dressings are defined by standards of identity (FDA, 1978a,b).

The safety of these products relates directly to the pH (4.1 or below) and the acetic acid content (approximately 0.3-1.2%) of the moisture phase. Egg is the sensitive ingredient in mayonnaise and salad dressings because of the potential for *Salmonella* contamination from this source. However, salmonellae, if present, in properly prepared products die in a matter of days due to the low pH and the acetic acid content. Also, growth of *Clostridium botulinum*, *Clostridium perfringens*, *Bacillus cereus*, and *Staphylococcus aureus* is prevented. Thus the hazard presented by properly prepared products is remote.

Unfortunately, the federal standards of identity for mayonnaise and for salad dressings do not specify a pH of 4.1 or below for either of these products. In the case of mayonnaise, the acidity of vinegar or of vinegar diluted with water that is used in its preparation must be not less than 2.5% calculated as acetic acid. Presumably a pH of 4.1 in the aqueous phase of a properly formulated product would be assured. No specific concentration of acetic acid is specified in the standard of identity for salad dressings nor is a pH level specified. Thus, assurance of safety depends primarily upon the manufacturer's understanding of the necessity to produce a product having a pH of 4.1 or below. Neither standard of identity as presently written would guarantee that such a pH level would be obtained.

In some mayonnaise manufactured in Europe the acidifying agent is lemon or lime juice or hydrochloric acid instead of vinegar (acetic acid). Citric and hydrochloric acids are far less active than acetic acid against microorganisms.

In 1976 the World Health Organization cooperated with the Spanish authorities in investigating outbreaks of salmonellosis among passengers on four flights between Las Palmas, in the Canary Islands, and Helsinki. The flights were provisioned with egg mayonnaise. *Salmonella typhimurium* was isolated from several patients and one food handler and a batch of mayonnaise used for one of the meals. Many hundreds of victims were severely ill; there were six deaths (Davies and Wahba, 1976).

The hazards of improperly prepared mayonnaise are further illustrated by the following: In Denmark in 1975 mayonnaise from a salad factory caused approximatey 10,000 cases of salmonellosis. A circular was prepared by the Danish Administration recommending procedures for preparing mayonnaise so that the pH of the product would be lower than 4.5. These recommendations involved a certain proportion of egg yolk in vinegar and a holding time before use of either room temperature for four days or 40°C (104°F) for at least two hours. Since then no cases of salmonellosis caused by commercially prepared mayonnaise have occurred in Denmark (B. Simonsen, 1980. Personal communication). For a description of additional Danish outbreaks, see ICMSF (1980).

Mayonnaise and salad dressings are subject to microbial spoilage (Smittle, 1977; ICMSF, 1980). Generally, yeasts and lactobacilli are the spoilage organisms of concern. They may be introduced originally from contaminated ingredients. Small numbers of them usually are held in check by the acidity of the finished product. However, faulty sanitary practices during manufacture, i.e., failure to properly clean and sanitize pumps, mixing and filling equipment, and other product contact surfaces, may easily introduce numbers sufficiently great to bring about spoilage. Frequently, however, malfunctions of equipment rather than improper cleaning may be the direct cause of spoilage. For example, a faulty seal or gasket on a pump or filler may lead to accumulation of product behind the pump or filler housing. The normal sanitation procedures would require that the face of the pump or filler be cleaned and sanitized, the assumption being made that the portion of the equipment behind the face is sealed by a properly functioning gasket. With malfunction, product accumulates behind the face and may result in inoculation of the product with inordinately high numbers of spoilage organisms despite adequate normal cleaning. In this type of operation, periodic breakdown of equipment to determine the proper function, i.e., preventive maintenance, is a critical control point. Thus, the critical control points are equipment sanitation and, particularly, the proper functioning of the equipment. The latter can best be controlled by periodic breakdown of various key pieces of equipment to verify their proper functioning.

Peanut Butter

The federal standard of identity for peanut butter (FDA, 1978c) requires that it be made from ground shelled roasted peanuts to which may be added suitable seasoning and stabilizing ingredients not to exceed 10% by weight of the finished product. The fat content must not exceed 55%. The water content is less than 1%. For a review of the microbiology of peanut butter, see ICMSF (1980).

Lack of available moisture (low a_w) in peanut butter prevents growth of microorganisms in the product. Thus, foodborne illness caused by toxigenic microorganisms such as S. aureus, C. perfringens, C. botulinum, and B. cereus is precluded.

Occasionally Salmonella as well as other microorganisms occur in peanut butter, although no foodborne illness outbreaks have been reported. The source of contaminating organisms is almost always raw peanuts, which may contain Salmonella and a variety of other microorganisms, some of which are of public health concern. The roasting process destroys Salmonella, as well as other non-sporeforming bacteria. If, however, cross-contamination between the raw and roasted peanuts were to occur, it would not be catastrophic, since the occasional Salmonella (much as in inert material) would be "diluted out" in the finished product since the moisture content of the finished product is sufficiently low as to prevent Salmonella growth. Problems arise when processing equipment used after the roaster process is wet-cleaned or if moisture is not completely controlled in the processing equipment, i.e., condensate from pipes or leaking water valves permitting water to accumulate on floors or on the surfaces of equipment, which would permit Salmonella growth.

Control of the processing environment is the primary critical control point in the manufacture of peanut butter. This control requires physical separation of raw and roasted peanuts to prevent contamination of the processing environment with microorganisms present in the raw peanuts (in particular Salmonella). It requires further the complete control of moisture in the processing environment. If wet cleanup becomes necessary, this must be undertaken with extreme care, with provision being made to rapidly dry areas that have been subject to cleaning and sanitizing.

Yet another concern is the occurrence of aflatoxin in the raw peanuts. Control is generally accomplished by pretesting incoming shipments of raw peanuts and rejecting those showing aflatoxin levels greater than the accepted level (20 ppb). Further control is generally exercised by electronic sorting of the roasted peanuts, a process that tends to eliminate peanuts with high levels of aflatoxin.

Although the likelihood of peanut butter being involved in *Salmonella* outbreaks appears remote, manufacturers would be well advised to routinely test production batches for *Salmonella*. Plant guidelines for aerobic plate count, coliform, and *Escherichia coli* can be useful as indicators of cross-contamination.

Margarine and Butter

For a review of the microbiology of these products see ICMSF (1980). The microbiological stability of margarine and butter is dependent upon heat treatment (pasteurization) of the ingredients, prevention of postpasteurization contamination and minute dispersion of water droplets in the fat (continuous) phase of the finished products. In the case of margarine, stability is further enhanced by certain preservatives that are permitted by the standard of identity for this product (FDA, 1978d). Failure to achieve the above conditions may lead to growth of spoilage organisms as well as pathogens. Reported outbreaks involving these products are rare.

Whipped butter and high moisture margarines are more susceptible to microbial growth due primarily to poorer dispersion of water in the fat phase. Two recent staphylococcal foodborne illness outbreaks due to whipped butter have occurred (CDC, 1970, 1977). Studies that have demonstrated the ability of *S. aureus* to grow in mildly salted whipped butter (Minor and Marth, 1972) point up the hazard that this product may present. Current technology of butter and margarine manufacture can virtually assure a relatively stable product with excellent keeping quality. On occasion movement of butter or margarine from refrigerated to warmer environments may lead to the deposition of moisture on exposed surfaces. This can result in development of mold.

Need for Microbiological Criteria

Mayonnaise and Salad Dressings

There is little if any justification for imposing a microbiological criterion for *Salmonella* or for any other pathogen. However, control of pH is critical to the safety of these products. In view of the many different manufacturers of mayonnaise and salad dressings and especially the ever increasing types of salad dressings available to the public, it would seem prudent to amend the standards of identity for these products to include a requirement for a pH of 4.1 or below in the aqueous phase.

Microbiological guidelines applicable at critical control points of manufacture should be useful. In addition to the APC, yeasts and molds and lactobacilli counts are applicable to evaluate plant sanitation and to detect potential spoilage problems (Kurtsman and Smittle, 1984). Direct microscopic examination of product is useful when product spoilage is being investigated.

Peanut Butter

A standard with respect to *Salmonella* would be applicable for peanut butter, this being a product that is generally consumed without cooking and is, indeed, a product that is apt to be consumed by the very young and the aged, groups highly susceptible to *Salmonella* infection.

Margarine and Butter

The rarity of involvement in outbreaks indicates that little would be served by imposing any regulatory criteria for butter and margarine, not withstanding the current USDA recommended criteria (see Chapter 8, Table 8-4). However, in-plant guidelines for APC and for *S. aureus*, particularly in the case of whipped butter, should be applied at critical control points of manufacture.

Where Criteria Should Be Applied

Microbiological guidelines are most usefully applied at the processing plant level at the critical control points for each of the products as identified earlier in this section.

References

CDC (Center for Disease Control)
    1970   Staphylococcal food poisoning traced to butter—Alabama. Morb. Mort. Weekly Rpt. 19:271.
    1977   Presumed staphylococcal food poisoning associated with whipped butter. Morb. Mort. Weekly Rpt. 26:268.
Davies, R. F., and A. H. Wahba
    1976   *Salmonella* infections of charter flight passengers. Report on a visit to Spain (Canary Islands) February 26th–March 2, 1976. Copenhagen: World Health Organization, Regional Office, Europe.
FDA (Food and Drug Administration)
    1978a   Mayonnaise. Code of Federal Regulations 21 CFR 169.140.
    1978b   Salad Dressings. Code of Federal Regulations 21 CFR 169.150. Washington, D.C.: U.S. Government Printing Office.

1978c   Peanut Butter. Code of Federal Regulations 21 CFR 164.150. Washington, D.C.: U.S. Government Printing Office.

1978d   Margarine. Code of Federal Regulations 21 CFR 166.110. Washington, D.C.: U.S. Government Printing Office.

ICMSF (International Commission on Microbiological Specifications for Foods).

1980   Microbial Ecology of Foods. Vol. 2. Food Commodities. New York: Academic Press.

Kurtzman, C. P., and R. B. Smittle

1984   Salad dressings. In Compendium of Methods for the Microbiological Examination of Foods. 2nd Ed. M. L. Speck, ed. Washington, D.C.: APHA.

Minor, T. E., and E. H. Marth

1972   *Staphylococcus aureus* and enterotoxin A in cream and butter. J. Dairy Sci. 55:1410–1414.

Smittle, R. B.

1977   Microbiology of mayonnaise and salad dressing: A review. J. Food Prot. 40:415–422.

O. SUGAR, COCOA, CHOCOLATE, AND CONFECTIONERIES

Sensitivity of Products Relative to Safety and Quality

These products have been involved only infrequently in foodborne disease outbreaks (ICMSF, 1980). Although the risks are low, the potential of such products to lead to major outbreaks cannot be ignored. Witness to this was the 1973-1974 outbreak of salmonellosis involving chocolate candy (D'Aoust, 1977).

Microbial spoilage of these commodities is rare due to low water activities, although specific problems involving yeasts, molds, and sporeformers have been documented (ICMSF, 1980). The HACCP system should be applied in the production of cocoa, chocolate products, and confections. Critical control points should be monitored microbiologically when indicated.

Sugar

Because of the source and nature of sugar, microorganisms are intrinsically present. These organisms include thermophilic sporeformers such as *Bacillus stearothermophilus*, *Bacillus coagulans*, and *Clostridium thermosaccharolyticum*. The spores of these organisms, while generally innocuous under usual storage conditions, have proved to be a nuisance to the canning industry. Thus, the National Food Processors Association (NCA, 1972) and other groups have developed specifications for bacterial spores in sugar. Liquid sugar is likely to give rise to problems with growth of osmophilic yeasts.

Cocoa and Chocolate Products

The predominant microorganisms in cocoa are *Bacillus*, yeasts, and molds (Gabis et al., 1970; ICMSF, 1980). The number of these organisms depends on the inherent contamination and control of the process. The level of heat-resistant spores found in cocoa (Gabis et al., 1970) should be controlled because they may cause spoilage in high moisture products where cocoa is an ingredient, for example, chocolate milk.

Salmonella in cocoa (Collins-Thompson et al., 1978; D'Aoust, 1977) make it a sensitive ingredient. When contaminated, the numbers of salmonellae are usually low, less than 1/g (D'Aoust, 1977; ICMSF, 1980). Milk chocolate made from contaminated cocoa was responsible for over 200 cases in 1973-1974. In this outbreak, the contaminated chocolate contained 20-90 cells of *S. eastbourne* per 100 g (D'Aoust et al., 1975; Craven et al., 1975). Thus, low levels of *Salmonella* can cause human infection (see Chapter 4, Table 4-3).

Organisms capable of surviving the processes used in chocolate manufacture belong primarily to the genus *Bacillus* (Barrile et al., 1971; Collins-Thompson et al., 1981). The key to low spore counts in chocolate appears to be the quality of the cocoa bean. The low water activity of chocolate does not permit outgrowth of the contaminating organisms but may give rise to spoilage problems when chocolate is used as an ingredient in foods with higher water activities. Sources of *Salmonella* in chocolate have been traced back to cocoa (D'Aoust, 1977) and milk powder. The final heating (conching) cannot be relied upon to kill all *Salmonella* in the product.

There are no steps in the manufacturing operation that assure destruction of microorganisms. The water activities of both the ingredients and the finished chocolate preclude microbial growth. Wet cleaning should not be employed in chocolate and confectionery manufacture.

Confectionery

The multitude of ingredients in confectionery including sugar, milk products, egg albumin, gums, nuts, fruits, and spices can give rise to microbial spoilage problems. Many of these are kept in check, however, as a result of low water activity. Fondants and other products vulnerable to spoilage have water activities in the 0.75-0.85 range. The spoilage of such products is usually caused by osmophilic yeasts (ICMSF, 1980). Residual lipolytic enzymes of microbial origin may give rise to soapy off-flavors in chocolate-containing confectionery after extended storage.

While sugar has not been shown to be a source of *Salmonella*, other confectionery ingredients such as dried eggs, milk, coconut, and gelatin are classified as critical raw materials because they may contain *Salmonella* (D'Aoust, 1977). Also, there are no steps in most confectionery processing to destroy these microorganisms.

Another safety concern with confectionery is the presence of mycotoxins in nuts. Confectionery products containing aflatoxin-contaminated nuts in excess of aflatoxin standards are subject to regulatory action. Since it is impossible to remove these toxins by heating, the raw ingredients should be inspected for mycotoxins as part of an ongoing HACCP program (see part S of this chapter).

Needs for Microbiological Criteria and Where Criteria Should Be Applied

Sugar

Microbiological criteria are important for sugar to be used as an ingredient in the canning, beverage, and confectionery industries. The canning industry has specifications for thermophilic, flat-sour, and sulfide spoilage spores (NCA, 1972). The bottling industry has developed criteria for mesophilic bacteria, yeasts, and molds (National Soft Drink Association, 1975). The specification for sugar to be used in soft drinks are ≤ 10 yeasts and ≤ 10 molds per 10 grams of sugar (Anonymous, 1971). These specifications appear adequate for the purposes intended. In the manufacture of confectioneries, liquid sugar is a critical control point because of the potential for growth of osmophilic yeasts. Therefore, microbiological criteria are applicable as part of a HACCP program.

Cocoa and Chocolate

Various microbiological criteria are useful (ICMSF, 1980). For example, specifications for ingredients of retorted products such as cocoa beverages should include limits for thermophilic spores (NCA, 1972).

It is appropriate to examine cocoa and chocolate for *Salmonella*. Sampling plans should be based upon the intended use of these products (NRC, 1969).

The HACCP program is recommended for chocolate production. Raw material inspection and testing to ensure that the incoming ingredients are *Salmonella*-free are necessary components of the HACCP system as the usual processing steps will not destroy *Salmonella*. The plant environment must be maintained free of *Salmonella*. Appropriate points should be monitored by regular collection and analyses of environmental samples.

Confectionery

Microbiological criteria are appropriate when applied to ingredients used in confectionery products. Guidelines for osmophilic yeasts are applicable for soft-centered chocolates, which are particularly prone to fermentation. Critical ingredients such as cocoa, coconut, dried milk, and egg albumin should be examined for *Salmonella*. Tolerances for aflatoxins are applicable for products containing nuts (see part S). As with the production of chocolate products, the environment is a critical control point (see above).

References

Anonymous
  1971   Beverage Production and Plant Operation. Washington, D.C.: National Soft Drink Association.
Barrile, J. C., K. Ostovar, and P. G. Keeney
  1971   Microflora of cocoa beans before and after roasting at 150°C. J. Milk Food Technol. 34: 369-371.
Collins-Thompson, D. L., K. F. Weiss, G. W. Riedel, and S. Charbonneau
  1978   Sampling plans and guidelines for domestic and imported cocoa from a Canadian national microbiological survey. Can. Inst. Food Sci. Technol. J. 11: 177-179.
Collins-Thompson, D. L., K. F. Weiss, G. W. Riedel, and C. B. Cushing
  1981   Survey of and microbiological guidelines for chocolate and chocolate products in Canada. Can. Inst. Food Sci. Technol. J. 14: 203-208.
Craven, P. C., D. C. Mackel, W. B. Baine, W. H. Barker, E. J. Gangarosa, M. Goldfield, H. Rosenfeld, R. Altman, G. Lachapelle, J. W. Davies, and R. C. Swanson
  1975   International outbreak of *Salmonella eastbourne* infection traced to contaminated chocolate. Lancet 1: 788-793.
D'Aoust, J. Y.
  1977   Salmonella and the chocolate industry. A review. J. Food Prot. 40: 718-727.
D'Aoust, J. Y., B. J. Aris, P. Thisdele, A. Durante, N. Brisson, D. Dragon, G. Lachapelle, M. Johnston, and R. Laidley
  1975   *Salmonella eastbourne* outbreak associated with chocolate. Can. Inst. Food Sci. Technol. J. 8:181-184.
Gabis, D. A., B. E. Langlois, and A. W. Rudnick
  1970   Microbiological examination of cocoa powder. Appl. Microbiol. 20: 644-645.
ICMSF (International Commission on Microbiological Specifications for Foods)
  1980   Sugar, cocoa, chocolate, and confectioneries. Pp. 778-821 in Microbial Ecology of Foods. Vol. 2. Food Commodities. New York: Academic Press.
National Soft Drink Association
  1975   Quality Specifications and Test Procedures for Bottlers: Granulated and Liquid Sugar. Washington, D.C.: National Soft Drink Association.
NCA (National Canners Association)
  1972   Bacterial Standards for Sugar. June 1972. Revised. Washington, D.C.: NCA.
NRC (National Research Council)
  1969   An Evaluation of the *Salmonella* Problem. Committee on *Salmonella*. Publication 1683. Washington, D.C.: National Academy of Sciences.

P. SPICES

Spices are the dried parts of plants which are used mainly as flavoring agents for foods. Some, such as black pepper in a household shaker, may be added to a food immediately before consumption (table spice), while others may be used as ingredients of foods that will receive further processing.

Sensitivity of Products Relative to Safety and Quality

As raw agricultural commodities, uncleaned and untreated spices commonly contain high microbial populations (APHA, 1976; ICMSF, 1980; Julseth and Deibel, 1974; Schwab et al., 1982). Spice-bearing plants are exposed to a wide variety of microorganisms from the environment in which they are grown and harvested. Furthermore, during drying, often a simple procedure utilizing the sun, significant microbial growth may occur. Numerous species of bacteria, yeasts, and molds constitute the normal microflora of dried spices (Christensen et al., 1967; Julseth and Deibel, 1974; Schwab et al., 1982), although aerobic sporeforming bacteria usually predominate (APHA, 1976; ICMSF, 1980). While bacteria generally are not responsible for the spoilage of spices, growth of fungi during storage and shipping may result in the development of off-flavors and in the production of undesirable enzymes (ICMSF, 1980).

Spices can be a source of spoilage microorganisms when they are used as seasonings for processed foods. For example, they may introduce heat-resistant spores into canned foods and a variety of spoilage bacteria into refrigerated products such as processed meats (ICMSF, 1980).

Bacteria of public health significance, e.g., *Clostridium perfringens* (Krishnaswamy et al., 1971; Leitao et al., 1975; Powers et al., 1975), *Bacillus cereus* (Kim and Goepfert, 1971; Powers et al., 1976), *Escherichia coli* (Kadis et al., 1971), *Staphylococcus aureus* (Julseth and Deibel, 1974; Schwab et al., 1982) and *Salmonella* (ICMSF, 1980; Laidley et al., 1974; Health and Welfare Canada, 1983) may be present but usually in low numbers. Mycotoxin-generating molds also have been isolated from spices (Christensen et al., 1967) and low levels of aflatoxin, usually under 10 μg/kg, have been detected (Scott and Kennedy, 1975).

Although contaminated spices have not been major causes of foodborne disease, a potential hazard exists, especially if the spice is to be used as a table condiment. Contaminated pepper, for example, was responsible for at least 126 cases of salmonellosis (CDC, 1982).

Need for Microbiological Criteria

The end use for a spice will determine the type of criterion that might be needed. Table spices and those used as ingredients of processed foods that do not receive a subsequent lethal treatment should be free of infectious pathogens such as *Salmonella*; therefore they should be tested for this pathogen.

Guidelines may be useful for monitoring processes applied to spices, in particular the treatment used to destroy much of the intrinsic microflora. Exposure to ethylene oxide gas is the common process, although there is concern at present about some of the products that are formed. The Environmental Protection Agency has set residue tolerances of 50 ppm ethylene oxide in treated spices (EPA, 1982). Treatment of spices with ionizing irradiations, a maximum of 1 megarad, has recently been approved (FDA, 1983).

References

APHA (American Public Health Association)
   1976   Compendium of Methods for the Microbiological Examination of Foods. M. L. Speck, ed. Washington, D.C.: APHA.
CDC (Centers for Disease Control)
   1982   Outbreak of *Salmonella oranienburg*-Norway. Morb. Mort. Weekly Rpt. 31(48):655-656.
Christensen, C. M., H. A. Fanse, G. H. Nelson, F. Bates, and C. J. Mirocha
   1967   Microflora of black and red pepper. Appl. Microbiol. 15:622-626.
EPA (U.S. Environmental Protection Agency)
   1982   Ethylene oxide; tolerances for residues. Code of Federal Regulations 40 CFR 180.151.
FDA (Food and Drug Administration)
   1983   Irradiation in the production, processing and handling of food. Final rule. Federal Register (48) 129:30613-30614. July 5.
Health and Welfare Canada
   1983   *Salmonella* in spices and chocolate. Canada Diseases Weekly Report 9(9):35-36.
ICMSF (International Commission on Microbiological Specifications for Foods)
   1980   Microbial Ecology of Foods. Vol. 2. Food Commodities. New York: Academic Press.
Julseth, R. M., and R. H. Deibel
   1974   Microbial profile of selected spices and herbs at import. J. Milk Food Technol. 37:414-419.
Kadis, V. M., D. A. Hill, and K. S. Pennifold
   1971   Bacterial content of gravy bases and gravies obtained in restaurants. Can. Inst. Food Technol. J. 4:130-132.
Kim, H. U., and J. M. Goepfert
   1971   Occurrence of *Bacillus cereus* in selected dry food products. J. Milk Food Technol. 34:12-15.
Krishnaswamy, M. A., J. D. Patel, and N. Parthasarathy
   1971   Enumeration of microorganism in spices and spice mixtures. J. Food Sci. Technol. 8:191-194.

Laidley, R., S. Handzel, D. Severs, and R. Butler
    1974   *Salmonella weltevreden* outbreaks associated with contaminated pepper. Epidemiol.
           Bull. 18:62. Ottawa: Dept. Natl. Health Welfare.
Leitao, M. F., I. Delazari, and H. Mazzoni
    1975   Microbiology of dehydrated foods (Coletanea Inst. Technol. Aliment. 5:223-241).
           Tech. Abstr. from Food Science 7, 9 B72.
Powers, E. M., R. Lawyer, and Y. Masuoka
    1975   Microbiology of processed spices. J. Milk Food Technol. 38:683-687.
Powers, E. M., T. G. Latt, and T. Brown
    1976   Incidence and levels of *Bacillus cereus* in processed spices. J. Milk Food Technol.
           39:668-670.
Schwab, A. H., A. D. Harpestad, A. Swartzentruber, J. M. Lanier, B. A. Wentz, A. P. Duran,
R. J. Barnard, and R. B. Read, Jr.
    1982   Microbiological quality of some spices and herbs in retail markets. Appl. Environ.
           Microbiol. 44:627-630.
Scott, P. M., and B.P.C. Kennedy
    1975   The analysis of spices and herbs for aflatoxins. Can. Inst. Food Sci. Technol. J.
           8:124-125.

Q. YEASTS

Sensitivity of Products Relative to Safety and Quality

Baker's yeast is grown in open fermentors and thus during propagation may be contaminated with low numbers of lactic acid bacteria and sometimes with coliforms including *Escherichia coli* (Reed and Peppler, 1973). Following the fermentation, the cells are centrifuged and washed several times and then concentrated to about 30% solids using presses or filters. The yeast may then be packaged and marketed as compressed yeast cake or it may be dried at a low temperature to produce active dry yeast. A third product is nutritional yeast, which consists of cells killed by drying at high temperatures on drum dryers.

Both live yeast and nutritional yeast have on occasion been contaminated with salmonellae (NRC, 1975). They may not be present in the fermentors but can be introduced at subsequent processing steps. The dead yeast cells that collect on equipment surfaces constitute an excellent growth medium for bacteria and thus soiled equipment may be a significant source of contamination (Reed and Peppler, 1973). Since nutritional yeast is heated to a high temperature during drum drying, the presence of viable salmonellae represents contamination following this treatment.

The spores of certain bacilli are another concern because their introduction into dough may result in ropy bread.

Need for Microbiological Criteria

Many yeast companies have established internal guidelines for levels of bacteria, wild yeasts, and molds. These guidelines aid in assessing conditions of sanitation in the fermentors and during subsequent processing.

The testing of yeast products for *Salmonella* is appropriate, and specific methods have been developed (FDA, 1978). The presence of the pathogen in nutritional yeast is of special concern since this food may not be heated prior to consumption. Baking, on the other hand, would destroy the salmonellae introduced with the active dry or compressed yeast.

References

FDA (Food and Drug Administration)
   1978   FDA Bacteriological Analytical Manual. Washington, D.C.: Association of Official Analytical Chemists.
NRC (National Research Council)
   1975   Prevention of Microbial and Parasitic Hazards Associated with Processed Foods: A Guide for the Food Processor. Committee on Food Protection. Washington, D.C.: National Academy of Sciences.
Reed, G., and H. J. Peppler
   1973   Yeast Technology. Westport, Conn.: AVI Publishing.

R.   FORMULATED FOODS

Sensitivity of Products Relative to Safety and Quality

Formulated foods have been described as commercially prepared, ready-to-cook or ready-to-eat foods containing major ingredients from two or more commodity categories (ICMSF, 1985). The potential hazards of the major ingredients of these foods are discussed in other sections of this chapter. The combining of these ingredients into a single product presents not only the original hazards of each ingredient, but also the possibility of magnified or additional hazards due to further handling, process innovations, or modification of the environment. For example, the chicken, gravy, vegetables, and spices in a chicken potpie carry their own hazards and also carry additional potential hazards due to increased handling, possible temperature abuse during the time spent in such handling, and the possibility that a microbiological situation of no concern in the original ingredients is of concern in the formulated food. Beef and chicken potpies have been the cause of botulism as a result of gross abuse by the consumer when heated pies were held at room or slightly higher temperatures for extensive periods of time (CDC, 1960; State of California, 1975, 1976).

Formulated foods have increased in number, diversity, and volume to meet the public's desire for more convenience. Today less food is being prepared from the basic ingredients in the home kitchen where it is likely to be consumed soon thereafter and where any outbreaks are likely to be limited to a small number of consumers. In contrast, increased amounts of food are now produced in factories and held for some time in distribution channels before they are eaten. Under these conditions there is increased potential for abuse and any foodborne illnesses will most likely affect a much larger number of consumers.

The responsibility for preserving safety and keeping quality of foods lies with the processor or formulator of the food. As a result of the increased number and volume of formulated foods, this responsibility has shifted somewhat from the individual in the home to the commercial processor. Because of large differences in composition, preparation, and storage of the many formulated foods, each formulated food or group of foods presents particular circumstances relative to assessment of needs for microbiological criteria (see Chapter 2). Criteria for some formulated foods have been discussed by the ICMSF (1984). However, no general all-product criteria can be developed. Instead, the potential hazards of each product or group of products must be identified and appropriately monitored if microbial growth and resulting health hazard or spoilage are to be prevented during the time the product is under producer control or in appropriate storage. The HACCP systems may include control points in addition to those developed for the separate ingredients. (See for example the discussion of critical control points for frozen foods by Peterson and Gunnerson, 1974.)

Means of preventing growth during storage depend on the conditions of processing, the temperature of storage, and the composition of the product. For example, some formulated foods, e.g., beef stew, liquid infant formula, chili, and tamales, are sterilized in a sealed container. These products are shelf-stable and need no more microbiological criteria than do other low-acid canned foods (see part J).

Other formulated foods are simple blends of dry ingredients, e.g., dried infant formula, soup mix, or cake mix. These foods also are shelf-stable, but they can be hazardous if an ingredient is contaminated with a pathogenic organism such as *Salmonella*. Both the FDA and the international Codex Alimentarius Commission recognize the need for the imposition of stringent standards on formulated foods designed for use by high-risk populations. The FDA is the more stringent of the two in the application of microbiological criteria to this broad group of products.

The FDA prescribed (FDA, 1978) analytical procedures for ingredients such as dried yeast, cheese, and pasta frequently used in blended formulated foods. While proper use of such formulated foods or their ingredients would destroy salmonellae, regulatory concern with respect to cross-contamination or inadequate heat treatment exists. Numerous recalls of dried blended soups and other foods have occurred and standards or implied standards for salmonellae have been imposed.

The Codex Alimentarius Committee on Food Hygiene concluded that microbiological criteria are not justified in the case of dried soup mixes. However, the committee has established microbiological end product specifications for some products that do require special attention either because they contain pathogenic organisms that may survive cooking procedures or because they are typically eaten by highly susceptible persons such as the very young, the aged, or those who are ill (Codex Alimentarius Commission, 1979a). These products include coated or filled dried shelf-stable biscuits for which criteria for coliforms and *Salmonella* were imposed, and also dried and instant products requiring reconstitution and dried products requiring heating to boiling before consumption for which criteria for APC, coliforms, and *Salmonella* were established.

A few formulated foods can be stored at room temperature because of their high acidity, e.g., mustard dressings, or their low water activity, e.g., certain pastries with butter cream fillings (see part M).

Most formulated foods are preserved by storage at low temperatures. Some are simply refrigerated, e.g., meat and seafood salads and sandwiches, but the majority are frozen, e.g., dishes such as meat potpies, egg rolls, pizza, and enchiladas. Microbiological hazards are diminished if the products are thoroughly heated before consumption.

An Example: Ready-to-eat Salads

Ready-to-eat salads are one class of formulated foods for which microbiological criteria are often considered. Most, but not all, of these salads have four characteristics in common: (1) they contain at least one raw ingredient, (2) they are ready-to-eat when purchased, (3) they are exposed to contamination during preparation, and (4) they are normally preserved by refrigeration but often suffer temperature abuse. Clearly, products with these characteristics are potential public health problems. Particularly vulnerable are those ready-to-eat salads containing high-protein foods such as diced or chopped meat, seafood, poultry, cheese, boiled eggs, and/or cooked potatoes. Salads made of diced ham, chicken, egg, or potato have been responsible for many outbreaks of foodborne disease during the past several decades (see, for example, CDC, 1981). Salads composed of raw celery, onion, peppers, carrots, or other vegetables are less likely to present microbial hazards. Other types of salads include diced fruit, gelatin with marshmallows, cooked macaroni with cheese or canned peas, and shredded cabbage (cole slaw). The variations in composition are almost limitless.

The microbial content of salads (or delicatessen foods, as they are sometimes called) has received a great deal of attention from regulatory agencies. Several microbiological criteria in the form of standards or guidelines have been established (Wehr, 1982). Unfortunately, these criteria usually do not reflect the basic differences between products. It is common for an agency to specify a single set of limits and requirements for all salads regardless of the composition of each. For example, the APC limit for all types of salads may be to not exceed 100,000 per gram while the coliform count may be to not exceed 100 per gram. Criteria such as these which fail to recognize the wide diversity of ingredients that go into salads are ill-advised. The natural microflora of raw vegetables, for example, can easily exceed 1,000,000 per gram. These organisms are perfectly harmless, yet salad manufacturers may have to soak vegetables in chlorine solution in order to meet an arbitrary limit of 100,000 per gram. For the same reason, a manufacturer may have to use processed cheese with typically lower counts rather than natural cheese in order to meet a general microbiological criterion. On the other hand, a limit of 100,000 per gram may be high for gelatin salads or other products made entirely of cooked ingredients.

In summary, then, microbiological criteria may be useful in revealing health hazards and breaches of good food-handling practice with certain types of salad items. Both the criteria and the types of salads to which they are applied must be carefully selected if they are to be meaningful. The current practice of applying the same criteria to all salads regardless of composition and potential hazard of each salad type reveals a lack of understanding of both the potential health hazards of salads and of appropriate solutions.

Need for Microbiological Criteria

Owing to the wide diversity of composition, preparation, and storage conditions, it is not possible to develop a single set of microbiological criteria that are suitable for all formulated foods. However, criteria have been established and are appropriate for certain classes of formulated foods as discussed above. Establishment of criteria should be preceded by consideration of the product as outlined in the foregoing section so as to decide what, if any, microbiological criteria would offer protection against health hazards and poor quality.

Assessment of Information Necessary for Establishment of a Criterion if One Seems To Be Indicated

Factors that determine the potential usefulness of microbiological criteria with formulated foods include:

1. The nature and extent of contamination: Ingredients that are traditionally associated with salmonellae, for example, should be subjected to routine testing for these organisms, especially if the product is likely to be consumed without thorough cooking.

2. Likelihood of contamination during preparation: Any product that is subjected to handling can be expected to contain a few coagulase-positive staphylococci; excessive numbers suggest breaches of good manufacturing practice.

3. Bactericidal treatment(s) during processing: Commercial pasteurization or sterilization will eliminate all pathogenic organisms from a food. Hence, the application of microbiological criteria to products that have undergone a terminal heat treatment usually is not cost-effective. Efficacy of heating can better be monitored by measuring temperature or enzyme destruction or by other appropriate means. Microbiological criteria may be appropriate, however, if there is opportunity for recontamination with pathogens after heating.

4. Likelihood of growth during storage: Under proper conditions of storage, microorganisms do not grow in a canned (heat sterilized), frozen, or dried product. In fact, bacteria gradually die off during frozen or dry storage. Abuses such as thawing and holding prior to refreezing or inadvertent moistening of a dry product may allow microbial growth. The occurrence of such abuse is sporadic and may occur in any of a number of places in the distribution system. Therefore, routine application of microbiological criteria is not an effective way to detect specific abuse situations. In the production of refrigerated formulated foods, microbiological guidelines can be usefully applied by the processor to assess potential shelf-life. However, the application of such criteria after the product has left the processing facility is not recommended.

5. Susceptibility of consumer: The very young, the aged, and the infirm are known to be more susceptible to infection by salmonellae and other pathogens than are healthy adults. Therefore, special care must be taken with foods intended for infants, hospital patients, residents of nursing homes, and other highly susceptible groups of people at elevated risk.

Microbiological criteria often are appropriate for these foods. (For further discussion, see Chapter 3 and Codex Alimentarius Commission, 1979b.)

References

CDC (Centers for Disease Control)
1960 Botulism. Morb. Mort. Weekly Rpt. 9:2.
1981 Foodborne Disease Outbreaks. Annual Summary 1979. Atlanta: Centers for Disease Control.
Codex Alimentarius Commission
1979a Microbiological specifications for foods for infants and children. Alinorm 79/13. Appendix V.
1979b Code of Hygienic Practices for Infants and Children, Appendix V. Report of the 16th Session of the Codex Committee on Food Hygiene, Codex Alimentarius Commission. Rome: Food and Agriculture Organization.
FDA (Food and Drug Administration)
1978 FDA Bacteriological Analytical Manual. Washington, D.C.: Association of Official Analytical Chemists.
ICMSF (International Commission on Microbiological Specifications for Foods)
1985 Formulated foods. In Microorganisms in Foods. 2. Sampling for microbiological analyses: Principles and specific applications. 2nd Ed. In preparation.
Peterson, A. C., and R. E. Gunnerson
1974 Microbiological critical control points in frozen foods. Food Technol. 28 (9):37–44.
State of California (Department of Health Services)
1975 Botulism—home canned figs and chicken pot pie. Calif. Morbidity. No. 46.
1976 Type A botulism associated with commercial pot pie. Calif. Morbidity. No. 51.
Wehr, H. M.
1982 Attitudes and policies of governmental agencies on microbial criteria for foods—an update. Food Technol. 36(9):45–54,92.

S. NUTS

Sensitivity of Products Relative to Safety and Quality

The meats of tree nuts are usually sterile when in the intact shell. Microbial contamination may occur during their harvest, transport, and processing (Hall, 1971; Hyndman, 1963; King et al., 1970; Kokal and Thorpe, 1969; Meyer and Vaughn, 1969). Microorganisms may be introduced as a result of insect infestation, e.g., immature almonds are attacked by the navel orange worm. The shells of tree nuts may be contaminated with enteric organisms, especially if they come in contact with the ground. Permitting cattle and other animals to graze in nut groves increases the opportunity for contamination by fecal microorganisms; collecting the nuts on clean canvas minimizes this problem. Nuts exposed to water, either for washing or tempering, are prone to contamination, especially if there has been a separation of the sutures. Microorganisms present on the shell may also be introduced onto meats during the cracking operation. Bacterial growth on nut meats is rarely a problem due to their low a_w. An exception is the coconut, which may develop leaks, become contaminated, and then support growth of various species, including salmonellae, in the coconut milk (Schaffner et al., 1967). When present, salmonellae may survive the drying process given to coconut meat. Elimination of the pathogen depends upon pasteurization in hot water prior to drying.

Peanuts (*Arachis hypogaea*) are subject to contamination from soil fungi, including species that produce aflatoxins. Mold growth may occur prior to harvest or when the peanuts have been dried insufficiently or stored under humid conditions (Marth and Calanog, 1976). Tree nuts such as pecans, almonds, pistachios, and Brazil nuts also may contain aflatoxins. The molds often are introduced via insect penetration.

Need for Microbiological Criteria

Nut meats are used primarily as ingredients of foods such as bakery products. Because they can be a source of spoilage organisms, purchase specifications for nut meats may contain limits on the microorganisms of concern such as molds.

Epidemiological evidence indicates that nut meats are not a significant vehicle of foodborne disease. However, a microbiological standard does exist in that the Food and Drug Administration has taken the position that the presence of *Escherichia coli* on nut meats is evidence of filth and thus adulteration; apparently growers and processors usually can produce a product that is free of this organism.

Salmonellae have been a problem in dried coconut; therefore, these products should be tested for this pathogen. The presence of aflatoxins in nut meats is a chronic problem, especially in peanuts and peanut products. Standards that place limits on the permitted concentration of unavoidable toxins should be continued (see Chapter 8 and this chapter, part N).

References

Hall, H. E.
1971   The significance of *Escherichia coli* associated with nut meats. Food Technol. 25 (3):230-232.
Hyndman, J. B.
1963   Comparison of enterococci and coliform microorganisms in commercially produced pecan nut meats. Appl. Microbiol. 11:268-272.
King, A. D., Jr., M. J. Miller, and L. C. Eldridge
1970   Almond harvesting, processing, and microbial flora. Appl. Microbiol. 20:208-214.

Kokal, D., and D. W. Thorpe
1969   Occurrence of *Escherichia coli* in almonds of nonpareil variety. Food Technol. 23(2):93-98.

Marth, E. H., and B. G. Calanog
1976   Toxigenic fungi. In Food Microbiology: Public Health and Spoilage Aspects, M. P. DeFigueiredo and D. F. Splittstoesser, eds. Westport, Conn.: AVI Publishing.

Meyer, M. T., and R. H. Vaughn
1969   Incidence of *Escherichia coli* in black walnut meats. Appl. Microbiol. 18:925-931.

Schaffner, C. P., K. Mosbach, V. C. Bibit, and C. H. Watson
1967   Coconut and *Salmonella* infection. Appl. Microbiol. 15:471-475.

T. MISCELLANEOUS ADDITIVES

A number of food additives used by the food industry are derived from animals, plants, or microorganisms. Three of the larger classes of additives are gums, enzymes, and food colors. Only limited published information is available regarding the microbiology of these substances.

Sensitivity of Products Relative to Safety and Quality

Gums

Gums hydrate in water to form viscous solutions or dispersions and thus exhibit useful suspending, dispersion, and stabilizing properties. They function in foods as emulsifiers, gelling agents, binders, flocculating agents, film formers, foam stabilizers, release agents, and lubricants. With this range of functional properties, they are widely used in dairy products, sauces, pie fillings, whipped toppings, salad dressings, puddings, and jellies.

The sources of these useful polysaccharides are the resinous exudates of trees (acacia, karaya, tragacanth), seeds (locust bean, guar), seaweed (agar, alginates, carrageenan), and microorganisms (xanthan). Starches and pectins from plants and gelatin from animals (Cottrell and Baird, 1980) are also used. Synthetic hydrocolloids include starch derivatives and modified celluloses (Whistler and Zysk, 1978).

The highest microbial populations in the major botanical gums (about 10^8/g) have been found in raw, unprocessed acacia, carrageenan, and tragacanth (Souw and Rehm, 1975, 1976). Pretreated products such as alginates, carrageenan powder, locust bean gum, and guar flour yielded lower counts. The predominant organisms in the unprocessed gums were the *Bacillus* species and *Streptococcus faecalis; Escherichia coli,* however, was not recovered. Coagulase-positive staphylococci with counts of up to 10^5/g have been found in tragacanth and locust bean; *Clostridium perfringens* has been recovered from these two gums as well as from acacia.

Most gums will support bacterial growth when sufficient moisture is present. Enzymes secreted by *Bacillus* species can degrade gels and gum solutions reducing viscosity. Gums most susceptible to degradation are tragacanth, acacia, karaya, guar, locust bean, carrageenan, and sodium alginates (Souw and Rehm, 1975, 1976).

Enzymes

The enzymes added to foods consist mainly of carbohydrases (amylase, cellulase, invertase, pectinase, etc.) and proteases (e.g., papain and rennet). Plants, animals, and microorganisms are sources of the enzymes.

Little is known about the microbiology of enzyme preparations. Animal and microbial rennets, the enzymes whose microbiology has been studied most extensively, may yield high counts but appear to be free of pathogenic bacteria (de Becze, 1970). Never has a health problem been traced to the use of an enzyme per se in food processing (Pariza and Foster, 1983).

Colors

Natural colors, including annatto, anthocyanins, beet red, carotene, carmine, and saffron, have long been added to foods. Except for carmine, which comes from an insect, these colors are derived from plants. They are extracted into oil or aqueous systems from seeds, skins, or flowers.

There are virtually no published data about the microbiological quality of natural food colors. Some anthocyanins have limited antimicrobial activity and thus may restrict growth of certain microorganisms. The one recorded disease outbreak traced to a food color was due to salmonellae in carmine. *Salmonella cubana* was found to be responsible although additional samples of insects contained *Salmonella newport* and *Salmonella enteritidis* (Lang et al., 1967).

Need for Microbiological Criteria

Since many of these additives are raw agricultural products, the usual indices such as APCs usually would be of little value. The type of criteria that might be applied would depend upon end use of the additive. For example, additives to be used in canned foods should not be a significant source of heat-resistant bacterial spores. At present there is little published information to suggest that microbiological criteria would be useful for most gums, enzymes, and colors. This also was the conclusion of a committee of FAO/WHO who examined the subject a number of years ago (de Becze, 1970).

References

Cottrell, I. W., and J. K. Baird
  1980   Gums. Pp. 45–66 in Vol. 12 of Kirk-Othmer Encyclopedia of Chemical Technology, 3rd Ed. New York: John Wiley and Sons.
de Becze, G. I.
  1970   Food enzymes. Critical Reviews in Food Technology 1(4): 479–518.
Lang, D. J., L. J. Kunz, A. R. Martin, S. A. Schroeder, and L. A. Thomson
  1967   Carmine as a source of nosocomial salmonellosis. N. Eng. J. Med. 276:829–832.
Pariza, M. W., and E. M. Foster
  1983   Determining the safety of enzymes used in food processing. J. Food Prot. 46:453–468.
Souw, P., and H. J. Rehm
  1975   IV. Microbiological degradation of three plant exudates and two seaweed extracts. Z. Lebensm. Unters.-Forsch. 159(5): 297–304.
  1976   V. Degradation of the galactomannans guar gum and locust bean gum by different bacilli. European J. Appl. Microbiol. 2: 47–58.
Whistler, R. L., and J. R. Zysk
  1978   Carbohydrates. Pp. 535–555 in Vol. 4 of Kirk-Othmer Encyclopedia of Chemical Technology, 3rd Ed. New York: John Wiley and Sons.

U.   BOTTLED WATER, PROCESSING WATER, AND ICE

Sensitivity of Products Relative to Safety and Quality

Drinking water has been and still is an important vehicle for transmitting disease-causing agents (bacteria, viruses, parasites, chemicals) to man. From 1977-1981, 189 outbreaks of water-related diseases involving an estimated 49,453 persons occurred in the United States (CDC, 1979, 1980, 1981, 1982 a,b). As for foodborne disease outbreaks, these figures should not be the basis for firm conclusions about the true incidence of waterborne disease outbreaks as it is most likely many times greater than that reported. Of the 189 outbreaks, 100 (53%) were of unknown etiology and were designated "acute gastrointestinal illness" (AGI). The remaining 89 (47%) outbreaks were of a confirmed etiology: *Giardia* (31), chemical (27), *Shigella* (9), Norwalk agent (7), *Salmonella* (5), *Campylobacter* (3), Parvovirus-like agent (3), hepatitis A (2), *Vibrio cholerae* O1 (1), and Rotavirus (1). In none of these outbreaks, however, were bottled waters identified as vehicles.

Public interest in pure, better-tasting water has created a large demand for bottled drinking water. Bottled water is defined by FDA (1982a) as water that is sealed in bottles or other containers and intended for human consumption.

The following types of bottled drinking water are available (APHA, 1984):

1. *Spring or Well Water*. This water is taken directly from a spring or well and bottled with minimum treatment.

2. *Specially Prepared Drinking Water*. This is water in which the mineral content has been adjusted and controlled to improve the taste. The source may be a public water supply or a well.

3. *Purified Water*. This water conforms to the United States Pharmacopeia standard (USP, 1980) for purified water with minerals removed to less than 10 mg/l. Water can be "purified" by distillation, ion-exchange treatment, or reverse osmosis. Method of preparation must be indicated. Only water prepared by distillation can be called "distilled water."

4. *Fluoridated Water*. Fluoride has been added to drinking water at the optimum concentration as set forth in the FDA Quality Standards (FDA, 1982a).

No definition or quality standard for "mineral" water has yet been established in the United States.

In view of the potential for water-related illnesses in humans, it is essential that bottled water be from a safe source (spring, artesian well, drilled well, municipal water supply, or other source) and that it be processed, bottled, held, and transported under sanitary conditions.

Water containing small numbers of enteric pathogens can cause disease in humans, whereas the same organisms ingested with food may require larger quantities of bacteria. Small amounts of water taken between meals pass the pyloric area with very little delay. Under such conditions enteric pathogens are hardly exposed to the bactericidal effect of gastric juice and reach the duodenum virtually unchanged (Levine and Nalin, 1976; Mossel and Oei, 1975). When the same bacteria are ingested with solid food, intragastric retention times are considerable. This results in a reduction in viable bacterial cells in individuals with normal gastric secretions.

In the United States, few published data are available on the microbiological condition of bottled drinking water or on the incidence of human disease outbreaks resulting from their use. According to two reports (EPA, 1972; Geldreich et al., 1975), the bacteriological quality of freshly bottled water varied greatly from brand to brand and from sample to sample within brand. Only 10% of samples had an initial APC greater than 500/ml. Coliforms were detected in 6 of 129 samples but only two of these samples exceeded the USPHS Drinking Water Standards. One of these samples also contained fecal coliforms and the other contained *Pseudomonas aeru-*

ginosa. During storage of bottled water pulsating changes in aerobic plate counts frequently occurred. Over 90% of counts of 10,000 bacteriological analyses of bottled water in California in 1977 were less than 100 per ml at time of bottling (Sheneman, 1983). Over 99.8% of these samples were free of coliforms.

Although there is no epidemiological evidence that bottled water processed in the United States has been a public health problem, bottled water has been cited as a cause of human disease in other parts of the world. For example, bottled noncarbonated mineral water was implicated as one of the primary vehicles involved in a cholera epidemic in Portugal in 1974 (Blake et al., 1977).

FDA microbiological standards for bottled water (FDA, 1982a) are based on the presence of coliforms. With the multiple tube fermentation method not more than one unit in a sampling of 10 (subsamples) shall have a MPN of 2.2 or more coliforms per 100 ml and no analytical unit shall have a MPN of 9.2 or more coliforms per 100 ml. With the membrane filter method, not more than one of the analytical units in the sample shall have 4.0 or more coliforms per 100 ml and the arithmetic mean of the coliform density of the sample shall not exceed one coliform per 100 ml.

The FDA GMPs for bottled water (FDA, 1982b) require coliform analysis at least once a week of a representative sample from a batch or segment of a continuous production run for each type of bottled drinking water produced during a day's production. Additionally, source water obtained from other than public water systems is to be sampled and analyzed for coliforms at least once each week. In addition, at least once each three months, a bacteriological swab and/or rinse count should be made from at least four containers and closures selected just before filling and sealing. No more than one of the four samples may exceed more than one bacterium per ml of capacity or one colony per cm^2 of surface area. All samples shall be free of coliforms.

In addition to the federal standards, state and local microbiological criteria and good manufacturing practice codes exist to monitor the production, processing, and distribution of bottled drinking water (Wehr, 1982). To promote high standards of quality in the bottled water industry, the International Bottled Water Association has published a technical manual containing a quality control program to assure compliance with FDA standards (IBWA, 1983). The American Sanitation Institute (ASI) inspects all IBWA-member plants for conformance with the regulations.

The indigenous microflora of bottled drinking water usually consists of gram-negative bacteria belonging to genera such as *Pseudomonas*, *Cytophaga*, *Flavobacterium*, and *Alcaligenes*. Although no total count is specified, good-quality drinking water at time of bottling usually contains less than 100 bacteria per ml (APHA, 1984). Higher initial counts represent a lack of good manufacturing practices. The presence of coliform bacteria in bottled water indicates either a lack of good manufacturing practices and/or a potential health problem. Ozone may be applied as a disinfectant just prior to bottling. Some surviving bacteria may multiply in the water after the ozone has dissipated.

No one microorganism or group of microorganisms can serve as an ideal indicator of pollution of various types of water. Although many organisms such as *Aeromonas*, *Streptococcus*, *Escherichia coli*, fecal coliforms, coliforms, sulfite-reducing *Clostridium*, *P. aeruginosa*, *Vibrio*, and *E. coli* phages have been suggested as potential indicator organisms of drinking water safety, total coliforms appear at the present to be the best indicator organisms (Ptak and Ginsberg, 1977).

Processing Water and Ice

Water is used extensively in the food-processing industry. It comes in direct contact with major food commodities such as meat, poultry, fish, fruits, vegetables, and cheese curd during washing or chilling operations. In addition, water is used in the cleanup operations of equipment and utensils that come in contact with food. Water also is used as an ingredient in the preparation of foods. Ice is used widely to chill foods such as fish and poultry and is added to some foods as in the preparation of some processed meats. In many food-processing industries, water is chlorinated to control levels of microorganisms, for example in cooling water of canning plants. Chlorination of processing water requires an understanding of needed chlorine concentration, effect of water characteristics such as pH on available chlorine, and proper testing procedures to periodically examine for available chlorine (FPI, 1982).

Water used in food production and processing can be a source of spoilage microorganisms and, if obtained from a nonpotable source or subsequently contaminated, it can be a source of pathogens. Several outbreaks of foodborne disease have been associated with or traced to the use of contaminated water, e.g., salmonellosis from fish (Gangarosa et al., 1968), typhoid fever from canned corned beef (Howie et al., 1968), and yersiniosis from tofu (Nolan et al., 1982).

Need for Microbiological Criteria

There is no epidemiological evidence to indicate that bottled water as available currently in retail channels offers a significant health hazard to the American public. Therefore, there appears to be little evidence of need for additional or modifications of criteria currently in FDA regulations. However, the commercial vending of bottled water including import supplies and the variety of sources from which water for bottling is obtained has proliferated. These recent increases suggest that a periodic reassessment should be made of practices in this industry relative to the microbiological quality and safety of bottled water offered to the public.

Water or ice that comes in contact with or becomes part of a food should be from a potable supply and the microbiological criteria for them should meet the standards set for drinking water (Greenberg et al., 1981).

Where Criteria Should Be Applied

Microbiological examination of bottled drinking water for compliance with standards or guidelines should be carried out on samples collected at the processing plant. Examination of samples for APC at the retail level has little merit.

References

APHA (American Public Health Association)
  1984   Compendium of Methods for the Microbiological Examination of Foods. 2nd Ed.,
          M. L. Speck, ed. Washington, D.C.: APHA.
Blake, P. A., M. L. Rosenberg, J. Florencia, J. B. Costa, L. D. P. Quintino, and E. J. Gangarosa
  1977   Cholera in Portugal, 1974. II. Transmission by bottled mineral water. Am. J. Epi-
          demiol. 105:344–348.
CDC (Centers for Disease Control)
  1979   Foodborne and Waterborne Disease Outbreaks. Annual summary 1977. Atlanta: Cen-
          ter for Disease Control.
  1980   Water-related Disease Outbreaks. Annual Summary 1978. Atlanta: Centers for Disease
          Control.
  1981   Water-related Disease Outbreaks. Annual Summary 1979. Atlanta: Centers for Disease
          Control.
  1982a   Water-related Disease Outbreaks. Annual Summary 1980. Atlanta: Centers for Disease
          Control.
  1982b   Water-related Disease Outbreaks. Annual Summary 1981. Atlanta: Centers for Disease
          Control.
EPA (U.S. Environmental Protection Agency)
  1972   Bottled water study. A pilot survey of water bottlers and bottled water. Washington,
          D.C.: Water Supply Division, EPA.
FDA (Food and Drug Administration)
  1982a   Quality standards for foods with no identity standards, bottled water. Code of Federal
          Regulations 21 CFR 103 (as corrected in Federal Register 47(205):47003–47004.)
  1982b   Processing and bottling of bottled drinking water. Code of Federal Regulations 21
          CFR 129.

FPI (The Food Processors Institute)
  1982   Canned Foods, Principles of Thermoprocess Control, Acidification and Container Closure Evaluation, 4th Ed. Washington, D.C.: FPI.
Gangarosa, E. J., A. L. Bisno, E. R. Eichner, M. D. Treger, M. Goldfield, W. E. DeWitt, T. Fodor, S. M. Fish, W. J. Dougherty, J. B. Murphy, J. Feldman, and H. Vogel
  1968   Epidemic of febrile gastroenteritis due to *Salmonella java* traced to smoked whitefish. Am. J. Pub. Health 58:114–121.
Geldreich, E. E., H. D. Nash, D. J. Reasoner, and R. H. Taylor
  1975   The necessity of controlling bacterial populations in potable waters—Bottled water and emergency water supplies. J. Amer. Water Works Assoc. 67:117–124.
Greenberg, A. E., J. J. Conners, D. Jenkins, and M. A. H. Franson
  1981   Standard Methods for the Examination of Water and Wastewater, 15th Ed. Washington, D.C.: American Public Health Association.
Howie, J. W.
  1968   Typhoid in Aberdeen, 1964. J. Appl. Bacteriol. 31:171–178.
IBWA (International Bottled Water Association)
  1983   International Bottled Water Association Technical Bulletin, Winter. Alexandria, Va.: IBWA.
Levine, R. J., and D. R. Nalin
  1976   Cholera is primarily waterborne in Bangladesh. Lancet 2:1305.
Mossel, D. A. A., and H. Y. Oei
  1975   Person-to-person transmission of enteric bacterial infection. Lancet 1:751.
Nolan, C., N. Harris, J. Ballard, J. Allard, and J. Kobayashi
  1982   Outbreak of *Yersinia enterocolitica*—Washington State. Morb. Mort. Weekly Rpt. 31:562–564.
Ptak, D. J., and W. Ginsberg
  1977   Bacterial indicators of drinking water quality. Pp. 218–221 in Bacterial Indicators/ Health Hazards Associated with Water. Spc. Techn. Publ. 635. Philadelphia: American Society for Testing and Materials.
Sheneman, J.
  1983   Memorandum from the California Food and Drug Section. Water bottling plants bacteriological analysis summary. In International Bottled Water Association, Technical Bulletin, Winter. Alexandria, Va.: IBWA.
USP (United States Pharmacopeia)
  1980   Purified water. P. 851 in The United States Pharmacopeia. Rockville, Maryland: U.S. Pharmacopeial Convention.
Wehr, H. M.
  1982   Attitudes and policies of governmental agencies on microbial criteria for foods—an update. Food Technol. 36(9):45–54, 92.

V. PET FOODS

Companion animals of man have been a source of diseases, including salmonellosis, in humans (Morse and Duncan, 1974, 1975; Morse et al., 1976; Pace et al., 1977) and contaminated pet foods have at times been incriminated as the original cause (Pace et al., 1977). Interest in the microbiology of these foods is influenced by the above and the fact that certain pet foods, mainly canned products, are at times consumed by humans.

Sensitivity of Products Relative to Safety and Quality

Although the true incidence of salmonellosis in animals is unknown (NRC, 1969), *Salmonella* are widely distributed in warm- and cold-blooded species and have been isolated from dogs, cats, horses, caged birds, turtles, frogs, skunks, raccoons, opossums, and others. The role of pets in the distribution of *Salmonella* has been recognized in a report by the Committee on *Salmonella* (NRC, 1969):

Of the many routes by which man can acquire salmonellosis, special mention should be made of household pets, including dogs, cats, turtles, chicks and ducklings.

Pet animals can become infected with *Salmonella* by a wide variety of routes, e.g., through coprophagy, by direct contact with infected animals, through eating diseased carrion and wildlife, and by the consumption of contaminated pet food. The latter is probably the least important source since the present day incidence of *Salmonella* in commercial pet food is very low (Pace et al., 1977).

Pet foods, which are sold predominantly for dogs and cats, may be marketed as canned, intermediate moisture (a_w 0.80-0.90), or dried products. Canned pet foods are terminally heat processed in hermetically sealed containers and are commercially sterile. They are subject to the regulations for low-acid canned foods and when in compliance are not of public health concern. Intermediate moisture pet foods and the dry products are given a heat process, generally during extrusion and pelleting, that will destroy the vegetative cells of pathogenic bacteria. The prevention of recontamination following heating, then, is the critical control step in their processing. Monitoring of environmental samples as well as finished product for *Salmonella* is thus important.

Recontamination of dry pet food with *Salmonella* is of special concern because water is often added to the food prior to feeding. Significant growth of the pathogen can occur if the food is held at ambient temperature for an extended time period following rehydration. A potential would then exist not only for infection of the pet but for cross-contamination of household items such as equipment, utensils, and human foods.

Need for Microbiological Criteria

Canned pet foods are subject to the regulations for low-acid foods and thus the main applications of criteria are to assure that ingredients are free of bacterial spores that might survive the thermal process.

Dry and intermediate moisture pet foods should be free of *Salmonella*, and a standard exists for this pathogen (U.S. Congress, 1980). Specifications and guidelines for these products are especially useful if applied at critical control points identified within a HACCP system. Guidelines and specifications serve to:

1. assess suitability, including safety, of incoming ingredients (The elimination of salmonellae from feed ingredients, particularly those of animal origin, would greatly reduce the occurrence of these organisms in finished pet foods, but this goal does not appear to be readily attainable at this time [USDA, 1978].);
2. identify acceptable ingredient suppliers;
3. assess control effectiveness at critical control points in manufacturing;
4. determine the acceptability of a finished product.

Information Necessary for Establishment of a Criterion if One Seems To Be Indicated

Extensive information is available regarding those feed ingredients that may be contaminated with *Salmonella* (ICMSF, 1980) and therefore may require specifications that limit this pathogen. Information is also available on the occurrence of *Salmonella* in pets (Morse, 1978), and in pet foods (D'Aoust, 1978; ICMSF, 1980; Pace et al., 1977). It is advisable for pet food manufacturers to conduct appropriate microbiological surveillance studies that will generate the information required for the development of guidelines.

Where Criteria Should Be Applied

Analyses for salmonellae might be conducted on the packaged product. Guidelines and specifications would best be applied at the plant processing level as components of an ongoing HACCP program. Their application at critical control points and on the finished product should assist in minimizing the contamination of pet foods with undesirable microorganisms.

References

D'Aoust, J. Y.
    1978   *Salmonella* in commercial pet foods. Can. Vet. J. 19:99-100.
ICMSF (International Commission on Microbiological Specifications for Foods)
    1980   Microbial Ecology of Foods. Vol 2. Food Commodities. New York: Academic Press.
Morse, E. V.
    1978   Salmonellosis and pet animals. In Proceedings of the Salmonellosis Seminar. Washington, D.C.: U.S. Department of Agriculture.

Morse, E. V., and M. A. Duncan
    1974   Salmonellosis—An environmental health problem. J. Am. Vet. Med. Assoc. 165:1015-1019.
    1975   Canine salmonellosis: Prevalence, epizootiology, signs, and public health significance. J. Am. Vet. Med. Assoc. 167:817-820.
Morse, E. V., M. A. Duncan, D. A. Estep, W. A. Riggs, and B. O. Blackburn
    1976   Canine salmonellosis: A review and report of dog to child transmission of *Salmonella enteritidis*. Am. J. Publ. Health 66:82-84.
NRC (National Research Council)
    1969   An Evaluation of the *Salmonella* Problem. Committee on *Salmonella*. Washington, D.C.: National Academy of Sciences.
Pace, P. J., K. J. Silver, and H. J. Wisniewski
    1977   *Salmonella* in commercially produced dried dog food: Possible relationship to a human infection caused by *Salmonella enteritidis* serotype Havana. J. Food Prot. 40(5):317-321.
U.S. Congress
    1980   Federal Food, Drug and Cosmetic Act, as amended. Washington, D.C.: U.S. Govt. Printing Office.
USDA (U.S. Department of Agriculture)
    1978   Recommendations for Reduction and Control of Salmonellosis. A Report of the U.S. Advisory Committee on *Salmonella*. Washington, D.C.: USDA.

10

Expansion of the HACCP System in Food Protection Programs

This subcommittee embraces the Hazard Analyses Critical Control Point (HACCP) concept as an effective and rational approach to the assurance of safety and to the prevention or delay of spoilage in foods (see Chapter 1 and Appendix G). In the application of HACCP the use of microbiological criteria is at times the most effective means of monitoring critical control points. In other instances, monitoring of critical control points can best be accomplished through the use of physical and chemical tests, visual observations, and sensory evaluations. Thus, microbiological criteria may play an important role or no role at all depending upon the nature of the food or the process. The applicability of microbiological criteria to the monitoring of critical control points in the production of various food commodities is discussed in detail in Chapter 9.

FACTORS TO BE CONSIDERED
FOR IMPLEMENTATION OF HACCP

Initially, HACCP was established by the FDA as an approach to the control of microbiological hazards in the mushroom-canning industry. After considerable refinement, the FDA applied HACCP to all low-acid canned foods; this approach to the control of microbiological hazards in low-acid canned foods was then mandated by federal regulations (FDA, 1973a,b).

The application of HACCP as a means of controlling microbiological hazards in low-acid canned foods has been successful for a number of reasons:

1. *Industry and government, working cooperatively, identified and developed monitoring procedures for critical control points in the production of this class of foods.* The procedures included details with respect to the frequency with which the tests should be performed, the keeping of records, and the actions to be taken when monitoring results indicated lack of compliance, i.e., failure at a critical control point.

2. *The FDA required that operators of retorts, aseptic processing packaging systems, product formulating systems, and container closure inspectors be under the supervision of a person who had satisfactorily completed the prescribed course approved by the FDA Commissioner.*

3. *FDA inspectors were trained in the elements of the HACCP system.* As a result, FDA inspectors became knowledgeable of the critical control points in the production of these products. At the time of plant inspections, major emphasis was placed upon review of monitoring results.

4. *The use of the HACCP system was mandated by federal regulation.*

The four points below are of considerable importance if the HACCP system is to be more broadly applied in the food industry:

1. *The hazard analysis of a food process requires technical sophistication as does the identification of critical control points and the establishment of effective monitoring programs.* Assistance from experts from disciplines other than microbiology may be required. The large, technically sophisticated processor may have personnel capable of accomplishing these tasks, whereas smaller operators are less likely to have them. The HACCP system as it has been applied to low-acid canned foods evolved as a result of joint industry/government cooperation. For it to be applied effectively in other areas, similar cooperative efforts will be required. This need not necessarily require industry/government collaboration, but the appropriate technical manpower can be mobilized within segments of the industry. This could be done through various industry trade associations. For example, the American Meat Institute (AMI, 1982) published guidelines for the production of dry and semidry sausages. Technical expertise for the establishment of these guidelines came from within the industry, and there seems little doubt that they will be acceptable to the USDA, the organization responsible for regulating these products.

If only the technically sophisticated companies within a given segment of the food industry apply the HACCP system, then the value of an industry-wide application to the production of a given product or products will be lost. For this reason organized technical input by industry is essential.

From the pooling of industry and government manpower, specific codes of Good Manufacturing Practices should evolve. These are needed since, as indicated in Chapter 1, "umbrella" codes are non-specific and vague to the degree that the courts have held that they do not have the force of law (*U.S.* v. *An Article of Food*, 1972).

If technical manpower is not utilized to establish HACCP systems within various segments of the food industry, then the weak links within a given segment will be the technically unsophisticated companies. The argument may be made that use of the HACCP system would place such companies at a competitive disadvantage. On the other hand, their failure to utilize HACCP would tend to result in greater exposure of their products to microbiological hazards. The greatest cost/benefit advantage would accrue if all producers within a given industry were applying HACCP principles in the control of their products and if regulators were judging manufacturing practices according to the HACCP principles, i.e., review of the results of monitoring critical control points.

2. *Those responsible for regulation must be trained in the concepts of the HACCP system.* FDA inspectors were so trained in the HACCP approach as applied to low-acid canned foods. Furthermore, they received training in application of the HACCP approach to the regulation of other types of foods. However, HACCP inspections with respect to other foods were optional. In fact, there have been no formal personnel training sessions by FDA since 1975. As a result of the optional status of HACCP inspections and the failure to train personnel, the HACCP approach to regulatory control has fallen into disuse in the United States (except for its application to low-acid canned foods, where it is mandated by law).

3. *The successful use of the HACCP approach to the control of low-acid canned foods was due in part to the mandatory training of various categories of food processing technicians.* Courses at selected universities were established by the FDA for this purpose. If HACCP is expanded, it will necessitate similar training of individuals in other segments of the industry. This training could be undertaken by industry, perhaps through trade associations or other appropriate organizations within various segments of the industry. Again, technical input could come from the technically sophisticated segments within a given industry.

4. *An important factor contributing to the successful application of HACCP in the low-acid canned food industry was mandatory use of this system.* For HACCP use to be broadly realized, it is likely that the utilization of this system will have to be required by regulation. It would thus be mandated that food processors establish monitoring programs relating to critical control points affecting the microbiological safety or quality of their products, such points having been established by hazard analysis. Quality attributes other than those relating to microbiological hazards would not be subject to such regulation. The regulation would require only a statement to identify the basic elements of the HACCP system including a provision requiring that the appropriate records be readily available to representatives of regulatory agencies. Details of the mechanism of applying the HACCP system should be the prerogative of the food establishment.

PROBLEMS ASSOCIATED WITH IMPLEMENTATION OF THE HACCP APPROACH

It was thought that the HACCP concept, so successfully applied to low-acid canned foods, would find its place in other segments of the industry, and that companies producing a given product or group of similar products would apply the system and identify critical control points and appropriate monitoring procedures. The regulatory inspectors would initially review the plant control protocols and satisfy themselves that the critical control points in a given program had been properly identified and that appropriate monitoring systems had been established. Regulatory emphasis would next be focused on a review of monitoring results that, if satisfactory, would correctly lead the inspector to conclude that the foods of concern were being produced under adequate microbiological control. This then would prevent the inspector from duplicating control efforts and would permit him to proceed elsewhere to make evaluations, thus providing more efficient use of inspectional personnel. Herein resides the cost/benefit value of the HACCP approach in regulatory control.

From a regulatory standpoint, a complete familiarity with and understanding of processes and product flows would greatly aid agency assessment of the effectiveness of a food firm's programs designed to assure product safety and quality. However, it is nearly impossible for any one regulatory inspector to have an intimate knowledge of every type of food-processing system. Utilization of HACCP as an integral part of the regulatory process would do much to obviate need for an investigator to know everything about the intricacies of a firm's processing systems. The net result would be cost-effective and less time-consuming and more meaningful to the regulatory evaluation of a firm's ability to assure safe and wholesome products.

In the past, adversary attitudes and lack of cooperation between regulatory agencies and the food industry have presented a serious hindrance to achievement of common goals of food quality and safety assurance. Regulatory agencies and the food industry have failed to recognize their responsibilities in areas of mutual concern and failed to capitalize on the special abilities and expertise which each can provide. They have failed to work in concert in an atmosphere of mutual respect, understanding, and trust to achieve these common objectives.

A particularly sensitive issue in this regard relates to access to industry records. Industry recognizes that records of observations are needed for meaningful food protection, e.g., monitoring results from critical control points. But identification of which records are relevant for regulatory purpose is an issue of major disagreement between regulatory agencies and the food industry. Much of the information in question may relate to manufacturing practices that may be proprietary in nature. The regulator should have access to monitoring results on critical control points and the action taken when limits are exceeded.

The issue of access to records should be reviewed and resolved so that the food industry's apprehensions are allayed and regulatory agencies have the necessary assistance for effective execution of their responsibilities. The adversary atmosphere that has historically existed is counterproductive to both the processor and the regulator and is the most serious impediment to the expansion of the HACCP concept. There should be no need for regulatory access to proprietary information having no relevance to food safety or quality. There is no fundamental reason why the broad application of HACCP throughout the food industry should not occur. The cost/benefit ratio is highly advantageous.

The technical expertise necessary to establish HACCP systems in various phases of the food industry must come from various experts within the involved industries. Considerations by these experts would result in identification of appropriate critical control points, monitoring systems, and acceptable (and relevant) recordkeeping systems that should be accessible to regulatory authorities. Regulatory officials should have the option to assess the appropriateness of the selected critical control points, the adequacy of the monitoring system, and the actions taken when limits are exceeded. Essential to the implementation of the HACCP system is the adequate training of inspectors.

THE NEED FOR APPLICATION OF HACCP
AT ALL POINTS IN THE FOOD CHAIN

The foregoing discussion has focused upon the application of HACCP in food-processing facilities; however, the concept is applicable at all points in the food chain. A few examples follow.

1. Diseased meat animals constitute a health hazard. The critical control point identified by the USDA is at the processing plant prior to slaughter, and it is monitored by *ante mortem* inspection by veterinary authorities.
2. Antibiotic residues in milk constitute a health hazard to sensitized individuals in the human population. Furthermore, such residues may prevent desired acid production in milk used to manufacture cheese. This may lead to spoilage or to health hazards such as the formation of *Staphylococcus* enterotoxin. These hazards may be monitored by analysis of milk samples at the farm level or in the processing plant.
3. Hazardous pesticide residues in fruits and vegetables can be monitored at appropriate points by chemical tests.
4. Storage of improperly dried grain at the farm or elevator level may cause spoilage and/or the hazard of mycotoxin formation. Critical control points can be monitored by appropriate tests to assure proper moisture control.
5. Microbiological hazards can arise during shipment of both perishable and shelf-stable foods from the processing plant to storage warehouses (see Chapter 9). For example, critical control points in the shipment of carcass meat include the internal temperature of the carcasses at the time of loading, the temperature of the air circulating in the transportation vehicle, the spacing of the carcasses, the air movement within the transportation vehicle, and the temperature of that air throughout the shipment. These critical control points can be monitored by physical tests, e.g., recording thermometers and visual observations.

   In the shipment of shelf-stable products, the cleanliness of vehicles may affect the safety and quality of goods being shipped and thus is a critical control point. This should be monitored before loading by visual inspection. Such inspection should include determination of general cleanliness, the absence of insect and rodent problems, and the soundness of the transportation vehicle.
6. Improper warehousing frequently leads to product recalls due to storage of foods under insanitary conditions. These problems can

be circumvented by appropriate monitoring of identified critical control points in the storage facility, for example, the monitoring of insect and rodent control programs.

7. At the retail level abuse of perishable foods, such as meats, poultry, and fish may lead to health and spoilage hazards. Storage temperature is a critical control point, as is the method of loading retail cases, for these may greatly influence temperature distribution. Hazards are created by cross-contamination. Cleanliness of equipment is a critical control point.

At no point in the food chain is there greater need for control over microbiological hazards than in food service establishments and in homes. Even if all those responsible for food production, from the farmer to the retailer, are successful in the control of microbiological hazards, the ultimate user of food products is generally responsible for foodborne diseases as a result of improper handling and storage practices. Table 10-1 dramatically illustrates this point. It will be noted that approximately 97% of foodborne disease outbreaks reported to the Centers for Disease Control over a 5-year period were traced to mishandling in food service establishments and in homes. The relationships shown in Table 10-1 are undoubtedly skewed. Foodborne disease outbreaks are poorly reported. Isolated incidents occurring in homes are far less likely to be noted than are large outbreaks traced to food service establishments. Furthermore, the figure for the proportion of outbreaks traced to food-processing plants is undoubtedly in error "on the high side," since such outbreaks are more likely to come to the attention of regulatory authorities. The conclusion is clear: most foodborne illness is caused by those who prepare foods in homes and food service establishments. If foods are not properly handled at these two points, foodborne illness is inevitable; thus, this nullifies to a large extent preventive measures that may have been applied earlier in

TABLE 10-1   Foodborne Disease Outbreaks Classified by Place of Mishandling Foods, United States, 1974 to 1978

Place	Number of Outbreaks	Percent of Known Places
Food service establishment	1,285	77
Homes	327	20
Food processing plants	52	3
Other/unknown/unspecified	615	—
TOTAL	2,279	100

SOURCE: Bryan, 1982, p. 67.

the food chain, e.g., at processing plants and in distribution channels. No dramatic decrease in the incidence of foodborne disease can be expected until those who prepare and handle foods in homes and food service establishments become knowledgeable in the principles of proper food handling and apply these principles.

Factors contributing to foodborne disease outbreaks are summarized in Table 10-2. The ultimate consumer of food must, in most cases, "further process" the products of the food industry, such processing being done in a kitchen of a home or a food service establishment. The factors listed in Table 10-2 include processing errors most frequently made at these points.

The HACCP approach is applicable to the control of microbiological hazards in food service establishments just as it is at previous links in the food chain. The use of the HACCP system in food service establishments has been studied extensively by Bryan (1982) (Table 10-3). The hazards, critical control points, and monitoring procedures applicable to food service establishments have been set forth in considerable detail. An extensive bibliography relating to the use of HACCP in controlling microbiological hazards in a number of specific foods prepared in food service establishments is also given. No attempt will be made to summarize these studies.

TABLE 10-2 Factors Contributing to Outbreaks of Foodborne Disease, United States, 1961 to 1976

Factors	Percentages[a]
Improper cooling	46
Lapse of a day or more between preparing and serving	21
Colonized persons touching cooked foods	20
Inadequate thermal processing, canning, or cooking	16
Improper hot storage	16
Inadequate reheating	12
Contaminated raw food	11
Cross-contamination	7
Improper cleaning of equipment	7
Obtaining foods from unsafe sources	5
Use of leftovers	4

NOTE: Other factors were faulty fermentations, toxic species of plants or mushrooms mistaken for edible varieties, poor dry storage practices, storing high-acid foods in toxic containers, incidental additives, and intentional additives (for example, MSG).

[a]Percentages exceed 100 because foodborne diseases have multiple causation: foods must become contaminated, contaminants may survive processes, and frequently bacterial pathogens multiply to reach large numbers or to produce toxins.

SOURCE: Bryan, 1978.

TABLE 10-3 Hazards, Critical Control Points, Preventive Measures, and Monitoring Procedures of Food Service Operations

Operational Step	Hazards	Critical Control Point	Relative Importance	Preventive Measures	Monitoring Procedures
Purchasing and receiving	Pathogens on raw foods or ingredients.	Incoming food.	*	Separate raw- and cooked-food operations and foods.	Probably none practicable because many raw foods are contaminated with a variety of foodborne pathogens. *Measurement:* Collect samples and test for pathogens to determine whether foods contain high numbers of pathogens (seldom practical).
	Processed foods contaminated with large numbers of pathogens.	Incoming food; food in distribution or after processing.	**	Reject foods, change supplier, reprocess.	*Measurement:* Collect samples and test to determine whether foods exceed purchase specifications.
	Foods have microbial counts that exceed purchase specifications.	Incoming food.	*	Formulate microbiological purchase specifications and analyze foods for compliance.	*Observation:* Check labels, tags, and perhaps purchase records to determine whether foods such as milk and processed eggs are from pasteurized sources and shellfish, meat, and ice are from approved sources.
	Foods obtained from unsafe source.	Food at source.	**	Obtain foods from ''approved'' sources.	*Observation:* Observe condition of food and package. *Measurement:* Measure a_w, pH, temperature (depending on product and process) of food.
	Product's shelf-life is less than would be expected if processed and stored according to good commercial practice.	Food during processing, storage, and distribution.	*	Process and store foods effectively.	
	Foods show signs of spoilage.	Incoming food.	*	Reject; discard.	*Observation:* Observe condition of food and container.

Storing incoming foods Frozen storage	Thawing because of power failures or improper frozen food storage or transport.	*	Thawed food.	Keep frozen foods frozen; maintain product temperature at or below 7°C (45°F) after thawing.	*Observation:* See that foods are frozen and remain so. *Measurement:* Measure temperature of freezing unit to determine whether it is −17°C (0°F); drill into frozen food and measure temperature to determine whether it is frozen.
	Prolonged storage.	*	Interval between freezing and use of food.	Rotate stock; use before detrimental effects occur.	*Observation:* Compare date of processing, if known; expiration date, if known; or date of storage with date of use; look at texture of product.
	Foods show signs of spoilage.	*	Usually thawed food.	Discard.	*Observation:* Observe condition of food for slime, mold, gas formation, off-odor, freezer burn, etc., that are characteristic of spoilage.
Refrigerated storage	Spoilage due to prolonged storage.	**	Temperature of refrigerator air.	Maintain temperature of chilled food below 7°C (45°F) preferably near 1°C (33°F).	*Measurement:* Insert thermometer into food that has been in refrigerator for several hours to get stabilized refrigerator temperature; measuring air temperature is of little value because it fluctuates greatly as doors are opened or hot foods are put into refrigerator. *Observation:* Observe condition of stored food for slime, mold, gas formation, off-odor, etc., that are characteristic of spoilage.

TABLE 10-3 (Continued)

Operational Step	Hazards	Critical Control Point	Relative Importance	Preventive Measures	Monitoring Procedures
	Cross-contamination.	Storage practices in refrigerators.	**	Separate refrigerators for raw foods and for cooked foods; separate areas in the same refrigerator for cooked and raw foods; put cooked foods on higher shelves than raw foods, if they are in the same area; cover foods or wrap foods (note: cooling may be impeded by lids).	*Observation:* Observe storage practices in refrigerator to see whether there are likely routes of contamination.
Dry storage	Physical breaks in package.	Relative humidity of storage facility.	*	Handle carefully; repackage; store in dry area.	*Observation:* Look at integrity of package and for entry of moisture.
	High moisture in environment.	Food product during storage.	*	Maintain low a_w.	*Measurement:* Measure a_w of food.
	Poisonous substances contaminate foods.	Storage practices in storerooms.	**	Store poisons in separate area from foods.	*Observation:* Look for presence of poisons (pesticides and cleaning agents) in food storage areas.
	Insects or rodents contaminate foods.	Storage practices; physical attributes of storage area.	*	Protect storage area from entrance of insects and rodents; vector control when applicable.	*Observation:* Look for presence of screens, pipe flanges, and other devices that will effectively keep insects and rodents out of storage areas. Also, look to see whether there is spillage that vectors can use as food or harborage; and look for evidence of vectors.

			Factors	Control measures	Monitoring
	Sewage contaminates food.	**	Storage practices; physical attributes of storage area.	Protect storage from sewage drippage or backflow.	*Observation:* Look for evidence of leaking sewer pipes; look for evidence of sewage backflow.
	Excessive heat damages food.	*	Storage practices; physical attributes of storage area.	Protect foods from excessive heat; adequate air circulation.	*Observation:* Look for evidence of heat sources (heated pipes, sunlight); poor air circulation; foods on floor or against wall.
Preprocessing	First step of cross-contamination; workers' hands and clothing become contaminated with foodborne pathogens.	**	Handling of raw foods of animal origin.	Wash hands after handling raw foods of animal origin.	*Observation:* Look to see whether workers wash their hands after handling raw foods of animal origin (raw meat or raw poultry or raw fish, shellfish, marine crustacea, or egg shells). *Microbiological testing:* Sample workers' hands and test rinses or swabs for pathogens.
	First step of cross-contamination; equipment and utensil surfaces become contaminated with foodborne pathogens.	**	Equipment surfaces that contact raw foods.	Clean and disinfect utensils and equipment; separate raw food areas and operations from cooked food areas and operations.	*Observation:* Observe flow of raw foods to see if they go into areas used for cooked foods. Look to see whether equipment and utensils (e.g., cutting boards, table tops, grinders, slicers, knives, cleavers) that are used for raw foods are washed and disinfected after use, before use for other foods. *Microbiological testing:* Sample equipment surfaces with rodac (replicate organism detection and counting) contact plates or swabs and test for pathogens, fecal indicator organisms, or aerobic plate count.

TABLE 10-3 (Continued)

Operational Step	Hazards	Critical Control Point	Relative Importance	Preventive Measures	Monitoring Procedures
	First step of cross-contamination; rags and sponges become contaminated with foodborne pathogens.	Rags and sponges used to clean areas and to process raw food preparation areas.	**	Use separate sponges, rags, cloths in raw food area from those used in cooked food areas.	*Observation:* Observe pattern of use of sponges, rags, and cloths that are used to wipe equipment and surfaces or any area where raw foods are processed.
Storing foods that are not to be cooked	Growth of bacteria during room temperature storage.	Time foods were exposed to room temperatures.	***	Refrigerate foods to be served cold immediately after preparation.	*Observation:* Look to see whether foods that will either not receive further cooking or are to be served cold are kept at room temperature or whether they are refrigerated.
	High-acid foods (usually liquids) stored in metal containers (which are either made of or coated with toxic heavy metals—zinc, cadmium, copper, antimony, lead).	High-acid foods stored in metal containers; metal containers used to store or prepare foods.	**	Do not store high-acid liquid or solid foods in metal containers that are either made of or coated with toxic heavy metals.	*Observation:* Look to see whether high-acid liquid or solid foods are stored in metal containers either made of or coated with toxic heavy metals. *Measurement:* Check pH of food in above-mentioned containers.
Cooking	Survival of pathogens because of inadequate cooking (internal time-temperature exposure fails to kill pathogens).	Temperature of food at completion of cooking or at completion of post-oven rise period.	**	Cook potentially contaminated foods thoroughly; eat cooked food immediately after cooking.	*Measurement:* Insert thermometer into geometric center of poultry and pork products upon removal from oven and leave in center until temperature rise begins to decline. Beef surfaces and poultry surfaces should reach 74°C (165°F); pork should reach at least 66°C (150°F). If temperatures reach 72°C (160°F) or

Operation	Hazard	What to monitor	Risk	Control	Monitoring
Holding cooked foods	Lapse of several hours between cooking and serving; if storage practices are poor, bacteria multiply.	Foods after cooking.	****	Eat cooked foods immediately after cooking or hold cooked foods hot (see hot holding), or rapidly chill cooked foods (see cooling).	higher, there is no need to collect samples of such foods for microbiological testing at this step of the operation. *Microbiological testing:* Sample food before and after cooking and test for change in quantity of microorganisms to determine whether the heat process (time-temperature exposure) was effective. *Observation:* See that cooked foods are either eaten soon after cooking, held hot, or rapidly chilled.
Hot holding	Growth of bacteria when temperatures are too low; unenjoyable eating temperature.	Temperature of cooked food during hot storage.	****	Hold cooked foods at temperatures higher than pathogenic bacteria multiply.	*Measurement:* Insert thermometer into geometric center (and upper portion) of steam-table held foods to see whether temperatures are 55°C (130°F) or higher. No need to sample if temperature of food is 55°C (130°F) or above.
Room-temperature holding	Rapid growth of bacteria.	Temperature of cooked food during room-temperature storage.	*****	Never hold cooked foods at room temperature for more than one-half hour and then only for tempering or to steam-out before chilling or during slicing or other	*Microbiological testing:* Sample and test for quantity of microorganisms present. *Observation:* Look to see whether cooked foods are kept at room temperature.

TABLE 10-3 (Continued)

Operational Step	Hazards	Critical Control Point	Relative Importance	Preventive Measures	Monitoring Procedures
				preparation. Hold foods at temperatures higher than pathogenic bacteria multiply or rapidly chill foods.	
Handling cooked foods	Contaminated by workers during handling.	Cooked foods during preparing, slicing, cutting, grinding, chopping, or otherwise handling or while in contact with equipment.	****	Do not touch cooked foods; use utensils to handle cooked foods.	*Observation:* Observe whether cooked foods are touched by workers or if poor personal hygiene or other poor food-handling practices might subject foods to contamination. *Microbiological testing:* Sample foods and test them for quantity of coagulase-positive staphylococci or *Escherichia coli*.
	Cross-contamination from foods of animal origin (via equipment, utensils, cleaning rags, or hands).	Cooked foods during handling and preparing.	***	Use cleaned and sanitized utensils or equipment to process, hold, or handle cooked foods. Use separate equipment and utensils for raw foods of animal origin than for cooked foods.	*Observation:* Look for possible routes of cross-contamination from raw foods of animal origin to cooked foods. *Microbiological testing:* Sample foods and test them for *E. coli* or *Salmonella*. *Microbiological testing:* Sample foods and test them for *Salmonella*, *E. coli*, or, in some cases, coliforms. Swab or press rodac plates on food-contact surfaces of cleaned equipment.

Cooling cooked foods	Growth of bacteria during long periods of room temperature cooling before refrigeration.	Temperature of food during cooling.	*****	Chill rapidly.	*Observation:* Look to see whether cooked food is stored at room temperature. *Measurement:* Insert thermometer into geometric center to determine whether cooked food temperature drops to 21°C (70°F) or below within two hours after cooling is initiated and that it continues to cool to 7°C (45°F) within another four hours.
	Growth of bacteria in large masses of foods during refrigerated storage.	Size of storage container.	*****	Store foods in shallow pans during refrigeration.	*Observation/Measurement:* Look in refrigerators to see whether any foods are stored in containers that are deeper than 4 in. (10 cm). (Also measure as mentioned above.)
	High temperatures of refrigerators conducive to more rapid bacterial growth.	Temperature of refrigerator air.	**	Set refrigerators to run at low temperature; unblock air circulation.	*Measurement:* Record temperature of refrigerator air but note that taking temperature of refrigerator air is of very limited value.
	Contamination of cooked foods from raw foods of animal origin during improper refrigerated storage.	Storage practices in refrigerators.	**	Cover refrigerated foods to prevent contamination but not to impede cooling; locate container so that contamination from direct contact or drippage is unlikely; store cooked foods in separate refrigerators or areas from raw foods.	*Observation:* Look at refrigerated foods to see whether any cooked foods are stored in a manner that could lead to contamination from foods of animal origin.

TABLE 10-3 (Continued)

Operational Step	Hazards	Critical Control Point	Relative Importance	Preventive Measures	Monitoring Procedures
Reheating	Survival of pathogens (perhaps large numbers that could multiply if storage were inadequate).	Temperature of reheated foods.	****	Reheat cooked, leftover foods thoroughly to at least 72°C (160°F) and sometimes to 74°C (165°F) (temperatures of geometric center; near surfaces if microwave reheating used).	*Measurement:* Insert thermometer into geometric center of reheated food to see whether it reached 72°C (160°F) or higher.
Cleaning and disinfection of equipment and utensils	Cross-contamination.	Equipment surfaces.	***	Clean equipment and utensils thoroughly. Disinfect cleaned and rinsed equipment and utensils.	*Observation:* Look at and feel surfaces of "cleaned" equipment to see whether they are clean to sight and touch. Seek evidence of cleaning schemes and sanitary maintenance schedules. Watch workers while they wash and disinfect equipment. *Measurement:* Test water temperatures, pressures, chemical concentrations, time of cycles of mechanical washing and sanitizing equipment and, when applicable, manual operations. Test temperature at surface of equipment being washed. *Microbiological testing:* Swab defined areas of cleaned equipment to see whether they comply with microbiological criteria for cleanliness

Workers and managers	Poor operational procedures leading to contamination of foods and survival or growth of food-borne pathogens in foods.	Procedures performed.	*****	Train and give certificates to managers and supervisors; train and supervise food workers.	*Observation:* Look for operations that contribute to food-borne diseases and for poor sanitation practices. *Measurement:* Test trainees at completion of training; inspect for changes in operational procedures before and after training.
	Contamination of foods by workers.	Disease control of workers.	****	Do not work when ill with diarrhea or colds or when infected with lesions containing pus.	*Observation:* Observe whether workers work when they have diarrhea, colds, or infected lesions.
	Contamination of foods by workers.	Personal hygiene practice of workers.	**	Practice personal hygiene.	*Observation:* Observe personal hygiene practices and ways foods are handled and whether hands are washed before beginning work, after going to the toilet, after touching raw meat, after coughing or sneezing.
					(less value than above observations and measurements).

SOURCE: Bryan, 1982.

The salient conclusion is that the HACCP system can be used in the facilities from which most reported outbreaks of foodborne disease arise.

The situation in the food service industry is analogous to that existing in the food-processing segment. Various codes of practice exist, but these contain vague terms subject to interpretation by inspectors and food service managers. As with processing codes little distinction is made between the important and unimportant, this leading to emphasis on practices of little significance and underemphasis on those with direct bearing on foodborne illnesses. A case in point is the USDHEW *Food Service Sanitation Manual* (FDA, 1976), which contains a model food service sanitation ordinance that has been adopted by many states and municipalities by reference. Unfortunately, those responsible for making inspections at the state and local levels often are ill-prepared to uniformly interpret the ordinance in terms of separation of the essential from the extraneous.

As with food-processing operations, the application of the HACCP concept in food service operations would identify the critical control points for appropriate monitoring and thereby place emphasis on factors most responsible for foodborne illness. The application of HACCP to food service operations would necessitate input from technical personnel within the industry as well as public health authorities. It would also require training of inspectors to this new approach. At the present time one of the greatest deficiencies in food service sanitation is the lack of adequate regulatory control. At the point from which most foodborne illness problems emanate there is the least degree of regulation. The use of the HACCP system would not obviate this problem, but it would greatly increase the efficiency and effectiveness of existing manpower for inspection.

The elements of HACCP that are applicable to food service establishments also apply to food handling in the home. As laws and regulations cannot be applied to practices within the home, the alternative is education in proper food-handling practices. Unfortunately, sporadic attempts to accomplish this have not been met with much success. For example, in April 1973 the Gallup Organization reported that, among women, 74% did not know what *Salmonella* is; 66% did not know how to minimize its spread; and 39% thought that raw meat and poultry are inspected for the presence of *Salmonella* by federal and state employees (GAO, 1974). Clearly, educational efforts have not been successful in reducing the incidence of foodborne illness, including salmonellosis, for its incidence has remained unchanged or perhaps increased somewhat (Silliker, 1980). One reason for lack of success of educational programs directed at adults may be the sporadic nature of educational efforts. Education and training for prevention of foodborne illness must be continuing processes. New personnel continuously enter the food-processing and food service industries and new homemakers continuously undertake food preparation in the home. These facts necessitate constant repetition of good food-handling educational programs. Perhaps positive effects, though long range, could be expected from educational programs directed toward tomorrow's homemakers, schoolchildren. Over a period of time they could become knowledgeable and perhaps even influence their elders in proper food-handling practices. Such programs are virtually nonexistent in the United States. In Denmark no formal education is directed toward the consumer, but there is an intensive program providing students in the seventh, eighth, ninth, and tenth grades with a course consisting of two hours per week covering food handling, food preparation, and cooking (Health/Agriculture/Industry Committee on *Salmonella*, 1979). Such an approach is worthy of consideration in the United States. Adequate teacher training is essential for its success.

COST/BENEFIT ASPECTS OF REGULATORY CONTROL THROUGH HACCP INSPECTIONS

The proper implementation of HACCP by the food industry would lead to more cost-effective and efficient regulatory control. At the present time the size of the food industry is so great as to make it physically impossible for the FDA and other regulatory agencies to inspect establishments under their control with sufficient frequency. With respect to FDA, HACCP systems would involve, primarily, review of monitoring results. If these appeared satisfactory, the inspectors would be free to place emphasis on other facilities. On-the-line inspections by USDA resident inspectors in the meat and poultry industry is labor-intensive and expensive. The Booze-Allen report on the USDA Meat and Poultry Inspection Program (Anonymous, 1977) recommended less on-the-line inspection. Application of the HACCP concept to meat and poultry inspection (see Chapter 9) would no doubt greatly increase the efficiency and effectiveness of this regulatory activity without compromising consumer safety.

Finally, emphasis on the principles of the HACCP system for application in food service establishments and in the home should measurably improve food sanitation practices at these two points in the food chain.

REFERENCES

AMI (American Meat Institute)
  1982 Good Manufacturing Practices I: Voluntary Guidelines for the Production of Dry Fermented Sausage. II: Voluntary Guidelines for the Production of Semi-dry Fermented Sausage. Washington, D.C.: American Meat Institute.

Anonymous
  1977   Study of the federal meat and poultry inspection system. Vols. 1, 2, 3. Submitted to USDA by Booze, Allen and Hamilton, June 13, 1977. Washington, D.C.
Bryan, F. L.
  1978   Factors that contribute to outbreaks of foodborne disease. J. Food Prot. 41:816–827.
  1982   Microbiological hazards of feeding systems. Pp. 64–80 in Microbiological Safety of Foods in Feeding Systems. Committee on Microbiology of Food, Advisory Board on Military Personnel Supplies, Commission on Engineering and Technical Systems, National Research Council. Washington, D.C.: National Academy Press.
FDA (Food and Drug Administration)
  1973a   Thermally processed low-acid foods packaged in hermetically sealed containers. Part 128B (recodified as Part 113), Federal Register 38(16) 2398–2410. Jan. 24.
  1973b   Emergency permit control. Part 90 (recodified as Part 109), Federal Register 38(92): 12716–12721. May 14.
  1976   Food Service Sanitation Manual. Model food service sanitation ordinance. Washington, D.C.: USDHEW/PHS/FDA.
GAO (U.S. General Accounting Office)
  1974   *Salmonella* in raw meat and poultry: An assessment of the problem. Report to Congress (B-164031(2)), July 22. Washington, D.C.
Health/Agriculture/Industry Committee on *Salmonella*
  1979   Report on the Scandinavian *Salmonella* control program in poultry with added observations from Finland, Germany and Switzerland. Ottawa, Canada.
Silliker, J. H.
  1980   Status of *Salmonella*—10 years later. J. Food Prot. 43:307–313.
U.S. v. An Article of Food
  1972   Pasteurized whole eggs, 339 F. Supp. 131 (N.D. Ga., 1972).

11
Plans of Action for Implementation of the HACCP System and of Microbiological Criteria for Foods and Food Ingredients

IMPLEMENTATION OF HACCP

Because the application of the HACCP system provides for the most specific and critical approach to the control of microbiological hazards presented by foods, use of this system should be required of industry. Accordingly, this subcommittee believes that government agencies responsible for control of microbiological hazards in foods should promulgate appropriate regulations that would require industry to utilize the HACCP system in their food protection programs.

The regulations should identify the basic elements of the HACCP system and provide for ready availability of industry monitoring records that relate to critical control points and other appropriate information for review by regulatory inspection personnel.

The regulations should not specify details of the application of the HACCP system. The development of such details should be the prerogative of industry.

The regulations should require adequate training of regulatory inspection personnel in the elements of the HACCP system so that their inspection activities focus on the review of monitoring records as the primary basis for assessing the adequacy of a food processor's control program.

The HACCP system should likewise be applied at points in the food-processing chain other than at the processing level, i.e., in production, storage, transport, retail sales, and at food service establishments.

Regulatory authorities should have the option of assessing the appropriateness of selected critical control points, the adequacy of the monitoring procedures and the actions taken when results of monitoring indicated the need for action.

IMPLEMENTATION OF MICROBIOLOGICAL CRITERIA FOR FOODS AND FOOD INGREDIENTS.

Introduction

This subcommittee believes that for the most part microbiological criteria can best be used as one of the components of the HACCP system for food protection, e.g., as one of the means of monitoring critical control points in food processing and distribution (see Chapter 10). However, microbiological criteria can be used independently of HACCP as a sole determinant of the acceptability of a food or a process, e.g., through attribute sampling and testing of finished products domestically produced and/or at point of import for presence of *Salmonella* or of staphylococcal enterotoxins. In any event, whether or not microbiological criteria are applied either through the HACCP system or independently, there are principles governing their development and application that must be adhered to if the criteria are to be meaningful in the interest of food protection. In the foregoing chapters of this report, the subcommittee has set forth these general principles. However, there is need for a plan of action that would be national in scope by which these general principles would be applied uniformly in the process of developing and implementing microbiological criteria. Toward this end the following is directed.

The Food Industry

The subcommittee wishes to emphasize that application of the HACCP system by industry is the most effective means of assuring the microbiological safety and quality of foods. However, it would be presumptuous to propose to industry the mechanism of a plan for development of microbiological criteria either as an integral part of the HACCP system or otherwise. The needs for microbiological criteria are far too varied, even within a single organization, for any other than corporate management to undertake that task. It is anticipated, however, that the principles and considerations set forth in this report will provide guidance to those commercial organizations that need to use microbiological criteria in their food safety and quality control programs. Since it is industry's responsibility to provide safe food of acceptable quality, it should be industry's prerogative to design and implement the means by which such responsibility can be met to the satisfaction of regulatory agencies, or more broadly, the consuming public.

Government Agencies

The primary purpose for use of microbiological criteria by regulatory agencies is to supplement other means they have of assuring that foods produced under their jurisdictions are safe and of acceptable quality (see Chapter 2) and to make certain that industry fulfills its responsibility. Since the processing and distribution of most foods fall under the regulatory jurisdiction of many state and municipal agencies, as well as being subject to federal regulations, there should exist a high degree of uniformity in the manner by which microbiological criteria (particularly those that pertain to finished product) are developed and implemented. Lack of such uniformity has resulted in the establishment of many criteria that are nonuniform, misapplied or unjustified, and highly controversial. Three examples will serve to illustrate:

1. *The current state of microbiological criteria established by state agencies:* Elsewhere (see Chapter 8) reference has been made to the surveys by Wehr (1982) of microbiological criteria for foods that currently are in effect in various states. Several observations immediately become apparent: (a) the great disparity among the states with respect to the foods for which microbiological criteria exist, (b) the variability of criteria applicable to the same food, (c) the impracticality of certain criteria, and (d) the large number of states that have not established microbiological criteria. The latter would seem to reflect indecision or indifference on the part of some as to the value of microbiological criteria in food protection programs.

2. *The Oregon experience:* Standards for fresh, frozen, and cooked or smoked meat products were promulgated by the state of Oregon in 1973. These standards did not fulfill the purposes for which they were established. They were unenforceable and created general adverse reaction. For these and other reasons, the standards were repealed in 1977 as "standards of quality, identity and composition." This unfortunate event caused confusion, ill will, and unwarranted costs. (For further discussion, see Chapter 9, part B.)

3. *FDA's microbiological quality standards:* FDA proposed to adopt microbiological criteria (under Section 401 of the Food, Drug and Cosmetic Act) designated as "standards of quality for foods for which there are no standards of identity" (see Chapter 2). This was an approach to expanding the agency's use of microbiological criteria. The proposal resulted in predominantly adverse reaction, as amply documented in the *Federal Register* and other publications. The standards were not purported to bear any relationship to safety.

Quality standards for four types of cream-type pies and food-grade gelatin were adopted but later, for various reasons, were withdrawn. However, FDA stated its intention to promulgate microbiological quality standards for other foods. Subsequently, due to lack of "sufficient resources to promulgate and enforce additional microbiological quality standard regulations," the agency stated its intention to "issue microbiological quality standards as recommendations or regulations as appropriate" and encouraged voluntary adoption by industry and state authorities of standards developed and recommended by the agency. Accordingly, standards for three seafood products (frozen fish sticks, fish cakes, and crab cakes) were recommended for adoption. The standards were based upon the results of national surveys of products obtained at retail outlets. At least 47 such product surveys have been made. However, to date no additional recommendations of microbiological quality standards have been issued. For further discussion of FDA's program for microbiological quality standards see Chapter 2.

Recently, FDA proposed microbiological defect action levels (presumably standards) for raw breaded shrimp (FDA, 1983). Comments on the proposal were invited. The criteria are based on the results of surveys at the plant level of 31 breaded-shrimp processors. Thus, the approach to the development of the microbiological defect levels was quite different from that used for the microbiological quality standards.

In retrospect, the turbulent history of FDA's attempt to promulgate microbiological quality standards leads to the conclusion that the effort has fallen far short of success. As for the proposed microbiological defect action levels, any conclusion as to success or failure is premature at this time.

In any event, the approach taken by FDA to expand its use of microbiological criteria was unilaterally conceived and pursued. In the early planning stages for the development of microbiological criteria there was little input from the various segments of industry, other federal agencies, state and municipal agencies, or others having a vital interest in any such undertaking. Had the agency enlisted these groups in the early planning stages in a coordinated effort, it is likely that needs for criteria would have been clearly delineated and justified and that chances for emergence of a successful program for an expansion of FDA's use of microbiological criteria for food would have been greatly enhanced.

There are excellent examples of successful multilateral programs that have been established in response to national needs relative to food safety.

Notable are the Cooperative Federal-State Program for Certification of Interstate Milk Shippers, the 3-A Sanitary Standards Program for sanitary design and operation of dairy equipment, the National Shellfish Sanitation Program (see Chapter 8), and the current good manufacturing regulation for low-acid canned foods. Also, the National Cooperative State/Federal Programs for the Eradication of Brucellosis and Tuberculosis in Cattle (see Chapter 4) were developed with broad participation of all concerned with the need for control of these diseases of cattle.

It is emphasized that especially in the development of the milk and shellfish programs, the 3-A Sanitary Standards and the low-acid GMPs, industry's participation was extensive. Much of the technical competence needed was provided by industry, and its voice was as influential as any in regard to regulatory requirements that were established.

It seems abundantly clear that the magnitude of the impact of the implementation by regulatory agencies of microbiological criteria for foods that would apply nationally would demand widespread participation by concerned groups in the development of the criteria. Such participation would tend to assure that the best interests of all were served and that general acceptance of the criteria would be forthcoming. It is logical that concerned federal agencies assume leadership in fostering a multilateral approach to development of microbiological criteria for foods. In fact, it is evident from the survey by Wehr (1978) that a preponderance of responses (50 of 64) received from states stated a preference for federal agencies to assume such leadership.

In view of the considerations given above, this subcommittee offers a plan for a national program for identification of foods for which microbiological criteria are needed, for development of criteria for those foods, and for appropriate implementation of such criteria in regulatory programs.

THE PLAN

1. The Bureau of Foods of the Food and Drug Administration, an appropriate subsidiary body of the Department of Agriculture, the National Marine Fisheries Service, and the U.S. Army Natick Research and Development Center, being the primary federal agencies having the responsibility of assuring that foods available to their constituencies are safe and of acceptable quality, jointly should establish an ad hoc Commission on Microbiological Criteria for Foods.
2. The objective of the commission should be to develop microbiological criteria for foods that will be responsive to need.
3. The Food and Drug Administration, having the broadest responsi-

bility for food protection among the federal agencies, should take the initiative to arrange with the cooperation of the other three agencies identified above for appointment of members to the commission.

4. Membership of the commission should consist of appropriate personnel selected from (a) each of the four above-mentioned federal agencies, (b) state and municipal food regulatory agencies, (c) the food industry, and (d) academia. The number of members on the commission should be kept to a minimum in the interest of expediency in reaching decisions and economy of operations.

5. Initially, the commission should address (a) the selection of foods and food ingredients on the basis of need for microbiological criteria that could effectively supplement and be incorporated in food protection programs of federal, state, and municipal food regulatory agencies (The selection process should include, but not be limited to, a review of foods for which criteria currently exist and an evaluation of the suitability of these criteria.), and (b) the development of criteria for each food for which it was determined that microbiological criteria would serve a useful purpose.

6. The commission should appoint expert working groups to carry out the tasks of selecting foods and of development of criteria. The expert working groups should present their recommendations to the commission.

7. The commission should present its recommendations to the federal agency having primary jurisdiction for the safety and quality of the food or food ingredient involved. The federal agency should take the necessary steps to promulgate regulations embodying the recommended criteria and to promote uniform adoption of the criteria by state and municipal regulatory agencies if it deems it appropriate to do so. Insofar as possible, the Department of Defense should utilize microbiological criteria recommended by the commission in developing military specifications for foods and food ingredients.

8. The development, review, and modification of microbiological criteria for foods is a continuing task. Therefore, as soon as the initial work of the commission has been set in motion, it should take the steps necessary to organize itself as a continuing body elected by vote or other suitable means of the participating groups indicated above, except that the representative of each federal agency should be appointed by an appropriate official of the respective agency. The subcommittee also suggests that the organizational structure of the several cooperative federal/state programs mentioned above be reviewed for guidance in this task.

9. Finally, the commission should address the continuing need for

research to (a) better understand the effects of current and emerging processing and distribution practices that may affect the microbial safety and quality of foods, and (b) improve and develop methods for the detection and enumeration of microorganisms and groups of microorganisms and their toxic agents that are important to the safety and quality of foods.

This subcommittee believes that the plan of action for implementation of the HACCP system provides for the most specific and critical approach to the control of microbiological hazards presented by foods. The plan of action for implementation of microbiological criteria that embodies the general principles and considerations presented in this report will lead to a coordinated national program for the establishment and application of microbiological criteria for foods that will enhance food protection programs of federal, state, and municipal agencies as well as those of the military and of industry. The subcommittee recommends that action be taken to implement these plans at the earliest opportunity.

REFERENCES

FDA (Food and Drug Administration)
1983   Raw breaded shrimp: Microbiological defect action levels. Federal Register 48(175):40563–40564.Sept. 8.
Wehr, H. M.
1978   Attitudes and policies of state governments. Food Technol. 32(1):63–67.
1982   Attitudes and policies of governmental agencies on microbiological criteria for foods—an update. Food Technol. 36(9):45–54, 92.

APPENDIXES

Appendix A

Summary Responses to Specific Contract Items

The following comprises summary responses to the explicit requests included in the Scope of Work as defined by the Contracting Agencies. The responses are addressed more comprehensively in Chapters 1-11 of this book.

I. The contractor will initiate a reevaluation of sampling plans employed for various classes of foods and food ingredients that are determining *Salmonella* presence in raw and finished food and food ingredients that are subject to *Salmonella* contamination.[1]

The Committee on *Salmonella* of the National Research Council (NRC, 1969) emphasized that the sale of foods containing salmonellae cannot be condoned but at the same time recognized that salmonellae can be found in many products if a sufficient number of tests are made. The report called attention to confusion and uncertainty that existed then in the food-processing industry due to lack of a definitive sampling and testing plan. The following question was posed: When should we stop testing and conclude that a product is *Salmonella*-free (which may simply mean that the contamination level is below the sensitivity of the sampling plan and the analytical procedure)?

In recognition of the fact that there is no way to be absolutely certain that a particular lot of nonsterile food is free of salmonellae, the Committee on *Salmonella* recommended two specific actions: (1) evolve a realistic

---

[1]Excluded from these considerations were raw meats and poultry from which, given existing technology, salmonellae cannot be eliminated.

assessment of the degree of hazard imposed by various foods, feeds, and drugs, and (2) develop sampling plans that will provide adequate assurance that the number of salmonellae present, if any, is below a statistically defined limit that offers minimal hazard to the consumer. The committee suggested a system by which the degree of hazard presented by any food could be assessed and it recommended a sampling and testing plan that could lead to a decision whether to accept or reject a particular lot of food.

Assessment of the degree of hazard presented by various foods was based upon three questions: (1) does the food contain a sensitive ingredient, (2) does the processing of the food include a controlled procedure that will destroy salmonellae, and (3) will salmonellae grow in the product if it is abused during distribution or after preparation for consumption? Based upon answers to the foregoing questions, eight different configurations of hazard characteristics are possible. These are delineated in Table A-1.

Five risk categories were recognized by the Committee on *Salmonella*:

Category I—foods that are intended for infants, aged, and the infirm, and that contain a sensitive ingredient.

Category II—foods with all three hazard characteristics.

Category III—foods with two hazard characteristics.

Category IV—foods with one hazard characteristic

Category V—foods with none of the three hazard characteristics.

TABLE A-1   Categories of Food Products Based on Product Hazard Characteristics

Type of Food	Hazard characteristic[a]			Category
	A	B	C	
Intended for infants, aged, and infirm	+	+ or 0	+ or 0	I
Intended for general use	+	+	+	II
	+	+	0	III
	+	0	+	III
	0	+	+	III
	+	0	0	IV
	0	+	0	IV
	0	0	+	IV
	0	0	0	V

[a]A = Product contains sensitive ingredient.
  B = No destructive step during manufacture.
  C = Likelihood for growth if abused.
  + = Hazard present; 0 = Hazard not present.

SOURCE: Olson, 1975.

The Committee on *Salmonella* recommended testing and acceptance criteria for "questioned" lots of food. These are summarized in Table A-2. Application of these criteria contemplates the collection of random sample units from the lot in question. Multiple 25-g analytical units, the number based upon the risk category of the product, are then analyzed for *Salmonella*. The intensity of sampling and analysis is related to the degree of risk (hazard category) presented by the product. The objective was to have a sampling and testing plan that would provide adequate assurance that the number of salmonellae, if present, would be below a statistically defined limit offering minimal hazard to the consumer. The limit for each category is given in the last column of Table A-2, i.e., 95% confidence that the *Salmonella* contamination level is no more than 1 in 500 g for Category I; no more than 1 in 250 g for Category II; and no more than 1 in 125 g for Categories III, IV, and V. It will be noted that within each category, two sampling plans are provided, one permitting acceptance only if all analytical units tested are found negative for *Salmonella*, the other permitting a single positive result. For example, for products in Category I, one sampling plan permits acceptance if each of 60 25-g analytical units is analyzed and found negative. The other sampling plan permits acceptance if one of 92 25-g units is positive. Justification for the two different sampling plans was based upon the fact that one positive result from 92 analytical units or zero positive results from 60 analytical units provides the same probability (95%) that the level of salmonellae as shown in the last column of Table A-2 is not exceeded.

It should be emphasized that the sampling and testing plan recommended by the Committee on *Salmonella* was intended for application to (1) processed foods or ingredients as contrasted to, e.g., raw meats and poultry; (2) lots that conform to specific criteria that establish their integrity; and (3) lots

TABLE A-2 Acceptance Criteria

Product Category	Number of Units Tested with No Positives	Number of Units Tested with No More than One Positive	Significance[a] 95% Probability of One Organism or Less in
I	60 (1,500 g)	92 (2,300 g)	500 g
II	29 (725 g)	48 (1,200 g)	250 g
III	13 (325 g)	22 (550 g)	125 g
IV	13 (325 g)	22 (550 g)	125 g
V[b]	13 (325 g)	22 (550 g)	125 g

[a]Accuracy of Attribute Sampling, USDA Consumer and Marketing Service, March 1966.
[b]Not normally applicable.

SOURCE: NRC, 1969.

that have been questioned because of the possible presence of salmonellae. The sampling plan was not designed or intended to replace routine surveillance operations, including testing, that a food manufacturer or a regulatory agency might employ. The plans were intended to be used in arriving at a final decision in order to accept or reject a particular lot in question.

After reviewing the report of the Committee on *Salmonella*, the FDA began to consider ways of responding to the various committee recommendations (Olson, 1975). It invited Dr. E. M. Foster, Director of the Food Research Institute, University of Wisconsin, to assemble a group of knowledgeable people representing both government and industry to develop a classification system and a sampling plan along the lines envisioned by the Committee on *Salmonella*. The Interagency-Industry Committee on *Salmonella* Control in Foods submitted its report to the FDA in October 1970, and the report was published in March 1971 (Foster, 1971). This report embraced the recommendations of the Committee on *Salmonella* both with respect to the establishment of categories of food products based upon product hazard characteristics and the sampling and analytical plans for determination of the acceptability of questioned lots. Further, it provided guidance on the assessment of hazard characteristics.

Subsequently FDA announced its position on *Salmonella* sampling and testing plans (Olson, 1975). Basically, FDA accepted the recommendations of the Committee on *Salmonella* (NRC, 1969) and the Interagency-Industry Committee (Foster, 1971) with the following exceptions. First, a sample lot would be accepted only if analyses of all analytical units were negative for salmonellae. The FDA position was that acceptance of any lot of food in which salmonellae were shown to be present would not be administratively feasible. Thus, the sampling plan shown in the second column of Table A-2 would be employed and the sampling plan shown in the third column (permitting a single positive among the analytical units tested) would not be utilized. Second, FDA provided for the compositing of multiple analytical units, the maximum size of a composite unit being 375 g. The composite unit was to consist of a series of 25-g analytical units. Finally, the FDA indicated that the acceptance criteria would be applied to any lot of product tested in connection with any of its surveillance or compliance programs. As previously noted, the two committees (NRC, 1969; Foster, 1971) had indicated that the sampling plan was not designed to replace routine surveillance operations, but was intended to be used in arriving at a final decision whether to accept or reject a particular lot in question. FDA's position on this point was made clear: ''If we sample a lot we question it; otherwise why sample it?''

The fourth edition of the *Bacteriological Analytical Manual for Foods*

(BAM) (FDA, 1976) reflected Olson's position paper (Olson, 1975). The classification of products by hazard categories and the attendant sampling plans were consistent with the report of the Committee on *Salmonella* and the recommendations of the Interagency-Industry Committee on *Salmonella* Control in Foods. Indeed, a vast number of industry quality control programs utilized the sampling plans routinely in their *Salmonella* control programs, not just for determining the status of suspect lots.

The fifth edition of the BAM (FDA, 1978), set forth a revised *Salmonella* sampling plan, one that departed radically from the recommendations of the Committee on *Salmonella*. Three categories of food were identified as follows:

Food Category I—foods that would normally be in Category II except they are intended for consumption by the aged, the infirm, and infants.

Food Category II—foods that would not normally be subjected to a process lethal to *Salmonella* between the time of sampling and consumption.

Food Category III—foods that would normally be subjected to a process lethal to *Salmonella* between the time of sampling and consumption. The following tabulation shows the number of sample units to be collected in each food category:

Food Category	Number of Sample Units
I	60
II	30
III	15

The categorization of foods and the sampling plans prescribed in the 1978 edition of the *Bacteriological Analytical Manual* depart both in philosophy and substance from those contained in the 1976 edition of the BAM. Likewise, of course, they depart from the recommendations of the NAS Committee on *Salmonella* and those of the Interagency-Industry Committee on *Salmonella* Control in Foods. The present system employed by the FDA for categorizing foods, as well as the sampling plans tied to such categorization, are unrelated to risk. The key issue, rather, is whether the food would normally be subjected to a process lethal to *Salmonella* between the time of sampling and consumption. This parameter played no role in the designation of food categories by the Committee on *Salmonella*, the recommendations of which were embraced by the Interagency-Industry Committee on *Salmonella* Control in Foods and the FDA. Ignored in the present classification system are: risk A: the product or an ingredient of the product has been identified as a significant potential source of salmonellae (i.e., it is "sensitive"); risk B: the *manufacturing* process does not include a controlled step that will destroy salmonellae; and risk C: there is a substantial likelihood of microbial growth if the product is mishandled or "abused" in distribution or consumer usage. The present system utilized by the FDA recognizes, only, that if a product were to be classified in "new" Category II, it would be classified in Category I if the product were to be consumed by high-risk groups. It is of interest to note that the Committee on *Salmonella* of the NAS classified any food consumed by high-risk groups in Category I if it contained a sensitive ingredient (risk factor A). Under the present system, such a product would be assigned to Category III if the food would normally be subjected to a process lethal to *Salmonella* between the time of sampling and consumption. Table A-3 lists examples of foods in Categories II and III as presented in the 1978 edition of the BAM. Table A-4 shows examples of "interesting shifts in classification" that have occurred as a result of the revised *Salmonella* sampling plan introduced in that edition.

It is difficult for this subcommittee to understand the rationale for the changes in food category classification and sampling plans between the 1976 and the 1978 editions of the BAM and thus, in effect, the rationale for the FDA rejection of the recommendations of the NRC Committee on *Salmonella*. In section A, Sampling Plans for *Salmonella* of Chapter 1 of the 1978 BAM the following statements are made: "Generally, the assignment of food categories has depended on the sensitivity of a consumer group (e.g., the aged, the infirm and infants), the history of the food, and whether there was a step lethal to *Salmonella* during the manufacturing process or in the home. Of these criteria the sensitivity of the consumer group and whether the food normally underwent a process lethal to *Salmonella* either at the manufacturing or consumer level appeared to be the most important considerations in the selection of a sampling plan. The history of the food would be more important in a decision on whether to sample rather than how many sample units to take." This subcommittee offers the following comments on these statements:

1. As stated, the sensitivity of the consumer group influences the assignment of food categories. But, as indicated above, the present FDA system would classify foods containing sensitive ingredients in Category III if such foods were normally subjected to a process lethal to *Salmonella* between the time of sampling and consumption. The NRC Committee on *Salmonella* would classify the same foods in Category I if they contained a sensitive ingredient regardless of their "normal" subsequent handling. The present FDA system simply assigns products in Category II to Category I if high-risk groups are involved. But if the same foods were "normally" subjected to a process lethal to *Salmonella* between the time of sampling

TABLE A-3   Food Categories II and III

Food Category II—Foods that would normally be subjected to a process lethal to *Salmonella* between the time of sampling and consumption.

Product Code	Food
03	Bread, rolls, buns, sugared breads, crackers, custard and cream-filled sweet goods
05	Breakfast cereals, ready-to-eat
07	Pretzels, chips, and specialty items
09	Butter and butter products; pasteurized milk and raw fluid milk and fluid milk products for consumption; pasteurized and unpasteurized concentrated liquid milk products for consumption; dried milk and dried milk products for consumption
12	Cheese and cheese products
13	Ice cream from pasteurized milk and related products that have been pasteurized; raw ice cream mix and related unpasteurized products for consumption
14	Pasteurized and unpasteurized imitation dairy products for consumption.
15	Pasteurized eggs, egg products from pasteurized eggs; unpasteurized eggs and egg products from unpasteurized eggs for consumption without further cooking
16	Canned and cured fish, vertebrates; other fish products; fresh and frozen raw oysters and raw clams, shellfish and crustacean products; smoked fish, shellfish, and crustaceans for consumption
17	Unflavored gelatin
20–22	Fresh, frozen, and canned fruits and juices, concentrates, and nectars; dried fruits for consumption; jams, jellies, preserves, and butters
23	Nuts and nut products for consumption
26	Oils consumed directly without further processing; oleomargarine
27	Dressings and condiments (including mayonnaise), salad dressing, vinegar
28	Spices, including salt; flavors and extracts
29	Soft drinks and water
30	Beverage bases
31	Coffee and tea
33	Candy, chewing gum
34	Chocolate and cocoa products
35	Pudding mixes not cooked prior to consumption, gelatin products
36	Syrups, sugars, and honey
38	Soups
39	Prepared salads

Food Category III—Foods that would normally be subjected to a process lethal to *Salmonella* between the time of sampling and consumption.

Product Code	Food
02	Whole grain, processed grain, and starch products for human use
04	Macaroni and noodle products
16	Fresh and frozen fish; vertebrates (except that eaten raw); fresh and frozen shellfish and crustaceans (except raw oysters and raw clams for consumption); other aquatic animals (including frog legs)
24	Fresh vegetables, frozen vegetables, dried vegetables, cured and processed vegetable products normally cooked before consumption
26	Vegetable oils, oil stock, and vegetable shortening
35	Dry dessert and pudding mixes that are cooked prior to consumption
37	Frozen dinners, multiple food dinners
45–46	Food chemicals (direct additives)

SOURCE: FDA, 1978.

TABLE A-4   Selected Examples of Categories—BAM
1976 vs. BAM 1978

Foods	BAM Classification	
	1976	1978
Salt, flavors and extracts, mayonnaise, fresh fruits and juices, jams, soft drinks, water, beverage bases, coffee, tea, snack items (dry), syrups.	CAT. III[b]	CAT. II[a]
Frozen dinners.	II	III
Fresh and frozen shellfish and crustaceans (ex. raw oysters and clams), other aquatic animals, fresh vegetables.	III	III

Sampling:
[a]Category II: Thirty 25-g samples.
[b]Category III: Fifteen 25-g samples.

SOURCE: Silliker, 1980.

and consumption, these foods would be assigned to Category III *regardless of the group at risk.*

2. The term ''history of the food'' is difficult for the subcommittee to interpret. One might equate this to a food with a history indicating it to be a *Salmonella* problem, i.e., a sensitive product. It is stated that the history of the food would be more important in a decision on *whether to sample* rather than on how many sample units to take. Thus, it would appear, and logic would dictate this, that one might be more concerned with a product in Category III (one containing a sensitive ingredient) than one in Category II. For example, one would certainly be more concerned with dry dessert and pudding mixes that are cooked prior to consumption or frozen dinners than with salad dressing or vinegar. Yet the former are classified in Category III and the latter in II. It seems, however, that to classify salad dressing and vinegar in Category II is ill-advised. These products are classified in Category II solely on the basis that they ''would not normally be subjected to a process lethal to *Salmonella* between the time of sampling and consumption.'' Vinegar, for example, clearly belongs in Category V (according to the report of the Committee on *Salmonella*), because (1) it contains no sensitive ingredient, (2) its acidity would destroy *Salmonella*, and (3) salmonellae are incapable of growth in the product. Yet the 1978 edition of the BAM would clearly place this product in Category II with a sampling plan ''twice as stringent'' as would be applied to dry dessert and pudding mixes or frozen dinners.

3. It is stated: ''Of these criteria, the sensitivity of the consumer group and whether the food normally underwent a process lethal to *Salmonella*

either at the manufacturing or consumer level appeared to be the most important considerations in selection of a sampling plan.'' The report of the Committee on *Salmonella* with reference to classification of food products according to risk is concerned with whether the manufacturing process does not include a controlled step that would destroy salmonellae. In this regard, the hazard relates to the manufacturing process, not to what occurs in the hands of the consumer. The report did recognize: "Obviously, the food or ingredient that will ultimately be used under conditions resulting in *Salmonella* destruction is far less hazardous than one that will be consumed without decontamination and quantitative guidelines take this into account. This does not ignore the danger of bringing the contaminated food into the kitchen or processing area but does recognize that the level of risk entailed is influenced by the ultimate usage.'' These considerations result, for example, in placing sensitive products, such as frozen dinners in Category III, even though such products contain (1) sensitive ingredients, (2) no final kill step at the manufacturing level, and (3) the potential of *Salmonella* growth if mishandled.

4. If "the history of food" is to be equated to whether it contains a "sensitive ingredient," then this characteristic of the product is not "more important in a decision on whether to sample rather than how many sample units to take," according to the recommendations of the Committee on *Salmonella*. It is, indeed, one of four factors that are considered in classification of a food into one of the five hazard categories. The others are the population at risk, whether the food is subject to a "pasteurizing" step at the manufacturing level, and whether *Salmonella* growth may occur in the product if it is mishandled. The present FDA scheme eliminates the "history of the food" as a determinant of the sampling plan when, indeed, the Committee on *Salmonella* gave equal weight to this and two other factors (kill step and potential of growth) in establishing its classification scheme.

This subcommittee supports the recommendations of the NRC Committee on *Salmonella* with respect to the classification of foods into five categories and the establishment of sampling plans, the stringency of which is related to the degree of hazard. It feels that the present FDA categorization of foods, and the sampling plans tied to these, ignore the recommendations of the NRC Committee on *Salmonella* and substitute these with a less effective system.

The recommendations of the NRC Committee on *Salmonella* not only were endorsed by the Interagency-Industry Committee on *Salmonella* Control in Foods and by the 1976 edition of the BAM but in addition by the International Commission on Microbiological Specifications for Foods (ICMSF, 1974).

II.   The contractor will evaluate whether or not suitable microbiological testing procedures and data bases have been developed and validated sufficiently to be useful for: regulatory purposes, for purchasing specifications, and/or for quality control purposes. If further work is indicated, the contractor will list priorities for the tasks that must be completed so that suitable microbiological tests and data bases will be available for the various purposes listed above.

Test procedures for pathogenic and indicator organisms are discussed and evaluated in Chapters 4 and 5 of this report. Adequate procedures are available for the aerobic plate count and the quantitation of coliform, fecal coliform, *Escherichia coli, Staphylococcus aureus, Clostridium perfringens*, enterococci, and yeasts and molds. Reliable procedures exist for the detection of *Salmonella*, staphylococcal enterotoxins, *C. perfringens* alpha toxin, and *Clostridium botulinum* toxins.

Additional satisfactory procedures are available (*Compendium of Methods for the Microbiological Examination of Foods*, APHA, 1984) for the direct microscopic count, and to detect and/or enumerate psychrotrophic, thermoduric, lipolytic, proteolytic, halophilic, osmophilic, pectinolytic, and acid-producing microorganisms, as well as for mesophilic aerobic sporeformers, mesophilic anaerobic sporeformers, aciduric flat-sour sporeformers, thermophilic flat-sour sporeformers, thermophilic anaerobic sporeformers, and sulfide spoilage sporeformers.

At present, *E. coli* is the most reliable bacterial indicator of fecal contamination. The standard enrichment-plating procedures routinely applied to detect and enumerate this organism in foods are time-consuming, laborious, and expensive, and there is some question about their accuracy. There are more rapid and accurate procedures for *E. coli* such as the Anderson-Baird-Parker direct plating method and recent modifications of this procedure.

Although existing procedures for *Bacillus cereus* and *Vibrio parahaemolyticus* seem to perform well in some laboratories, certain problems are encountered with these procedures. In the detection and enumeration of *B. cereus*, existing procedures do not always clearly separate this organism from other contaminants. In the case of *V. parahaemolyticus*, a recent study (ICMSF, in preparation) has revealed some inconsistencies regarding the MPN procedure.

Although rapid progress is being made, procedures for the detection of *Yersinia enterocolitica, Yersinia pseudotuberculosis*, and *Campylobacter fetus* subsp. *jejuni* (*Campylobacter jejuni/coli*) from foods require additional studies.

Continued studies are recommended for the detection and quantification of mycotoxins, particularly to develop more practical and precise methods. Similar recommendations are proposed for toxins important in certain fish and shellfish such as ciguatoxin, saxitoxins, and closely related toxins. One of the most severe problems related to microbiological criteria is the time necessary to obtain the results of microbiological test procedures. For this reason, additional studies are needed to develop microbiological techniques that require a minimum of time, are simple, sensitive, cost-effective, and usable on-site, in-process as part of microbiological control programs.

Microbiological criteria for viruses in foods are not feasible at the present time primarily because of lack of practical methods. Development of methods for the detection of viruses in foods that can cause human illness is highly recommended.

An evaluation of available data bases for microbiological criteria of various foods has been made in Chapter 9. Additional information related to this contract item can be found in Chapters 4, 5, and 9.

III. The contractor will determine the relative merits of: aerobic plate count, fecal coliform, coliform, *E. coli*, and coagulase-positive *Staphylococcus* procedures currently used to identify contamination of foods during and after processing.

In perishable foods, the aerobic plate count (APC) can reflect the microbial condition of the raw materials and ingredients used, the effectiveness of processing methods (for example heat treatment), the efficacy of cleaning and sanitation procedures employed, the microbiological condition of the processing equipment, and the conditions of storage (time-temperature abuse). One or more of these conditions, if not adequately controlled, can be responsible for higher than expected APC during and after processing. Thus, to identify a specific cause of contamination by the APC, it would be necessary to eliminate the other potential causes. Results of testing final products only do not tell which event(s) may have caused a high APC, but if used in conjunction with observations made during plant inspection they may provide information to make some inferences. To identify where contamination occurred, APCs of line samples before and after critical control points have merit. In shelf-stable foods that do not support microbial growth, results on finished products also will not give information about specific causes of high APC. Contamination, however, can be identified by APC as described for perishable foods. In fermented food, the APC offers no information about contamination.

From their original fecal, water, soil, or plant environment, coliform bacteria can reach the food processing and preparation environments and become established there. The principal value of determining coliform bacteria is as an index of postprocessing contamination of foods that are heat processed for safety. Coliform bacteria are used for this purpose, primarily because they are heat-sensitive organisms and a relatively simple test is available for their detection. *E. coli*, the most sensitive bacterial indicator of fecal contamination, is a member of the coliform group. Unfortunately, the fecal connotation of *E. coli* is often linked to any food in which coliform bacteria are found, most of the time inappropriately. Thus, the presence of coliform bacteria in food does not mean that there was necessarily fecal contamination or that pathogens are present. Small numbers of coliform bacteria are normally present in raw milk and on vegetables, meats, poultry, fish, and many other raw foods. These organisms are readily destroyed during heat processing of foods. The presence of coliforms in foods thus indicates either (1) presence of these organisms in a raw product that was not heat processed, (2) ineffective heat processing, and/or (3) contamination after heat processing by contact with contaminated equipment, utensils, or employees. Excessively high coliform counts may result from massive contamination, process failure, or from growth resulting from extended processing delays and/or from improper storage practices (time-temperature abuse). The use of the coliform count as an index of contamination requires a thorough knowledge of the significance of coliform bacteria in various foods and even in a single food at different stages of processing. In some cases, it may also require examination of line samples. For example, some coliform bacteria can be expected in raw milk. After proper pasteurization, the presence of coliform bacteria indicates postpasteurization contamination. Although this seldom poses a health hazard, the presence of coliforms may be indicative of contamination of the product with spoilage bacteria that could materially reduce shelf-life. Results of line samples are needed to identify the source of contamination.

The merit of the fecal coliform or *E. coli* count to identify contamination is subject to the same limitations as described above for the coliform count, although the possibility of direct or indirect involvement of fecal contamination becomes greater with a positive fecal coliform test and even greater when *E. coli* is detected. Without doubt, *E. coli* is presently the most reliable bacterial indicator of fecal contamination. If fecal coliforms in a food are used as an index of *E. coli* and thus as an index of fecal contamination, this relationship must be established for the product where fecal coliforms are used for this purpose. In summary, fecal coliform and *E. coli* counts are made for the purpose of determining fecal contamination; for post-heat treatment contamination, coliform determinations are more appropriate. The presence of coagulase-positive staphylococci in foods indicates that direct or indirect contamination resulted from either human or animal sources. Although some may survive mild heat processing, their presence in these foods usually represents postprocessing contamination. Small numbers, therefore, do indicate contamination, whereas large numbers usually result from time-temperature abuse and represent a more serious condition that eventually may pose a health hazard. If large numbers of staphylococci occur in a food as a result of growth, it usually occurs in a food that has been heat processed to eliminate competing organisms, thus with temperature abuse setting the stage for unrestricted growth of staphylococci. It is necessary, however, to point out that the absence or low numbers of coagulase-positive staphylococci in heated or fermented foods does not imply safety—they may have been destroyed during processing but their enterotoxins still may be active.

Additional information related to this contract item can be found in Chapters 4 and 5.

IV. The contractor will evaluate the optimal number of samples that should be taken from a lot of food to establish the number of indicator organisms present when the result is to be used for: (1) quality control purposes, (2) purchase specifications, and (3) regulatory purposes. The contractor shall include consideration of cost vs. benefit in determining the optimal number.

This contract item raises a number of interesting aspects to sampling. To evaluate the optimal number of samples for indicator organisms is not a simple process. The task is made more difficult if one has or uses three different sampling procedures, i.e., for quality control, purchase specifications, and regulatory purposes. From a philosophical point of view, it would be undesirable to suggest that such a procedure be adopted if one wishes to have the same level of confidence in each result. As a manufacturer, one would expect the same sensitivity in the microbiological testing program as that of the federal government, especially if court procedures were to be involved. Likewise, if one purchases raw material from a supplier at an agreed specification, one would like to know the risks involved in processing that material using the same sampling procedure as the supplier. Thus, the same method and sampling plan should be used for all three purposes.

The development of optimal number of samples has been dealt with in part in Chapter 6 and relates to the stringency of the sampling plan. The significance of indicator organisms varies with the food. The presence of these in a pasteurized food or shellfish means something different from their presence in raw foods like meat (see Chapter 5). The ICMSF concept of relating the stringency of the sampling plan to the degree of hazard is generally accepted as a useful and meaningful way of making such a selection. The number of analytical units examined (n) and the number of analytical units permitted to exceed the established limit (c) vary with the degree of hazard.

In summary, to determine optimal numbers of samples for indicator organisms, one needs to know:

1. degree of risk involved to the consumer
2. hazards involved
3. processing steps before eating
4. final use of food, i.e., cooking, storage, etc.

The cost-benefit consideration for indicator organisms follows the same concern as listed in item VIII of this Appendix. Current information is that 3-class plans can be used for indicator organisms.

Additional information also can be found in Chapter 6 of this report and in Chapter 1 of ICMSF (1974).

V. The contractor will determine the usefulness of a zero tolerance for such indicator organisms as *E. coli* and *S. aureus*; e.g., no *E. coli* in one gram.

For foods, *E. coli* is the best bacterial indicator of fecal contamination of relatively recent origin. Thus, the presence of *E. coli* in a food indicates the possibility that fecal contamination may have taken place and that other microorganisms of fecal origin, including pathogens, may be present. However, it does not imply that pathogens are present or, if present, the level of contamination. On the other hand, the absence of *E. coli* does not imply the absence of enteric pathogens. In many raw foods such as milk, fresh meats, and poultry small numbers of *E. coli* can be expected because of the close association of animals with fecally contaminated environments during production and the likelihood of spread to carcasses during slaughter-dressing operations. Because *E. coli* is relatively heat-sensitive, the presence of *E. coli* in a heat-processed food, such as cooked crabmeat, for example, indicates underprocessing and/or postprocessing contamination through equipment, utensils, by persons handling the cooked food, or from cross-contamination with raw foods. Occasionally a few of these organisms will reach the product even under reasonably good manufacturing practices. However, the criteria for heat-processed products should be strict. This can be achieved by proper selection of n, c, m, and M (see Chapter 6).

An evaluation of the usefulness of a zero tolerance for the indicator organism *E. coli*, i.e., less than one *E. coli* in one gram of food, requires an examination of the purpose of the microbiological limit and, most important, a recognition of the limitations of the analytical procedure. A microbiological limit of less than one *E. coli* per gram implies the use of a MPN procedure. The current AOAC MPN procedure for *E. coli* (AOAC, 1980) is laborious and requires several days to complete. More important, however, the limits in precision of the MPN procedure are often ignored when MPN values are interpreted. Even under the best of experimental conditions, there are distinct limitations to the precision of the MPN estimate. The MPN estimate is not one value but represents a range, the extent of which depends upon many factors, one of which is the number of tubes in a set. Woodward (1957) reported that for a 3-tube test the 95% confidence limits cover a 33-fold range from approximately 14% to 458% of the actual tabular MPN estimate. For a 5-tube multiple detection test, the 95% confidence limits cover a 13-fold range from approximately 24% to 324% of the MPN. In practice these intervals may be considerably larger than those calculated from standard MPN tables. For example, results on coliform determinations in peanut butter, dried buttermilk, and dried egg albumen (Silliker et al., 1979) indicated 95% confidence intervals for a single log value of ± 0.88, ± 1.03, and ± 0.87 log units respectively, indicating ranges of 1.76, 2.06, and 1.74. The average range for the three products was 1.85 and the average 95% confidence interval for a single log value, ± 0.925. Thus, in the application of a microbiological criterion involving a MPN procedure (including one of <1 *E. coli* per g) it is important to know the precision of the analytical method so that the criteria can be properly administered and interpreted.

A direct plating method (Anderson-Baird-Parker Method and modifications) is available that not only detects typical *E. coli* but also lactose-negative and anaerogenic indole-positive variants (Anderson and Baird-Parker, 1975; Holbrook et al., 1980; Mehlman, 1984; Rayman et al., 1979; Yoovidhya and Fleet, 1981). Modifications of this procedure include a resuscitation step to recover injured cells. Additional advantages of the direct plating method include availability of results in 24 hours compared to 4 days or longer using conventional MPN procedures, better recovery from frozen samples, decreased requirement for laboratory media, and decreased cost for technical personnel. In enumerating *E. coli* from raw meats (Rayman et al., 1979), the direct plating method yielded higher counts than the MPN method for frozen samples. For oysters (Yoovidhya and Fleet, 1981), the direct plating method was sensitive and accurate in the range of two to five *E. coli* cells per gram of oyster homogenate. By placing 1 ml of a 1:5 dilution of meat on duplicate filters a lower limit of detection of 2.5 cells per gram of meat could be reached (Rayman et al., 1979). With 1 ml of a 1:10 dilution, the lower limit of detection would be <10 per gram of food.

Small numbers of *S. aureus* are to be expected in foods that have been exposed to or handled by people. Large numbers (1,000 or more per gram of food) result either from extensive contamination or more likely from growth. The latter situation most often occurs in a food in which competing microorganisms have been destroyed by processing, with subsequent time-temperature abuse creating conditions for extensive growth of staphylococci. Although very high numbers (10^6 or higher per gram of food) indicate the possibility of presence of toxin, lower numbers do not imply absence of toxin because the number of viable cells may have decreased by some food-processing procedure such as heating. A few staphylococci are likely to reach foods even though good manufacturing practices were applied.

An evaluation of the usefulness of a zero tolerance for *S. aureus* in foods also requires a recognition of the purpose of the criterion and the precision of the analytical method. The purposes for examining foods or food ingredients for low levels (<100/g) of *S. aureus* include: to determine whether the food or ingredient is a potential source of enterotoxigenic *S. aureus* and/or to demonstrate postprocessing contamination, which usually is due to human contact with processed food or exposure of the food to inadequately sanitized food equipment surfaces. Detection and enumeration of relatively low numbers of *S. aureus* in foods is sometimes complicated by the presence of large numbers of other microorganisms and/or by the presence, particularly in processed foods, of injured (sublethally stressed) cells of *S. aureus*. Injured cells may not be recovered on media that are satisfactory for noninjured cells.

For a limit of <1 *S. aureus* per gram of food a MPN procedure is commonly used. The present AOAC MPN procedure (AOAC, 1980), which uses a 3-tube dilution procedure with trypticase soy broth containing 10% NaCl, has been shown to be inhibitory to injured cells of *S. aureus* (Brewer et al., 1977; Flowers et al., 1982; Flowers et al., 1977; Gray et al., 1974). Some work (Flowers et al., 1982; Giolitti and Cantoni, 1966) has shown that other enrichment broths such as that of Giolitti and Cantoni (1966) may be more productive. The basic limitations in the precision of the MPN procedures as described for *E. coli* also apply to MPN procedures for *S. aureus*. The direct plating method is another approach for the detection and enumeration of *S. aureus* in foods. Baird-Parker agar and some of the more recent modifications of this medium have proven to be superior to other selective media particularly by being less inhibitory to injured cells (Baird-Parker and Davenport, 1965; Devriese, 1981; Flowers et al., 1977; Gray et al., 1974; Idziak and Mossel, 1980; Rayman et al., 1978; Stiles and Clark, 1974; Tatini et al., 1984). Direct plating of a 0.1-ml portion of a 1:10 dilution of the sample on a single plate or a 1-ml portion divided equally over triplicate plates of Baird-Parker agar would allow estimates of <100 or <10/g, respectively. In view of the limitations associated with current MPN procedures for *S. aureus*, it is questionable whether the public health relevance of a processed food with levels of <100 or <10 *S. aureus* per gram as determined by a direct plating method (Baird-Parker agar) is significantly different from that of the same food in which the level was <1/g using a MPN technique. Taking into account the precision and accuracy of current MPN procedures, a microbiological limit of <1 *S. aureus* per gram of food does not appear meaningful. In conclusion, zero tolerances (<1/g of food) for either *E. coli* or *S. aureus* are meaningless unless they take into account the variability of the MPN procedures.

Additional information related to this contract item can be found in Chapters 4 and 5.

VI.   The contractor will determine whether aerobic plate count together with coliform or *E. coli* counts are complimentary or redundant for processed foods.

The same basic conditions may be responsible for higher than normal APC, coliform, or *E. coli* counts in processed foods, namely: inferior quality raw materials and ingredients, inadequate heat processing, post-heat processing contamination, and time-temperature abuse. However, this does not mean that these counts are affected to the same degree by these conditions. In a heat-processed food there may be some postprocessing contamination that does not result in significant changes in APC. However, the presence of a few coliforms may indicate that some lack of good manufacturing practices existed. For example, the presence of 1-10 coliform bacteria per ml of pasteurized milk still constitutes a legal product but this count should alert the processor that postpasteurization contamination has taken place.

As pointed out earlier (no. III in this appendix), a distinction should be made in the merits of the *E. coli* and coliform counts. *E. coli*, a member of the coliform group, is presently the most reliable bacterial indicator of fecal contamination. However, the presence of coliform bacteria in a processed food does not necessarily mean the presence of either *E. coli* or fecal contamination. For example, in Grade A pasteurized milk, the presence of a few coliform bacteria is unrelated to fecal contamination but results in most cases from contamination of improperly cleaned and sanitized equipment used to store, transport, or package the pasteurized product.

In northern Europe, the coliform test has been supplanted by the *Enterobacteriaceae* test, simply because this encompasses a larger group of organisms that share properties with the more restricted group of the coliforms. In summary, the three determinations clearly are not redundant.

Additional information related to this contract item can be found in Chapter 5.

VII.   The contractor will evaluate the public health relevance of *Salmonella* and other foodborne pathogens of similar resistance to heat in raw seafoods, in food-processing plants, in restaurants and in family kitchens.

Small numbers of a variety of pathogens such as *Salmonella, Yersinia, Campylobacter*, and *Vibrio* may be associated particularly with raw animal foods such as fresh raw meats, poultry, milk, or fish. For example, *Salmonella* with raw meats and poultry; *Yersinia* with raw meats, particularly pork; *Campylobacter* with raw milk and poultry; *V. parahaemolyticus* with seafood; and *V. cholerae* with shellfish. *S. aureus* can be readily transferred to foods as they are handled by people.

In most instances, foodborne illness resulting from the above-mentioned pathogens has its genesis in the occurrence of these organisms in raw foods of animal origin. For example, man becomes infected with *Salmonella*, in the vast majority of cases, because the potential occurrence of *Salmonella* in raw foods of animal origin is not taken into account although the routes and circumstances leading to human infection from such raw foods are fairly well understood. The incidence of foodborne illness caused by these pathogens will be reduced only if the potential presence of these organisms in raw foods of animal origin is taken into account and raw and processed animal foods are not mishandled. This involves application of the HACCP system at the food-processing plant and food service establishment (see Chapter 10). Thus, everyone throughout the entire food chain has to recognize the potential problems that these organisms can pose. Control of these organisms and hence elimination of public health hazards usually can be achieved (a) by proper heat processing of the food, and (b) by avoiding recontamination of the heat-processed food with the same or other pathogens from contaminated surfaces of equipment or utensils and through poor hygienic practices of food handlers. Application of proper refrigeration also is important in minimizing the hazard because in many foodborne disease outbreaks there is not only a history of contamination but also one of time-temperature abuse. Though low numbers of some pathogens may lead to illness, the likelihood of disease is greatly increased with increasing dosage.

In summary, a variety of pathogens can be expected as part of the normal flora of various raw foods of animal origin. They do pose definite health hazards in the entire food chain if proper preventive and control measures are not applied. Meat and poultry are the most important sources of foodborne illness in the United States, and failure to handle the raw and cooked materials properly in food-processing plants, food service operations, and in the home is the major cause of foodborne disease involving these foods in the U.S. Contamination of seafoods with pathogens of similar heat resistance as *Salmonella* do not cause, generally, the same foodborne disease problem in the United States as do red meat and poultry—though shellfish are not an insignificant source of other types of foodborne disease.

Additional information related to this contract item can be found in Chapters 4 and 9.

VIII. The contractor will define the purposes for microbiological criteria and will make cost vs. benefit assessment for their use in regulatory control of raw and heat-processed foods.

The overall purposes of microbiological criteria for foods have been discussed in Chapter 2. This contract item requests that purposes of criteria for (1) raw and (2) heat-processed foods be defined. The subcommittee's response to this contract item is presented in Chapters 2, 3, 10, and particularly in Chapter 9. No summary response can do justice to this contract item; thus only a few isolated examples are given below.

Raw Foods

The usefulness of criteria for raw foods will vary depending upon food type (see Chapters 3 and 9). For example, sound raw fruits and vegetables may harbor high populations of microorganisms. Within reason, however, these numbers have little relationship to quality or production practices. Even when eaten raw, they have not presented a serious health problem in the United States. The routine testing of these foods for viable microorganisms offers few benefits. Microbiological standards for raw meat and poultry would prevent neither spoilage nor foodborne illness. On the other hand, the application of criteria to raw foods such as shellfish can be extremely useful. Shellfish harvested from polluted waters present a potential public health problem because they often are eaten raw. Criteria that include limits on fecal indicator organisms provide a very necessary safeguard for this class of food.

Heat-Processed Foods

There are a variety of thermal processes for foods ranging from the pasteurization of wines at relatively low temperatures to the use of retorts for the commercial sterilization of low-acid canned vegetables. The usefulness of microbiological criteria for regulatory control will vary with the process and the type of food. The application of criteria to foods such as pasteurized milk and egg products aids in assessing adequacy of the process and in the detection of contamination following heat treatment (see Chapter 9, parts A and F). Guidelines are useful for frozen vegetables to detect poor manufacturing practices following blanching. If proper action is taken, application of microbiological criteria to precooked ready-to-eat products can lead to rejection of product that has the potential to cause a public health problem. Criteria based on microscopic mold counts for certain canned fruits and vegetables aid in detecting poor quality raw materials and insanitary processing lines.

Cost/Benefits

Foods most amenable to microbiological criteria are those that have relatively stable microbial populations such as certain dried, heat-processed, and frozen products.

Benefits to be derived from microbiological criteria and appropriate actions on test results include:

1. An improvement in food safety by rejecting unsafe product on the basis of detection of pathogens or toxins.

2. Results indicating poor manufacturing practices may lead to action resulting in good manufacturing practices (better sanitation, improved process control, and monitoring of critical control points).

A disadvantage to the expanded use of microbiological criteria for finished products is increased costs that undoubtedly would be passed on to the consumer. Two of the sources of the costs are:

1. The costs of conducting a greater number of analyses by the processor and by regulatory agencies.

2. An increased holding time becomes a disadvantage when the manufacturer must delay shipments pending availability of test results.

It is extremely difficult to make an accurate assessment of the cost/benefit of the use of microbiological criteria. A few attempts have been made to establish the economic losses of foodborne illness. For example, some information has been presented relative to the economic losses of human salmonellosis (NRC, 1969).

Additional information related to this contract item can be found in Chapters 2, 3, 9, and 10.

IX. The contractor will evaluate at which level in the food chain microbial pathogens should be tested for in foods, by food class.

As indicated previously, small numbers of certain pathogens can be expected on part of our raw foods of animal origin. With few exceptions there is little merit in testing these foods for pathogens. In some instances raw imported foods (shrimp and frog legs, for example) are tested for *Salmonella* to detect gross mismanagement of these foods or the harvesting from fecal-polluted waters. In the case of shellfish, the water and the product are checked for either coliform or fecal coliform bacteria, which are used as an index of potential fecal contamination. In processed foods, relevant tests for pathogens are best conducted at the processing level, before the foods leave the processing plant, or at least before control of the product is lost by the manufacturer in trade channels. In addition to microbiological tests to check for effective processing at critical control points, "control at source" requires that control be exercised over inspection and maintenance of equipment and practice of sanitation in the processing plant, i.e., HACCP supplemented with appropriate finished product testing. When conditions related to a food after it has left the processing plant result in the introduction of pathogens and/or growth of pathogens, and in some cases production of toxin, then tests for pathogens might be necessary during transportation, warehousing, or at the retail level. Tests for pathogens might even be appropriately made in food service establishments such as a large food preparation and catering establishment where mishandling may result in growth of pathogenic organisms and in some cases attendant toxin production. In most cases, "control at source" will be most effective, but for certain foods and in certain uses of foods it may be necessary to conduct tests for pathogenic microorganisms at other points in the food chain. Regulatory agencies might appropriately test foods at any point along the food chain.

The presence and growth of pathogens in a food depends upon many factors, including the nature and source of the food, the physical-chemical properties of the food, and the conditions of processing, packaging, storage, and distribution. Therefore, only those pathogens should be tested for that are of public health relevance in a particular food. Chapter 9 of this report presents the relevant pathogens for which specific groups of foods should be tested and at which level in the food chain tests should be applied.

X.   The contractor will examine relationships between food quality and microbiological characteristics and criteria of foods.

Food quality in the broad sense includes flavor, color, texture, nutritional value, and safety. At some point sufficient microbial growth will occur on a perishable food to affect its organoleptic properties, usually adversely. Volatile compounds may be generated that change flavor; pigments may be degraded or new colors produced; texture may be altered due to the activity of microbial proteases, pectinases, cellulases, and other hydrolytic enzymes; the utilization of food constituents and the release of metabolic products may influence nutritive properties.

The numbers needed to produce detectable changes will be influenced by food type and the predominant microorganisms. In terms of criteria established according to the principles of this report, the value of m represents levels consistent with Good Manufacturing Practices and is set at a level below that at which these characteristics become evident. The value of M relates to a point, and approaches to it, where the changes are or soon will be evident. Foods meeting these criteria will not show manifestations of quality deterioration (see Chapters 6 and 9).

When high microbial populations originate from contaminated equipment only, rather than from actual microbial growth on the food, fewer changes, either detectable or nondetectable, will occur. The types of microorganisms also can be important. Growth of lactic acid bacteria on meats, for example, produces less flavor change than comparable growth of certain pseudomonads.

While high counts may reflect lower quality or poor processing conditions, the opposite is not necessarily true. Low counts may result because the food was given a lethal treatment at a stage near the end of the process, or because many of the contaminating microorganisms had died off during storage of the food. The presence of pathogenic microorganisms, especially on ready-to-eat foods, is of course evidence of poor quality. The finding of excessive numbers of mold mycelia in certain foods such as catsup is evidence that it was made from raw materials containing rots. Additional information related to this contract item can be found in Chapters 2, 6, and 9.

XI. The contractor will evaluate at which level during harvesting, processing, storage, and distribution needed microbiological criteria can be best applied.

The objective of the criterion will determine when microbiological analyses should be performed.

If the criterion is a purchase specification that, for example, limits the number of heat-resistant mold spores in an ingredient, analyses usually are conducted by the purchaser when the shipment is first received at the plant. Frequently, the supplier analyzes the product before it is shipped to the purchaser.

If the criterion is a guideline designed to monitor a critical control point in a process, samples collected immediately after the unit operation might be analyzed.

If the objective is to assess good manufacturing practices, the level(s) at which microbiological testing should be conducted depends upon the processes to which such food is subjected. For some foods, microbiological testing of finished product after packaging may be appropriate to assess good manufacturing practices. With certain processes the analysis of the finished product would not be particularly useful to assess good manufacturing practices, for example, with a product subjected to a heat treatment. There are many situations where evaluating manufacturing practices would require microbiological testing at points other than finished products, for example, sanitary conditions of equipment.

If the concern is abuse or contamination during transport of the food or while it is held in the marketplace or food service establishment, samples collected at the retail level should be analyzed. Furthermore, samples may be collected to monitor critical control points in food service establishments as well as in processing plants. Additional information related to this contract item can be found in Chapters 2 and 9.

XII. The contractor will determine the validity of aerobic and coliform plate counts as indicators of insanitation and of time-temperature abuse of foods.

High aerobic plate counts (APCs) in finished products or in products during processing may be caused by either poor sanitation or time-temperature abuse or both. Several other conditions, however, may be involved, such as the quality of raw materials and ingredients and adequacy of a heat-processing procedure if one is used. Hence, the APC can be a valid indicator of insanitation or of time-temperature abuse (primarily in perishable foods) if other potential causes are eliminated. The relationship of APC to insanitation or to time-temperature abuse can be determined best by a thorough understanding of the microbiology of the product (hazard analysis) and examination of line samples taken at critical control points. For example, a high APC of packaged ground beef may have resulted from (a) poor-quality trimmings, (b) poor sanitation of equipment (for example, grinder), and (c) holding of the product for too long or at marginal temperatures at which normal aerobic, psychrotrophic, gram-negative rods continue to multiply.

Coliform bacteria are particularly valuable as indicators of postprocessing contamination of foods treated for safety. The validity of coliform counts as an indicator of insanitation and of time-temperature abuse requires a thorough understanding of the microbiology of a food. In some foods they have little relationship to the above-mentioned conditions, in others they have more. Coliforms can be a valid indicator of poor sanitation if it can be shown that their presence at a particular point in the processing and handling of a food is not expected or their numbers are at a level beyond what is considered normal. For example, small numbers of coliforms are common in raw milk, vegetables, and meats. Large numbers in raw milk indicate insanitation and likely time-temperature abuse. Even small numbers of coliforms in pasteurized milk indicate postpasteurization contamination. In heat-processed foods, the presence of coliforms indicates most likely contamination (poor sanitation) after heating that may be accentuated by time-temperature abuse of the food.

Additional information related to this contract item can be found in Chapter 5.

XIII. The contractor will determine the validity of aerobic and coliform counts as significant or useful indices as one facet of food ''quality.''

This question has been discussed extensively in Chapter 2 of this report. Appropriate sections are repeated here to emphasize certain aspects of this question.

The term quality as commonly applied to food summarizes its desirable characteristics. Quality of a food as perceived by the public can be described as a value related to flavor (taste and odor), color, and texture. It also includes imperceptible traits such as nutritional value and safety. Excluding safety and utility from this discussion, from the microbiological viewpoint quality includes: (a) shelf-life, as perceived by attributes such as flavor and appearance, and (b) adherence to Good Manufacturing Practices.

Each of these attributes is measurable to some extent microbiologically; the decisive question, however, is to what extent.

The ultimate shelf-life of a perishable food can be estimated to some degree through the application of microbiological criteria. Assuming that storage conditions are the same, a perishable food with a low number of spoilage microorganisms will have a longer shelf-life than the same product with larger numbers of such organisms. However, relationships between common microbiological parameters such as aerobic plate counts and coliform counts and the shelf-life of a food are inexact. Some types of microorganisms, because of enzyme systems acting upon the constituents of a food, cause marked changes in perceptible quality characteristics of a food while others are relatively inert biochemically and thus produce little change. In addition, the effect of certain levels and/or types of microorganisms on perceptible quality characteristics often differs from food to food and is also subject to changes in environmental conditions such as temperature and gaseous atmosphere.

Lack of adherence to Good Manufacturing Practices often can be related to APC and/or coliform counts in excess of those present in a food produced under good conditions. The use of poor-quality materials, inadequate heat processing, careless handling, or insanitation may result in a higher bacterial count in the finished product. This relationship may not always be valid, however, because a heat treatment or other lethal treatment in the process can cover up the grossest evidence of malpractice, and organisms may die off during storage of frozen, dried, or fermented foods. Low counts in a finished product or ingredient, therefore, do not necessarily indicate good manufacturing practices or even food safety. High aerobic plate counts, on the other hand, do not necessarily mean careless handling or lack of wholesomeness. For example, ground beef prepared from the trimmings from carcasses may yield a high aerobic plate count, but this may merely reflect the growth of harmless psychrotrophic bacteria during refrigerated storage. On the other hand, it could also represent poor sanitary conditions and/or time-temperature abuse.

The relationship between the microbiology of a food and adherence to good manufacturing practices must be established by conducting repeated surveys of processing lines to obtain statistically valid data. The critical control points must be identified and the microbiology of the food at the different stages of processing must be determined. Through these studies one can arrive for some foods at numbers and types of organisms that characterize the flora of a food produced under a given set of conditions, and thus provide a basis for the establishment of a microbiological criterion. Even then an allowance has to be made for variations because of differences in processing procedures and equipment. Finished foods that exceeded the criterion might reasonably be expected to have been mishandled somehow during production and/or storage.

In recent years microbiological quality standards (APC and coliform counts) have been proposed for various foods under Section 401 of the Food, Drug and Cosmetic Act. Recently, they have been recommended for frozen fish sticks, fish cakes, and crab cakes. This has been discussed extensively in Chapter 2.

Additional information related to this contract item can be found in Chapters 2 and 5.

REFERENCES

Anderson, J. M., and A. C. Baird-Parker
   1975   A rapid and direct plate method for enumerating *Escherichia coli* biotype 1 in food. J. Appl. Bacteriol. 39:111–117.
AOAC (Association of Official Analytical Chemists)
   1980   Official Methods of Analysis of the Association of Official Analytical Chemists. 13th Ed. W. Horwitz, ed., Washington, D.C.: AOAC.
Baird-Parker, A. C., and E. Davenport
   1965   The effect of recovery medium on isolation of *Staphylococcus aureus* after heat treatment and after storage of frozen or dried cells. J. Appl. Bacteriol. 28:390–402.
Brewer, D. G., S. E. Martin, and Z. J. Ordal
   1977   Beneficial effects of catalase or pyruvate in a most-probable-number technique for the detection of *Staphylococcus aureus*. Appl. Environ. Microbiol. 34:797–800.
Devriese, L. A.
   1981   Baird-Parker medium supplemented with acriflavine, polymyxins and sulphonamide for the selective isolation of *Staphylococcus aureus* from heavily contaminated materials. J. Appl. Bacteriol. 50:351–357.
FDA (Food and Drug Administration)
   1976   Bacteriological Analytical Manual for Foods. Washington, D.C.: Association of Official Analytical Chemists.
   1978   Bacteriological Analytical Manual for Foods. Washington, D.C.: Association of Official Analytical Chemists.
Flowers, R. S., D. A. Gabis, and J. H. Silliker
   1982   Examination of methods for detection of low numbers of *Staphylococcus aureus* in foods. American Public Health Association Project Progress Report, June, 1982.

Flowers, R. S., S. E. Martin, D. G. Brewer, and Z. J. Ordal
  1977   Catalase and enumeration of stressed *Staphylococcus aureus* cells. Appl. Environ. Microbiol. 33:1112–1117.
Foster, E. M.
  1971   The control of salmonellae in processed foods: A classification system and sampling plan. J. Assoc. Offic. Anal. Chem. 54:259–266.
Giolitti, G., and C. Cantoni
  1966   A medium for the isolation of staphylococci from foodstuffs. J. Appl. Bacteriol. 29:395–398.
Gray, R.J.H., M. A. Gaske, and Z. J. Ordal
  1974   Enumeration of thermally stressed *Staphylococcus aureus* MF-31. J. Food Sci. 39:844–846.
Holbrook, R., J. M. Anderson, and A. C. Baird-Parker
  1980   Modified direct plate method for counting *Escherichia coli* in foods. Food Technol. Austral. 32:78–83.
ICMSF (International Commission on Microbiological Specifications for Foods)
  1974   Microorganisms in Foods. 2. Sampling for microbiological analysis: Principles and specific applications. Toronto: University of Toronto Press.
Idziak, E. S., and D.A.A. Mossel
  1980   Enumeration of vital and thermally stressed *Staphylococcus aureus* in foods using Baird-Parker pig plasma agar (BPP). J. Appl. Bacteriol. 48:101–113.
Mehlman, I. J.
  1984   Coliforms, fecal coliforms, *Escherichia coli* and enteropathogenic *E. coli*. In Compendium of Methods for the Microbiological Examination of Foods. 2nd Ed. M. E. Speck, ed. Washington, D.C.: American Public Health Association.
NRC (National Research Council)
  1969   An Evaluation of the *Salmonella* Problem. Committee on *Salmonella*. Washington, D.C.: National Academy of Sciences.
Olson, J. C., Jr.
  1975   Development and present status of FDA *Salmonella* sampling and testing plans. J. Milk Food Technol. 38:369–371.
Rayman, M. K., J. J. Devoyod, U. Purvis, D. Kusch, J. Lanier, R. J. Gilbert, D. G. Till, and G. A. Jarvis
  1978   ICMSF methods studies. X. An international comparative study of four media for the enumeration of *Staphylococcus aureus* in foods. Can. J. Microbiol. 24:274–281.
Rayman, M. K., G. A. Jarvis, C. M. Davidson, S. Long, J. M. Allen, T. Tong, P. Dodsworth, S. McLaughlin, S. Greenberg, B. G. Shaw, H. J. Beckers, S. Qvist, P. M. Nottingham, and B. J. Stewart
  1979   ICMSF methods studies. XIII. An international comparative study of the MPN procedure and the Anderson-Baird-Parker direct plating method for the enumeration of *Escherichia coli* biotype 1 in raw meat. Can. J. Microbiol. 25:1321–1327.
Silliker, J. H.
  1980   Status of *Salmonella*—Ten years later. J. Food Prot. 43:307–313.
Silliker, J. H., D. A. Gabis, and A. May
  1979   ICMSF methods studies. XI. Collaborative/comparative studies on determination of coliforms using the most probable number procedure. J. Food Prot. 42:638–644.
Stiles, M. E., and P. C. Clark
  1974   The reliability of selective media for the enumeration of unheated and heated staphyloccoci. Can. J. Microbiol. 20:1735–1744.

Tatini, S. R., D. G. Hoover, and R.V.F. Lachica
  1984 Methods for the isolation and enumeration of *Staphylococcus aureus*. In Compendium of Methods for the Microbiological Examination of Foods. 2nd Ed. M. E. Speck, ed. Washington, D.C.: American Public Health Association.
Woodward, R. L.
  1957 How probable is the most probable number? J. Amer. Water Works Assoc. 49:1060–1068.
Yoovidhya, T., and G. H. Fleet
  1981 An evaluation of the A-1 most probable number and the Anderson and Baird-Parker plate count methods for enumerating *Escherichia coli* in the Sydney Rock oyster, *Crassostrea commercialis*. J. Appl. Bacteriol. 50:519–528.

Appendix B
General Principles for the Establishment and Application of Microbiological Criteria for Foods[1]

These general principles are intended to guide, primarily, Codex committees in the establishment and application of microbiological criteria, and to this end they contain definitions of mandatory and advisory criteria which relate specifically to the requirements of the Codex Alimentarius. They are also intended for application where microbiological criteria for foods are being developed.

1. DEFINITION OF MICROBIOLOGICAL CRITERIA FOR FOODS

A microbiological criterion as defined for Codex purposes, consists of:

1.1 a statement of the microorganisms and parasites of concern and/ or their toxins. For this purpose, microorganisms include bacteria, viruses, yeasts, and molds;

1.2 the analytical methods for their detection and quantification;

1.3 a plan defining the number of field samples to be taken, the size of the sample unit, and where and, if appropriate, when the samples are to be taken;

1.4 microbiological limits considered appropriate to the food; and

1.5 the number of sample units that should conform to these limits.

2. APPLICATION OF MICROBIOLOGICAL CRITERIA

Microbiological criteria, as defined for Codex purposes, fall into two main categories: (See also Section 5 for interpretation)

---

[1]Appendix II, 17th Session, Committee on Food Hygiene, Codex Alimentarius.

2.1 Mandatory criterion

2.1.1 *A microbiological standard* is a criterion contained in a Codex Alimentarius Standard. Wherever possible it should contain limits only for pathogenic microorganisms of public health significance in the food concerned. Limits for nonpathogenic microorganisms may be necessary and when these are included the provisions of paragraph 6.1 shall apply. A microbiological standard shall not be introduced *de novo* but shall be derived from microbiological end-product specifications which have accompanied Codes of Practice through the Codex Procedure and which have been extensively applied to the food.

2.2 Advisory criterion

An advisory criterion is one of two types contained in Codes of Practice.

2.2.1 *A microbiological end-product specification* is intended to increase assurance that the provisions of hygienic significance in the Code have been met. It may include microorganisms which are not of direct public health significance.

2.2.2 *A microbiological guideline* is applied at the establishment at a specified point during or after processing to monitor hygiene. It is intended to guide the manufacturer and is not intended for official control purposes. It may include microorganisms other than those regarded in 2.1.1 and 2.2.1.

3. PURPOSE OF MICROBIOLOGICAL CRITERIA FOR FOODS

3.1 The purpose of microbiological criteria for foods is to protect the health of the consumer by providing safe, sound and wholesome products and to meet the requirements of fair practices in trade.

4. GENERAL CONSIDERATIONS CONCERNING PRINCIPLES FOR ESTABLISHING AND APPLYING CRITERIA

4.1 The basis of control of microbiologically sensitive foods should be through the application of Codes of Practice. A microbiological criterion should be established and applied only where there is a definite need for it and where it can be shown to be effective and practical. Such need is demonstrated by epidemiological evidence that the particular food is a public health hazard, or where an assurance is required that the provisions of hygienic significance in the Code have been adhered to. The criterion should be technically attainable by good manufacturing practice so that it does not encourage the use of objectionable treatments in an attempt to reduce microorganisms to the acceptable level.

4.2 To fulfill the purposes of microbiological criteria, consideration should be given to

- the evidence of hazards to health;
- the microbiology of the raw material;
- the effect of processing on the microbiology of the food;
- the likelihood and consequences of microbial contamination and/or growth during subsequent handling and storage;
- the category of consumers at risk; and
- the cost/benefit ratio associated with the application of the criterion.

4.3 The number of samples tested shall be as stated in the sampling plan and shall not be exceeded.

4.4 To make the best use of limited resources of money and manpower, it is essential that only appropriate tests be applied to those foods and at those points during the processing and distribution of food that offer maximum benefit in providing the consumer with a safe, sound and wholesome food.

4.5 The need for inspection of the establishment including the production process should be considered.

5. INTERPRETATION OF RESULTS

5.1 When a product fails to meet a criterion, the action to be taken depends on the type of criterion and on the circumstances. If the limit exceeded is part of a standard, the product concerned must be rejected as unfit for its intended use; if it is part of an end-product specification, appropriate action should be taken to rectify the causative factor. It is optional whether any action is taken. When a limit in a guideline is exceeded, this should not necessarily result in rejection of product but should in general lead to the identification and correction of causative factors.

5.2 When product is rejected, there are in principle several options as to the action to be taken, depending on the findings and the circumstances. Such options include sorting, reprocessing (e.g., by heating), and destruction, and may need to be specified in the criterion. In deciding on the option the major consideration should be to keep to a minimum the risk that unacceptable food reaches the consumer. However, food must not be needlessly destroyed nor declared unfit for human consumption.

6. COMPONENTS OF A MICROBIOLOGICAL CRITERION

6.1 Microorganisms of importance in a particular food
  6.1.1 The microorganisms included in a criterion should be widely

accepted as relevant—as pathogens, as indicator organisms or as spoilage organisms—to the particular food and technology. Organisms whose significance in the food is in doubt should not be included in a criterion.

6.1.2 The mere finding, with a presence-absence test, of certain organisms which have caused foodborne illness (e.g., *Staphylococcus aureus, Clostridium perfringens* and *Vibrio parahaemolyticus*) does not necessarily indicate a hazard.

6.1.3 When choosing a test for an indicator organism, there should be a clear understanding as to whether the test for this organism is used to indicate an unsatisfactory manufacturing practice or whether it is used to indicate the possible presence of a pathogen. Where pathogens can be detected directly, a test for these should be used instead of tests for indicator organisms.

6.2 Microbiological methods

6.2.1 For use in a standard or end-product specification, methods elaborated by international organizations for a food or a group of foods should be preferred. For standards, and wherever possible for end-product specifications, only methods for which the reliability (accuracy, reproducibility, inter- and intra-laboratory variation) has been statistically established in comparative or collaborative studies in several laboratories should be used. While reference methods to be used in standards and end-product specifications should be the most sensitive and reproducible for the purpose, methods to be used in guidelines might often sacrifice to some degree sensitivity and reproducibility in the interests of speed and simplicity. They should, however, have been proved to give a sufficiently reliable estimate of the information needed.

6.2.2 When choosing a microbiological method as a reference method, consideration should be given to the universal availability of media, equipment, etc.

6.2.3 Methods which are applicable uniformly to various groups of commodities should be given preference over methods which apply only to individual commodities. Methods for testing rapidly perishable foods should be so designed that the results of microbiological examinations can be available before the foods are consumed or exceed their shelf-life.

6.3 Microbiological limits

6.3.1 Limits should be based on microbiological data appropriate to the food and to the kind of criterion in question. Limits for standards and end-product specifications should be based on data gathered at various stages of production, storage and distribution, while limits for guidelines could be based on data obtained from microbiological monitoring during production. The numerical limits should take into consideration the risk associated with the organisms likely to affect the acceptability of the food, and the conditions under which the food is expected to be handled and consumed. Numerical limits should also take account of the distribution of microorganisms in the food and the inherent variability of the analytical procedure.

6.3.2 If a criterion requires a particular microorganism not to be detected, the size of sample shall be indicated. It should be borne in mind that no feasible sampling plan can ensure complete absence of a particular organism.

6.3.3 Microbiological limits can be related only to the time and place of sampling and not to the presumed number of microorganisms at an earlier or a later stage. As good manufacturing practice aims at producing foods with microbiological characteristics significantly better than those required by public health considerations, a numerical limit in a guideline may be more stringent than in a standard or an end-product specification.

6.4 Sampling plans

6.4.1 A sampling plan is the particular choice of sampling procedure and the decision criteria to be applied to a lot, based on examination of a prescribed number of sample units by defined methods. Sampling plans should be administratively and economically feasible. In particular, sampling plans should take into account the heterogeneity of distribution of microorganisms. For standards and end-product specifications, 2- or 3-class attribute plans may find useful applications. (See ICMSF Book 2.)

6.4.2 Wherever possible, the confidence limits of the sampling plans should be given.

7. SAMPLING METHODS AND HANDLING OF SAMPLES

7.1 The sampling method shall be defined in the sampling plan. The time between field sampling and analysis should be as short as possible, and during transport to the laboratory the conditions (e.g., temperature) should be appropriate to the food, so that the results reflect—within the limitations given by the sampling plan—the microbiological conditions of the lot presented for inspection.

8. REPORTING

8.1 The test report shall give the information needed for complete identification of the sample, the results, and the test method.

9. PROVISIONS FOR RECONSIDERATION AT REGULAR INTERVALS

9.1 Criteria should be reviewed and if necessary revised at three year intervals after their adoption by the Codex Alimentarius Commission.

Appendix C

International Microbiological Specifications[1]

TABLE C-1 FAO/WHO Expert Consultation on Microbiological Specifications for Foods: Egg Products

Product	Test	n	c	m	M
Dried and frozen whole egg	Mesophilic aerobic bacteria	5	2	5×10^4	10^6
	Coliform	5	2	10	10^3
	Salmonella	10	0	0	—
Other egg products	*Salmonella*	10	0	0	—
Any egg product intended for special dietary purposes	*Salmonella*	30	0	0	—

SOURCE: CAC/RCP 15, 1976.

[1]See Chapter 6, page 134 for explanation of letter symbols.

372

TABLE C-2 FAO/WHO Expert Consultation on Microbiological Specifications for Foods: Foods for Infants and Children

Product	Test	Case	n	c	m	M
Dried biscuit						
plain	None	—	—	—	—	—
coated	Coliform	5	5	2	<3	20
	Salmonella	11	10	0	0	—
Dried instant	Mesophilic	6	5	2	10^3	10^4
products	aerobic bacteria					
	Coliform	6	5	1	<3	20
	Salmonella	12	60	0	0	—
Dried products	Mesophilic	4	5	3	10^4	10^5
requiring	aerobic bacteria					
heating before	Coliform	4	5	2	10	10^2
consumption	*Salmonella*	10	5	0	0	—

SOURCE: CAC/RCP 21, 1979.

TABLE C-3 FAO/WHO Expert Consultation on Microbiological Specifications for Foods: Precooked Frozen Shrimp and Prawns

Test	n	c	m	M
Mesophilic aerobic bacteria	5	2	10^5	10^6
Staphylococcus aureus	5	2	5×10^2	5×10^3
Salmonella	5	0	0	—

SOURCE: CAC/RCP 17, 1978.

TABLE C-4 FAO/WHO Expert Consultation on Microbiological Specifications for Foods: Ice Mixes

Test	n	c	m	M
Mesophilic aerobic bacteria	5	2	2.5×10^4	10^5
Coliform	5	2	10	10^2
Salmonella	10	0	0	—

SOURCE: Report of 2nd Joint FAO/WHO Expert Consultation, 1977.

TABLE C-5 FAO/WHO Expert Consultation on Microbiological Specifications for Foods: Edible Ices

Test	n	c	m	M
Mesophilic aerobic bacteria	5	2	5×10^4	2.5×10^5
Coliform	5	2	10^2	10^3
Salmonella	10	0	0	—

SOURCE: Report of 2nd Joint FAO/WHO Expert Consultation, 1977.

TABLE C-6 International Dairy Federation Proposed Microbiological Specifications for Dried Milk, 1982

Test	n	c	m	M
Mesophilic count	5	2	5×10^4	2×10^5
Coliforms	5	1	10	100
Salmonella	15	0	0	

SOURCE: IDF: D-Doc 90, 1982.

TABLE C-7 European Economic Community Standards for Caseins and Caseinates

Organism(s)	M (Maximum Allowable Concentration)
Total bacterial count	30,000/g
Thermophilic organisms	5,000/g
Coliforms	0(in 0.1g)

SOURCE: Regulation (EEC) No. 2940/73, O.J. No. L301/25.

TABLE C-8 European Economic Community Standards for Natural Mineral Waters

Organism(s)	M (Maximum Allowable Concentration)
Total count	20/ml at 37°C
	100/ml at 22°C
Parasites and pathogenic microorganisms	absent
E. coli, coliforms and fecal streptococci	absent in 250 ml
Sulphite-reducing anaerobes	absent in 50 ml
Pseudomonas aeruginosa	absent in 250 ml

SOURCE: Council Directive 15 July 1980 (BO/7/7/EEC), O.J. No. L229/1.

TABLE C-9 European Economic Community Standard for Water for Human Consumption

Organism(s)	m (Guide Level)	M (Maximum Allowable Concentration)
Total count	10/ml at 37°C	—
(tap water)	100/ml at 22°C	—
Total count	5/ml at 37°C	20
(bottled water)	20/ml at 22°C	100
Total coliforms	—	
Fecal coliforms	—	MPN ≤ 1
Fecal streptococci	—	
Sulphite-reducing clostridia	—	MPN ≤ 1
All pathogenic bacteria, viruses, algae, parasites	absent	

SOURCE: Council Directive 15 July 1980 (80/778/EEC), O.J. No. L229/11.

TABLE C-10 Microbiological Guidelines of Codex Standard for Natural Mineral Waters

Organism(s)	M (Maximum Allowable Concentration)
Aerobic mesophilic count at source	20/ml at 21°C (72 hrs) 5/ml at 37°C (24 hrs)
Aerobic mesophilic count after bottling	100/ml at 20–22°C (72 hrs) 20/ml at 37°C (24 hrs)
Coliforms (including E. coli)[a]	none in 250 ml (30–32°C and 44°C)
Fecal streptococci (Lancefield Group D)[a]	none in 250 ml
Sporulated sulphite-reducing anaerobes[a]	none in 50 ml
Pseudomonas aeruginosa, parasites and pathogenic microorganisms[a]	none in 250 ml

[a]Applies both at source and during marketing.

SOURCE: Appendix 1 CX/FH 79/4—ADD.1, 1979.

TABLE C-11 Proposed Guidelines for Drinking-Water Quality

Parameter/Organism	Value (number per 100 ml)	Remarks
I. Microbiological Quality		
Piped water supplies		
Treated water entering the distribution system		
Fecal coliforms	0	Turbidity < 1 NTU; for disinfection with chlorine, pH preferably < 8.0, free chlorine residual 0.2–0.5 mg/l following 30 minutes (minimum) contact.
Coliform organisms	0	
Untreated water entering the distribution system		
Fecal coliforms	0	
Coliform organisms	0	In 98% of samples examined throughout the year for large supplies with sufficient samples examined.
Coliform organisms	3	In occasional sample but not in consecutive samples.
Water in the distribution system		
Fecal coliforms	0	
Coliform organisms	0	In 95% of samples examined throughout the year for large supplies with sufficient samples examined.
Coliform organisms	3	In occasional sample but not in consecutive samples.
Unpiped water supplies		
Fecal coliforms	0	
Coliform organisms	10	Not occurring repeatedly. Repeated occurrence and failure to improve sanitary protection, alternate source to be found if possible.
Bottled drinking-water		
Fecal coliforms	0	
Coliform organisms	0	
Emergency water supplies		
Fecal coliforms	0	Advise public to boil water in case of failure to meet guideline values.
Coliform organisms	0	
Enterovirus	—	No guideline value set.
II. Biological Quality		
Protozoa (pathogenic)	—	No guideline value set.
Helminths (pathogenic)	—	No guideline value set.
Free-living organisms (algae, others)	—	No guideline value set.

SOURCE: EEP/82.39 (adapted).

Appendix D

Excerpts From the Regulations Pursuant to the Food and Drugs Act, a Statute of the Government of Canada

Regulation Number	Food	Regulation and Sampling Plan
1. B.04.010 (item f)	Cocoa	Cocoa or powdered cocoa shall be free from bacteria of the genus *Salmonella*, as determined by the official method. $n = 10$, $c = 0$, $m = 0$
2. B.04.011	Chocolate	No person shall sell chocolate, plain chocolate, bitter chocolate, chocolate liquor, sweet chocolate, sweet chocolate coating, milk chocolate, sweet milk chocolate, milk chocolate coating or sweet milk chocolate coating unless it is free from bacteria of the genus *Salmonella*, as determined by the official method. $n = 10$, $c = 0$, $m = 0$
3. B.08.014A	Skim milk powder	No person shall sell milk powder, whole milk powder, dry whole milk, powdered whole milk, skim milk powder or dry skim milk unless it is free from bacteria of the genus *Salmonella*, as determined by the official method. $n = 20$, $c = 0$, $m = 0$
4. B.08.016 (item e)	Flavoured milk	(Naming the flavour) milk may contain not more than 50,000 bacteria per cubic centimetre as determined by the official method. $n = 5$, $c = 2$, $m = 5 \times 10^4$, $M = 10^6$

n = number of sample units per lot
c = number of positive samples or marginal samples permitted
m − population level determining marginal acceptance
M − population level above which sample is unsatisfactory

Regulation Number	Food	Regulation and Sampling Plan
5. B.08.018 (item f)	Partly skimmed milk	(Naming the flavour) partly skimmed milk may contain not more than 50,000 bacteria per cubic centimetre as determined by the official method. $n = 5$, $c = 2$, $m = 5 \times 10^4$, $M = 10^6$
6. B.08.024	Milk for manufacture	No person shall sell milk for manufacture into dairy products if it contains more than a) 2,000,000 bacteria per millilitre, or b) 2 milligrams of sediment per 16 fluid ounces, as determined by the official method. $n = 5$, $c = 0$, $m = 2 \times 10^6$
7. B.08.026 (item g)	Skimmed milk with added milk solids	(Naming the flavour) partly skimmed milk with added milk solids may contain not more than 50,000 bacteria per cubic centimetre as determined by the official method. $n = 5$, $c = 2$, $m = 5 \times 10^4$, $M = 10^6$
8. B.08.048 (item 1a)	Cheese from pasteurized milk	No person shall sell cheese, including cheese curd, made from a pasteurized source if the cheese contains more than 100 *Escherichia coli* per gram as determined by the official method. $n = 5$, $c = 2$, $m = 100$, $M = 2,000$
9. B.08.048 (item 1b)	Cheese from pasteurized milk	No person shall sell cheese, including cheese curd, made from a pasteurized source if the cheese contains more than 100 *Staphylococcus aureus* per gram as determined by the official method. $n = 5$, $c = 2$, $m = 100$, $M = 10,000$
10. B.08.048 (item 2a)	Cheese from unpasteurized milk	No person shall sell cheese, including cheese curd, made from an unpasteurized source if the cheese contains more than 500 *Escherichia coli* per gram as determined by the official method. $n = 5$, $c = 2$, $m = 500$, $M = 2,000$

Regulation Number	Food	Regulation and Sampling Plan
11. B.08.048 (item 2b)	Cheese from unpasteurized milk	No person shall sell cheese, including cheese curd, made from an unpasteurized source if the cheese contains more than 1,000 *Staphylococcus aureus* per gram as determined by the official method. $n = 5$, $c = 2$, $m = 1,000$, $M = 10,000$
12. B.08.054	Cottage cheese	No person shall sell cottage cheese or creamed cottage cheese that contains more than 10 coliform bacteria per gram as determined by the official method. $n = 5$, $c = 1$, $m = 10$, $M = 1,000$
13. B.08.062 [item d(i)]	Ice cream	Ice cream shall contain not more than 100,000 bacteria per gram as determined by the official method. $n = 5$, $c = 2$, $m = 10^5$, $M = 10^6$
14. B.08.062 [item d(ii)]	Ice cream	Ice cream shall contain not more than 10 coliform organisms per gram as determined by the official method. $n = 5$, $c = 1$, $m = 10$, $M = 1,000$
15. B.08.072 [item d(i)]	Ice milk	Ice milk shall contain not more than 100,000 bacteria per gram as determined by the official method. $n = 5$, $c = 2$, $m = 100,000$, $M = 10^6$
16. B.08.072 [item d(ii)]	Ice milk	Ice milk shall contain not more than 10 coliform organisms per gram as determined by the official method. $n = 5$, $c = 1$, $m = 10$, $M = 1,000$
17. B.12.001 (item b)	Mineral or spring water	Water represented as mineral water or spring water shall not contain any coliform bacteria as determined by the official method, subject to the tolerances permitted therein. $n = 10$, $c = 1$, $m = 0$, $M = 10/100$ ml

Regulation Number	Food	Regulation and Sampling Plan
18. B.12.004 (item a)	Water in sealed containers	No person shall sell water in sealed containers, other than water represented as mineral water or spring water if it contains any coliform bacteria as determined by the official method, subject to the tolerances permitted therein. $n = 10$, $c = 1$, $m = 0$, $M = 10/100$ ml
19. B.12.004 (item b)	Water in sealed containers	No person shall sell water in sealed containers, other than water represented as mineral water or spring water if it contains more than 100 aerobic bacteria per milli-litre as determined by the official method, subject to the tolerances permitted therein. $n = 5$, $c = 2$, $m = 100$, $M = 10^4$
20. B.12.005 [item 1(a)]	Prepackaged ice	No person shall sell prepackaged ice if it contains any coliform bacteria as determined by the official method, subject to the tolerances permitted therein. $n = 10$, $c = 1$, $m = 0$, $M = 10/100$ ml
21. B.12.005 [item 2(a)]	Prepackaged ice	No person shall manufacture prepackaged ice for sale if the water from which it is made contains any coliform bacteria as determined by the official method, subject to the tolerances permitted therein. $n = 10$, $c = 1$, $m = 0$, $M = 10/100$ ml
22. B.21.027 [item c(ii)]	Fish protein	Fish protein shall not contain more than 10,000 bacteria per gram as determined by the official method. $n = 5$, $c = 1$, $m = 10^4$, $M = 5 \times 10^5$
23. B.21.027 [item c(iii)]	Fish protein	Fish protein shall not contain *Escherichia coli* as determined by the official method. $n = 5$, $c = 1$, $m = 0$, $M = 10$
24. B.14.061 (item b)	Edible bone meal or flour	Edible bone meal or edible bone flour shall contain not more than 1,000 bacteria per gram as determined by the official method. $n = 5$, $c = 1$, $m = 1,000$, $M = 10^5$

Regulation Number	Food	Regulation and Sampling Plan
25. B.14.061 (item c)	Edible bone meal or flour	Edible bone meal or edible bone flour shall contain no *Escherichia coli* as determined by the official method. $n = 5, c = 1, m = 0, M = 10$
26. B.14.062 [item d(i)]	Gelatin or edible gelatin	Gelatin or edible gelatin shall not contain more than 5,000 bacteria per gram as determined by the official method. $n = 5, c = 3, m = 5,000, M = 10^5$
27. B.14.062 [item d(ii)]	Gelatin or edible gelatin	Gelatin or edible gelatin shall not contain more than 10 coliform bacteria per gram as determined by the official method. $n = 5, c = 1, m = 10, M = 1,000$
28. B.14.062 [item d(iii)]	Gelatin or edible gelatin	Gelatin or edible gelatin shall not contain bacteria of the genus *Salmonella* as determined by the official method. $n = 10, c = 0, m = 0$
29. B.21.031	Froglegs	No person shall sell fresh or frozen froglegs unless they are free of the genus *Salmonella* as determined by the official method. $n = 5, c = 0, m = 0$
30. B.22.033	Egg product	No person shall sell any egg product for use as a food unless it is free from bacteria of the genus *Salmonella* as determined by the official method. $n = 10, c = 0, m = 0$
31. B.11.016	Tomatoes, tomato juice and vegetable juice	No person shall sell canned tomatoes, tomato juice or a vegetable juice that contains mould filaments in more than 25 percent of the microscopic fields when examined by the official method.
32. B.11.017	Tomato puree, paste, pulp or catsup	No person shall sell tomato puree, tomato paste, tomato pulp or tomato catsup that contains mould filaments in more than 50 percent of the microscopic fields when examined by the official method.

Regulation Number	Food	Regulation and Sampling Plan
33. B.08.007 (item a)	Sterilized milk	Sterilized milk shall be milk that has been heated without concentration or appreciable loss of volume to a temperature of at least 100°C for a length of time sufficient to kill all the organisms present.
34. B.08.043	Cheese	No manufacturer shall sell any cheese that is not made from a pasteurized source if it has been cut into smaller portions, unless a) it has been duly stored, or b) each portion of cut cheese is marked, branded or labelled with the date of the beginning of the manufacturing process. ["Stored" according to B.08.030 means to have been kept or held at a temperature of 2°C or more for a period of 60 days or more from the date of the beginning of the manufacturing process. The purpose is to allow for the die-off of pathogens if present.]
35. B.08.044 (item 1)	Cheese	Subject to B.08.044 item (2), no person shall sell cheese, including cheese curd, that is not made from a pasteurized source unless it has been stored (see definition of "stored" immediately above).
36. B.08.044 (item 2)	Cheese	Cheese, including cheese curd, that is not made from a pasteurized source may be used as an ingredient in any food providing such food is manufactured or processed so as to pasteurize the cheese in the manner described in the definition "pasteurized source." ["Pasteurized source" according to B.08.030 means milk, skim milk, cream, reconstituted milk powder, reconstituted skim milk powder or any combination thereof that has been pasteurized by being held at a temperature of not less than 61.6°C for a period of not less than 30 minutes, or for a time and temperature that is equivalent thereto in phosphatase destruction as determined by the official method.]

Regulation Number	Food	Regulation and Sampling Plan
37. B.08.046	Cheese	No person shall sell any whole cheese that has not been made from a pasteurized source unless there is stamped thereon the date of the beginning of the manufacturing process.
38. B.08.047	Cheese	Every manufacturer, wholesaler, or jobber who sells cheese not made from a pasteurized source and which has not been stored shall keep a record of a) the registered number of the cheese factory; b) the date of manufacture of the cheese; c) the vat number or vat numbers; d) the name and address of the person to whom the cheese is sold; and e) the weight sold from each vat for each lot of cheese sold.
39. B.14.013	Meat	No person shall sell a meat, meat by-product or preparation thereof, packed in a hermetically sealed container unless it has been heat processed after or at the time of sealing at a temperature and for a time sufficient to prevent the survival of any microorganisms capable of producing toxins.
40. B.14.014	Meat	Notwithstanding Section B.14.013 a meat, meat by-product or preparation thereof, packed in a hermetically sealed container that has not been processed as required by Section B.14.013 may be sold if a) it has been stored continuously under refrigeration, and the label carries a statement on the main panel to the effect that the product is perishable and must be kept refrigerated; b) it has been maintained continuously in the frozen state and the label carries a statement on the main panel to the effect that the product is perishable and must be kept frozen; c) it contains a Class I preservative or appropriate mixtures thereof in accordance with good manufacturing practice and has been heat processed after or at

Regulation Number	Food	Regulation and Sampling Plan
		the time of sealing at a temperature and for a time sufficient to prevent the formation of any bacterial toxins; d) it has been subjected to a dehydration procedure in accordance with good manufacturing practice; or e) it has a pH of 4.6 or less.
41. B.14.072	Meat	No person shall sell meat or a meat by-product that has been barbecued, roasted or broiled and is ready for consumption unless the cooked meat or meat by-product a) at all times (i) has a temperature of 40°F (4.4°C) or lower, or 140°F (60°C) or higher, or (ii) has been stored at an ambient temperature of 40°F (4.4°C) or lower, or 140°F (60°C) or higher; and b) carries on the main panel of the label a statement to the effect that the food must be stored at a temperature of 40°F (4.4°C) or lower, or 140°F (60°C) or higher.
42. B.22.026	Poultry	No person shall sell poultry, poultry meat or poultry meat by-product that has been barbecued, roasted or broiled and is ready for consumption unless the cooked poultry, poultry meat or poultry meat by-product a) at all times (i) has a temperature of 40°F (4.4°C) or lower, or 140°F (60°C) or higher, or (ii) has been stored at an ambient temperature of 40°F (4.4°C) or lower, or 140°F (60°C) or higher; and b) carries on the main panel of the label a statement to the effect that the food must be stored at a temperature of 40°F (4.4°C) or lower, or 140°F (60°C) or higher.
43. B.21.025	Fish	No person shall sell smoked marine and fresh water animals and their products or marine and fresh water animals and their products to which liquid smoke flavour has been added that is packed in a container sealed to exclude air unless it

Regulation Number	Food	Regulation and Sampling Plan
		a) has been heat processed after sealing at a temperature and for a time sufficient to destroy all spores of the species *Clostridium botulinum:* or
		b) contains not less than 9 percent salt, as determined by the official method; or
		c) is customarily cooked before eating; or
		d) is frozen and the label carries the following statement on the principal display panel in the same size type as used for the common name "Keep Frozen Prior to Use."
44. Table XI Part I, items P.1 and S.4 combined	(1) Potassium and/ or sodium nitrate in meat binder for dry sausage, preserved meat and preserved meat by-products prepared by slow cure processes	(1) When the meat binder is used in accordance with label instructions, whether potassium nitrate or sodium nitrate are used separately or in combination, the total amount of such nitrates thereby added to each batch of dry sausage, semi-dry sausage, preserved meat or preserved meat by-products shall not exceed 0.32 ounce per 100 pounds or 200 ppm calculated prior to any smoking, cooking or fermentation.
	(2) Potassium and/ or sodium nitrate in cover pickle and dry cure employed in the curing of preserved meat and preserved meat by-products prepared by slow cure processes	(2) When the cover pickle or dry cure is used in accordance with label instructions, whether potassium nitrate or sodium nitrate are used separately or in combination, the total amount of such nitrates thereby added to each batch of preserved meat or preserved meat by-products shall not exceed 0.32 ounce per 100 pounds or 200 ppm calculated prior to any smoking, cooking or fermentation.
	(3) Potassium and/ or sodium nitrate in dry sausage, semi-dry sausage, preserved meat and preserved meat by-products prepared by slow cure processes	(3) Whether potassium nitrate or sodium nitrate (is) are used separately or in combination, the total amount of such nitrates added to each batch of dry sausage, semi-dry sausage, preserved meat or preserved meat by-products shall not exceed 0.32 ounce per 100 pounds or 200 ppm, calculated prior to any smoking, cooking or fermentation.

Regulation Number	Food	Regulation and Sampling Plan
45. Table XI Part 1, items P.2 and S.5 combined	(1) Potassium nitrite and/or sodium nitrite in meat binder, pumping pickle, cover pickle and dry cure employed in the curing of preserved meat and preserved meat by-products	(1) When the meat binder, pumping pickle or dry cure is used in accordance with label instructions, whether potassium nitrite or sodium nitrite are used separately or in combination, the total amount of such nitrites thereby added to each batch of preserved meat or preserved meat by-products shall not exceed 0.32 ounce per 100 pounds or 200 ppm, calculated prior to any smoking, cooking or fermentation.
	(2) Preserved meat, except side bacon, and preserved meat by-products	(2) Whether potassium nitrite or sodium nitrite are used separately or in combination, the total amount of such nitrites added to each batch of preserved meat except side bacon or preserved meat by-products, shall not exceed 0.32 ounce per 100 pounds or 200 ppm, calculated prior to any smoking, cooking or fermentation.
	(3) Side bacon	(3) Whether potassium nitrite or sodium nitrite are used separately or in combination, the total amount of such nitrites added to each batch of side bacon shall not exceed 0.24 ounce per 100 pounds or 150 ppm, calculated prior to any smoking, cooking or fermentation.
	(4) Preserved poultry meat and preserved poultry meat by-products	(4) Whether potassium nitrite or sodium nitrite are used separately or in combination, the total amount of such nitrites added to each batch of preserved poultry meat or preserved poultry meat by-products shall not exceed 0.32 ounce per 110 pounds or 200 ppm, calculated prior to any smoking, cooking or fermentation.

Appendix E

Microbiological Criteria for Foods Purchased by the Military

TABLE E-1 Microbiological Criteria for Dehydrated Cooked Food

Item	Specification Number	Limit per gram	
		APC[a]	E. coli
Beef stew	MIL-B-43404D 1977		
Beef with rice	MIL-B-43750-F 1980		
Chicken and chicken products	MIL-C-43135H 1981		
Chicken, diced, compressed	MIL-C-44052 1981		
Chicken with rice	MIL-C-43289E 1980	Proposed criteria for these items[b]	
Chili con carne	MIL-C-43287F 1981	$n = 5$ $c = 1$	$n = 5$ $c = 1$
Escalloped potatoes with pork	MIL-E-43749F 1979	$m = 75,000$ $M = 150,000$	$m < 3$ $M \leq 20$
Hash, beef	MIL-H-43224G 1981		
Patties, pork	MIL-P-44069 1982		
Patties, beef	MIL-B-44078 1982		
Spaghetti with meat sauce	MIL-S-43275F 1979		

[a]Aerobic plate count.
[b]3-class attribute plan (ICMSF, 1974, 1985):
    n = number of sample units.
    c = number of marginal quality units allowed.
    m = bacterial count that separates good from marginal quality.
    M = bacterial count that separates marginal from defective quality.
        Values above M are unacceptable.

TABLE E-2 Microbiological Criteria[a] for Milk and Milk Products

Item	Specification Number	Maximum Count Per Gram (ml)				
		APC[b]	Coliforms	Salmonellae	Yeast and Molds	DMC[c]
Cream substitute, dry, or liquid, nondairy	MIL-C-43338E 1979	20,000	10	—	—	—
Flavored dairy drink, dry, chocolate-coffee flavored	MIL-F-35100B 1971	20,000	10	Neg[d]	—	—
Malted milk	C-M-50A 1971	30,000	10	—	—	—
Milk and milk products, fresh fluid, concentrated, and frozen	C-M-1678C 1977	20,000	10	—	—	—
Milk (plain or chocolate), cream, half and half, filled	MIL-M-35082B 1968	20,000	10	—	—	—
Milk fat	MIL-M-1036F 1976	5,000	10	—	20	—
Milk, nonfat, dry	C-M-350C 1977	—	—	Neg[d]	—	—
Milk, whole, dry	C-M-355B 1976	—	10	—	—	—
Premium		—	10	—	—	40,000,000
Extra grade		—	10	—	—	75,000,000
Milk, filled, dry, plain, or chocolate, fortified	MIL-M-43241A 1971	30,000	90	Neg[e]	—	—

[a]Sampling plan: MIL-STD-105.
[b]Aerobic plate count.
[c]Direct microscopic count.
[d]Negative per 100 grams.
[e]Negative per 25 grams.

TABLE E-3 Microbiological Criteria[a] for Miscellaneous Dairy Products and Water Ice

Item	Specification Number	Maximum Count Per Gram (ml)			
		APC[b]	Coliforms	Yeast and Molds	Salmonellae
Butter	C-B-801H 1974	≤ 100[c]	10	20	—
Buttermilk, fluid and milk, whole fresh, cultured	C-B-816G 1977	—	10	—	—
Cheese, cottage	C-C-281F 1974	≤ 100[d]	10	10	—
Cheese, processed, American, dehydrated	MIL-C-35053C 1977	50,000	90	—	—
Cream, sour, cultured or acidified	C-C-678D 1977	—	10	10	—
Ice cream mixes, dehydrated	EE-I-1699 1977	30,000	10	—	Neg/25g
Ice cream, regular, vanilla	EE-I-116E 1975	50,000	10	—	—
Ice cream, regular, chocolate and other flavors, fruits and nuts	EE-I-116E 1975	50,000	20	—	—
Ice milk	EE-I-116E 1975	50,000	10	—	—
Sherbert, regular	EE-I-116E 1975	50,000	10	—	—
Water ice	EE-I-116E 1975	50,000	10	—	—
Novelties: ice cream bars, sherbert/ice cream bar, frozen fudge bar, ice cream sandwich, ice cream cone (preformed)	EE-I-116E 1975	50,000	20	—	—

TABLE E-3 (Continued)

Item	Specification Number	Maximum Count Per Gram (ml)			
		APC[b]	Coliforms	Yeast and Molds	Salmonellae
Ice cream, mellorine and mellorine types, vanilla	EE-I-116E 1975	50,000	10	—	—
Ice cream, mellorine and mellorine types, chocolate and other flavors, fruits and nuts	EE-I-116E 1975	50,000	20	—	—
Ice milk, mellorine and mellorine types	EE-I-116E 1975	50,000	10	—	—
Sherbert, mellorine and mellorine types	EE-I-116E 1975	50,000	10	—	—

[a]Sampling plan: MIL-STD-105.
[b]Aerobic plate count.
[c]Proteolytic and lipolytic count.
[d]Psychrophiles.

TABLE E-4 Microbiological Criteria[a] for Frozen Egg and Egg Products and for Dehydrated Egg Mix

Item	Specification Number	Maximum Count Per Gram (ml)				Yeast and Molds
		APC[b]	Coliforms	Salmonellae[c]		
Frozen egg and egg products	C-E-230E 1977					
Whole egg, table grade		15,000	—	Neg		50
Whole eggs		50,000	—	Neg		50
Egg white		50,000	—	Neg		50
Egg yolk		50,000	—	Neg		50
Sugared yolk		50,000	—	Neg		50
Salted yolk		50,000	10	Neg		50
Egg mix dehydrated	MIL-E-43377C 1973	25,000		Neg		—

[a]Sampling plan: MIL-STD-105.
[b]Aerobic plate count.
[c]Per 25 grams.

TABLE E-5 Microbiological Criteria[a] for Ingredients for Canned Foods

| | Thermophilic Spore Count Per Gram | | Anaerobic H₂S-negative | Anaerobic H₂S-positive |
Ingredient	Aerobic	Flat-Sour		
Starches, flour cereals, alimentary pastes, sugars, and dry milk	n = 5[b] ≤ 150/10g[c] Mean ≤ 125/10g	n = 5 ≤ 75/10g[c] Mean ≤ 50/10g	n = 5 Negative samples ≥ 2 ≤ 4/6 positive tubes in each positive sample unit	n = 5 Negative samples ≥ 3 ≤ 5 spores/10g in each sample unit

[a]Standard no.: MIL-STD-900, 1981.
[b]n = sample unit.
[c]Each unit.

TABLE E-6 Microbiological Criteria[a] for Candy and Chocolate Confections

Item	Specification Number	Salmonellae[b]
Chocolate-coated (Type I); sugar, pan-coated confections: Chocolate discs (Type VI); enriched sweet chocolate with almonds, buttercrunch or toffee (Type VII); fudge bar, chocolate, survival (Type VIII)	Z-C-2104 1979	Negative

[a]Sampling plan: MIL-STD-105.
[b]Per 25 grams.

TABLE E-7 Microbiological Criteria[a] for Miscellaneous Foods

| Item | Specification Number | Maximum Count Per Gram (ml) | | | | Rope Spores | Aflatoxin (ppb) |
		APC[b]	Coliforms	Salmonellae			
Oysters, fresh (culled) and frozen, shucked	PP-O-956G 1976	500,000	230[c]				
Topping, dessert and bakery products, frozen or dehydrated	MIL-T-43856A 1978	10,000	10	Neg[d]			
Bakers yeast[e], compressed, Type I	EE-Y-131E 1975					100	
Bakers yeast[e], active, dry, Type II	EE-Y-131E 1975					200	
Peanut butter	Z-P-196E 1978						≦ 20

[a]Sampling plan: MIL-STD-105.
[b]Aerobic plate count.
[c]Fecal coliform/100g.
[d]Negative in 25 grams.
[e]Presently purchased by Commercial Item Description.

Appendix F

Raw Milk—An Editorial

RAW MILK: A CONTINUING VEHICLE FOR THE TRANSMISSION OF INFECTIOUS DISEASE AGENTS IN THE UNITED STATES*

To many infectious disease workers it appears incredible that in this day and age there should be a controversy over whether raw milk can serve as a vehicle of transmission for *Salmonella* and other human pathogens. However, the controversy is a very real one and has been present, albeit with different degrees of intensity, in various parts of the United States since the turn of the century.

Human milk is the most valuable single food for infants, and in its absence cow's milk is a good substitute. However, the shockingly poor level of sanitation in many commercial dairies during the latter part of the 19th century resulted in devastating outbreaks of infectious diseases; many infants and children died because of contaminated milk. An important initial response to these deplorable conditions in commercial dairies was the formulation, in 1893, of Medical Milk Commissions which established sanitary criteria for the maintenance of dairy herds and for the collection and handling of market milk. These criteria included standards for raw milk which was "certified" by the Commissions; such raw milk exists today under the copyrighted trademark "Certified Milk."[1]

The work of the Medical Milk Commissions was a positive step in

*This editorial is reprinted with permission from the *Journal of Infectious Diseases* 146(3):440–441, 1982. Published by The University of Chicago Press. Copyright © 1982 by The University of Chicago.

reducing contamination of commercial raw milk, but it was recognized by medical authorities that milk certification could not eliminate contamination. The underside of a cow is often caked with mud and manure so that, even if it is washed and wiped with several towels, the udders can hardly be considered clean enough (much less sterile) to collect milk for direct human consumption.

Pasteurization provided a means to prevent milk from transmitting infectious disease agents. In 1893, Nathan Straus, a layman who personally led the fight to have all milk in the United States pasteurized, established the first facility for the pasteurization of milk for infant feeding in New York City.[2] A battle between advocates of raw milk and pasteurized milk has raged since then.

Infectious disease epidemiologists have amply documented the health risks of raw milk (including certified raw milk); the raw milk industry has stressed the benefits of raw milk and minimized or denied any infectious disease hazards. Raw milk advocates perceive health benefits from the alleged "essential" enzymes, vitamins, and other undefined beneficial substances which they claim are destroyed by pasteurization. They also claim that pasteurization of the proteins in milk, together with homogenization, promote atherosclerosis. What has evolved is a virtual cult of advocacy for raw milk in which some believers absolutely deny any possible transmission of infectious disease agents by this so-called life-giving fluid. Other raw milk advocates concede possible "minuscule" contamination of raw milk on occasions with enteric pathogens such as *Salmonella* but cite older medical papers which state that huge doses of *Salmonella* ($\geq 10^6$ organisms) are necessary to cause human disease. Those who place such confidence in the safety of milk contaminated with *Salmonella* ignore the potential logarithmic growth of these bacteria in milk: an initially low level of contamination may, under suitable conditions, become very high in a few hours. Such misplaced confidence also ignores recent findings that contamination as low as one *Salmonella* organism/100g of food has resulted in human infection and disease.[3]

The raw milk industry believes that the abundant laboratory and epidemiologic data which associate raw milk with disease are, at best, contrived. Its concept of a milkborne outbreak is one in which virtually 100% of exposed persons develop severe illness. Raw milk advocates find incomprehensible those factors known to govern the transmission of infection by contaminated raw milk as well as those variables which significantly reduce the number of disease cases which come to public health recognition. These factors can be placed in several major groups.

Initially, there are varying levels of infection at the source. Cows suffer from enteric and mammary infections, and contamination of milk is a possibility at all times. After milking, variations in holding conditions and holding temperatures up to the time of consumption can lead to rapid growth of organisms. Equally important in determining whether disease may occur is the response of persons who consume contaminated raw milk. There are differences in the number of organisms ingested; host defenses, such as gastric acidity; transit time; and immune status. Finally, signs and symptoms of disease may vary widely as do patients in seeking medical care of physicians in determining medical diagnoses. Laboratory tests may or may not have been obtained for a given patient, and laboratories differ in their isolation and identification of pathogens. Ultimately, great variation exists in reporting and investigation of disease. Public health epidemiologists are convinced that many thousands of enteric infections due to raw milk contaminated with *Salmonella, Campylobacter,* and other enteric pathogens occur annually in the United States, but few of these infections are recognized or associated with raw milk.

The consistency of the findings of the Centers for Disease Control reported in this issue of the *Journal*[4] with previously published results in California[5] will likely be viewed by the unbelieving raw milk industry as further evidence of what is alleged to be a conspiracy among public health agencies to deny raw milk to those who want and need the ''elixir of life'' the industry sells. The report by Taylor et al.[4] does not present any new or startling findings and may be considered to be essentially preaching to the already converted. Infectious disease professionals consider the scientific case against raw milk to be irrefutable. Several national health organizations including the American Academy of Pediatrics, the Conference of State and Territorial Epidemiologists, the American Veterinary Medical Association, the U.S. Animal Health Association, and the National Association of State Public Health Veterinarians have adopted policy statements which recommend that milk and milk products for human consumption be pasteurized. In some 20 states where the sale of raw milk is legal, the American Veterinary Medical Association has recommended that raw milk carry a warning label: ''Not pasteurized and may contain organisms that cause human disease.'' Even with such a label, any batch of raw milk confirmed to be contaminated with *Salmonella* or other human pathogens must be promptly removed from commercial distribution and home refrigerators. To do any less would be to condone continuation of human exposure to known pathogens.

The raw milk industry has lost its suit in the scientific and medical courts, so it has now carried its case to the political and legal arenas, where it is a formidable opponent in what amounts to a court of last resort.[6] In these forums, the industry and its advocates cannot be lightly dismissed, especially in the current climate of heightened concern for personal liberties, freedom of choice, and frequent rejection of science. Infectious disease workers cannot rest on the accumulated scientific evidence alone since in the words of a modern epidemiologic sage "public policy is established by the public, not by scientists."[7] It is the responsibility of all health professionals to see that the public—and the policy makers—are adequately informed about the scientific findings so that public policy on raw milk may be compatible with scientific knowledge and protective of the public's health.

James Chin
Infectious Disease Section
California Department of Health Services
Berkeley, California

REFERENCES

1. Methods and standards for the production of certified milk. American Association of Medical Milk Commissions. Alpharetta, Georgia, 1976, 46 pp.

2. Straus, L. G. Disease in milk: the remedy pasteurization. The life work of Nathan Straus, 2nd ed. (Reprint ed. Arno Press, New York, 1977). E. P. Dutton, New York, 1917, 383 pp.

3. Fontaine, R. E. Cohen, M. L., Martin, W. T., Vernon, T. M. Epidemic salmonellosis from cheddar cheese: surveillance and prevention. Am. J. Epidemiol. 111:247–253, 1980.

4. Taylor, D. N., Bied, J. M., Munro, J. S. Feldman, R. A. *Salmonella dublin* infections in the United States, 1979–1980. J. Infect. Dis. 146:322–327, 1982.

5. Werner, S. B., Humphrey, G. L., Kamei, I. Association between raw milk and human *Salmonella dublin* infecton. Br. Med. J. 2:238–241, 1979.

6. Currier, R. W. Raw milk and human gastrointestinal disease: problems resulting from legalized sale of "certified raw milk." Journal of Public Health Policy 2:226–234, 1981.

7. Stallones, R. A. Epidemiology and public policy: pro- and anti-biotic. Am. J. Epidemiol. 115:485–491, 1982.

Appendix G
Report Of The WHO/ICMSF[1]
Meeting On Hazard Analysis:
Critical Control Point System
In Food Hygiene
Geneva, 9–10 June 1980

CONTENTS

---

[1]International Commission on Microbiological Specifications for Foods.

399

PREFACE

In view of the emphasis given to the application of Hazard Analysis Critical Control Point (HACCP) by the WHO Expert Committee on Microbiological Aspects of Food Hygiene (1976),[1] the World Health Organization proposed that this be further studied and practical guidelines elaborated for its use in both developed and developing countries.

The purposes of this meeting were: (1) to review the literature relating to HACCP; (2) to collect information on the practical use of the system; (3) to assess its practical use in developing as well as in developed countries; and (4) to prepare a guide for this system, particularly for its potential use in developing countries.

I. INTRODUCTION

Microbiological hazards in food, which may result in either human illness or food spoilage, are well documented. In terms of human morbidity alone, the importance of microbiological hazards exceeds that of the other health hazards associated with foods, such as pesticide residues, food additives, chemical toxicants, and natural poisons or toxic substances.

---

[1]WHO Technical Report Series, No. 598, 1976.

While incidence data are incomplete, available information provides considerable cause for concern (Todd, 1978; Vernon, 1977).

Numerous microbiological agents of food-borne disease have been identified (WHO, 1976; Speck, 1976; ICMSF, 1978), and factors that influence the occurrence, development and control of hazardous numbers or concentrations of these agents in foods have been described (ICMSF, 1980a, b). Although the epidemiology and control of many food-borne disease-causing agents have been described in considerable detail, the role of other agents is yet to be determined (Riemann & Bryan, 1979).

With regard to food spoilage, the literature is replete with studies dealing with the nature, causes and control of microbiological spoilage or deterioration of many food commodities (ICMSF, 1980b). As a consequence, specific spoilage problems have been identified, and the principles on which control programmes can be based have been established. Nevertheless, the economic losses continue to be enormous.

New and modified technologies may introduce additional opportunities for the entry of microbiological contaminants and for their survival or proliferation along the food chain, which may require new approaches to hazard control.

The places in the food chain where foods may be mishandled are numerous. Three such places are food processing or manufacturing plants, food service establishments (e.g., restaurants, cafeterias, and institutional kitchens), and homes. Available surveillance data indicate that the incidence of food-borne disease outbreaks caused by mishandling foods in food processing plants is very much lower than mishandling foods in food service establishments or in the home (Health and Welfare Canada, 1976-1979; United States Department of Health, Education, and Welfare, 1975-1979). However, whilst the number of outbreaks attributed to faulty processing is relatively few, the potential for involving large numbers of persons is high, particularly for foods distributed regionally, nationally or internationally. Therefore, rigorous and continuing applicaton of control measures to prevent food-borne illness and food spoilage arising as a result of poor processing or manufacturing practice is necessary.

II. CONTROL OPTIONS

Traditionally, three principal means have been used by governmental agencies and commercial organizations to control microbiological hazards of foods. These are education and training (A), inspection of facilities and operations (B), and microbiological testing (C). Sophisticated programmes utilize combinations of all three approaches.

A. Education and training

Education and training programmes for the control of microbial hazards of foods are directed primarily towards developing an understanding of the causes of microbial contamination, including the survival and/or growth of the contaminants. An appreciation of personal hygiene, community sanitation and food hygiene should be acquired during primary and secondary education. The extent of training required depends upon the technical complexity of the food operations and the level of responsibility of the individuals involved. Broad in-depth training may be necessary for some, e.g., supervisory personnel; for others, training may relate only to some specific aspects of a food operation. Trained personnel should be able to select and apply control measures that are essential for providing safe products of acceptable quality.

B. Inspection of facilities and operations

Inspection of facilities and equipment and observations of hygienic practices of personnel which are often required by regulatory authorities are commonly used to check adherence to good food handling practices. Such practices may be those considered essential by the inspector, or they may be specified in various advisory or mandatory documents, such as Good Manufacturing Practice (GMP) guidelines, Codes of Hygienic Practice (such as those developed by the Codex Alimentarius Food Hygiene Committee), or food control laws, ordinances or regulations. Unfortunately, such documents often contain vague terms, such as "satisfactory," "adequate," "acceptable," "if necessary," "suitable," relative to some stated requirement, without specifying what is considered to be in compliance with the requirement. This lack of specificity, or some indication of the relative importance of the requirement, leaves the interpretation of compliance solely to the discretion of the inspector. Lack of discrimination between important and relatively unimportant requirements may result in overemphasis upon unnecessary or relatively minor requirements and thus increase costs without significantly reducing hazards. Also, requirements that are critical to the safety of the product may be overlooked or underestimated.

C. Microbiological testing or examination

Samples of ingredients, materials obtained from selected points during the course of processing or handling, and the final product are sometimes examined for microorganisms. Such sampling and testing assist in determining adherence to good manufacturing, handling and distribution practices. In some instances, foods are examined for specific pathogens or their toxins (e.g., salmonellae or staphylococcal enterotoxins). More often, however, examinations are made to detect either organisms that are indicative of the possible presence of pathogens or spoilage or for specific spoilage organisms. Microbiological criteria (i.e., standards, specifications, and guidelines) that state acceptable numerical limits for microorganisms in foods are useful to government and industry. Principles of sampling and the establishment and application of microbiological criteria have been proposed (FAO/WHO, 1979), and sampling plans, test procedures, and decision criteria (limits) for many foods have been suggested (ICMSF, 1974).

D.   A modified approach

Whilst the above control options are widely applied, singly or in combination, there is little epidemiological evidence of their effectiveness, as the incidence of food-borne disease remains high even in the developed countries that apply these measures. Concern over apparent lack of success in this respect, as well as the need to reduce costs associated with assuring the safety and quality of foods, has led to the development of a more rational approach based on the Hazard Analysis Critical Control Point (HACCP) system. This HACCP concept, first presented at the 1971 National Conference on Food Protection (United States Department of Health, Education, and Welfare, 1972), was originally developed for use in food processing establishments (Kaufmann & Schaffner, 1974), but it has been extended more recently to food service establishments (Bobeng & David, 1977; Bryan & McKinley, 1979; Bryan, 1980), and to the home (Zottola & Wolf, 1980).

III.   HAZARD ANALYSIS CRITICAL CONTROL POINT (HACCP) SYSTEM

The Hazard Analysis Critical Control Point (HACCP) system consists of: (1) an assessment of hazards associated with growing, harvesting, processing/manufacturing, distribution, marketing, preparation and/or use of a given raw material or food product[1]; (2) determination of critical

---

[1]"Hazards" include contamination of food with unacceptable levels of food-borne disease-causing microorganisms and/or contamination with spoilage organisms to the extent that hazards occur within the expected shelf life or use of the product.

control points required to control any identified hazard(s)[2]; and (3) establishment of procedures to monitor critical control points.[3] Basically, the HACCP system provides a more specific and critical approach to the control of microbiological hazards than that achievable by traditional inspection and quality control procedures.

A. Hazard analysis

A hazard analysis consists of an evaluation of all procedures concerned with the production, distribution, and use of raw materials and food products: (1) to identify potentially hazardous raw materials and foods that may contain poisonous substances, pathogens, or large numbers of food spoilage microorganisms, and/or that can support microbial growth; (2) to find sources and specific points of contamination by observing each step in the food chain; and (3) to determine the potential for microorganisms to survive or multiply during production, processing, distribution, storage, and preparation for consumption.

The participants did not deal with HACCP in growing and harvesting areas but thoroughly discussed the application of this system in processing plants, food service establishments and the home.

1. In food processing plants

A hazard analysis should be carried out on all existing products and on any new products that a processor intends to manufacture. Changes in raw materials used, product formulation, processing, packaging, distribution, or intended use of the product should indicate the need for re-analysis of hazards, because such changes could adversely affect safety or shelf life. Microbiological hazards will vary from one product to another, depending upon the raw materials, the processing procedures, the manner in which the finished product is marketed, and its ultimate use. They may vary from one food processing plant to another producing the same product and therefore must be determined by observations and investigations of the particular processing plant.

Hazards caused by microbiological contamination of raw materials must be evaluated. In some cases, microbiological safety and shelf life depend

---

[2]"Critical control point" is a location or a process which, if not correctly controlled, could lead to contamination with foodborne pathogens or spoilage microorganisms or their survival or unacceptable growth.

[3]"Monitoring" is the checking or verifying that the processing or handling procedure at the critical control point is properly carried out.

almost entirely on the selection of microbiologically suitable raw materials. For example, in the manufacture of dry blended products which are reconstituted without further heating, processing cannot be relied upon to eliminate contamination present in raw materials. Also, the stability of low-acid canned foods is dependent upon control of the level of thermophilic spore-forming bacteria in the ingredients.

Food products manufactured from raw materials of animal origin should receive special attention because they are the main source of different food-borne diseases in man (salmonellosis, campylobacteriosis, yersiniosis). Other food products that can be assumed to be contaminated with pathogenic microorganisms are of vegetable origin. Such ingredients must be carefully considered in a hazard assessment of processes that utilize them.

Many of the processes used in food manufacture, such as heat treatment, acidulation, fermentation, and salting, will destroy or inhibit the growth of harmful microorganisms. However, other procedures, such as cooling of cooked products, boning of cooked meats, chilling of cans after sterilization in retorts, and slicing of processed meats, may add harmful microorganisms. Hazards associated with these procedures must be evaluated, and the consequences of failure of processing steps designed to destroy or inhibit harmful microorganisms must be understood. For example, the failure of a starter culture to initiate acid production promptly may permit the growth of staphylococci and enterotoxin production during the manufacture of cheese or fermented meats. Failure to allow for the equilibration of pH in an acidified canned food during pasteurization could result in growth of *Clostridium botulinum* spores. Similarly, failure to "vent" a retort properly prior to heat processing could result in cold spots, thus leading to under-processing and failure to destroy *C. botulinum*.

The physicochemical characteristics of a finished product that influence growth, death, or survival of microorganisms should be identified. These include such factors as water activity, pH, the presence of preservatives, the packaging system, and the gaseous environment within it. If interactions between various physical and chemical agents are relied on for safety, e.g., a_w and pH, pH and preservatives, packaging and gas atmosphere, fermentation and pH reduction, then these factors must be defined in terms of their influence on the microbial flora during processing, distribution, storage, and use by the consumer.

Hazard analysis should include an evaluation of the potential of the food processing plant environment as a source of contamination to the finished product. For example:

• To what extent is there opportunity for cross-contamination between contaminated raw materials and finished goods?

• Is air movement away from finished goods and toward raw materials?
• Are there steps, such as the manual handling of products that are eaten without further cooking, where employees could contaminate the finished product with pathogenic microorganisms?
• Is the cooling water of satisfactory microbiological quality?

2. In food service establishments

Each phase of food preparation operations—from taking delivery of foods to serving—should be examined step by step for sources or means of contamination, possibilities of the contaminants surviving heating processes, and likelihood of microbial growth. Particular attention should be given to foods and food preparation procedures that are known from epidemiological studies to be a hazard (Bryan, 1978; ICMSF, 1980b). A few examples are as follows:

Raw meat, poultry, eggs, fish and rice are frequently contaminated with food-borne pathogens when they reach food service establishments. For example, poultry frequently harbours salmonellae which may be spread to surfaces of equipment, to the hands of workers and to other materials. The possibility of cross-contamination to cooked foods must be checked during hazard analyses. For products eaten raw, such as certain fish (common in Japan), oysters, clams, etc., hazard analyses must concentrate on chilling practices before and after these products arrive at the establishment.

If frozen turkeys are not completely thawed before cooking, salmonellae may survive the cooking process. Also, the interiors of rolled roasts, meat loaves and various ground meat products may contain food-borne pathogens. The significance of such contamination must be considered in any hazard analysis of a food service operation which offers these products. Therefore the thoroughness of cooking these products must be evaluated.

Food handlers constitute a hazard. Cooked ingredients in potato salad, for instance, can be contaminated by persons during peeling, slicing, chopping or mixing operations in its preparation. Hazard analysis should therefore include observations of food handling and hand-washing practices of the kitchen staff.

Epidemiological information indicates that the most important factors contributing to the occurrence of food-borne disease outbreaks are related to operations that follow cooking. For instance, rice becomes hazardous after cooking when it is left unrefrigerated for several hours or stored in large masses in large pots overnight. These conditions may permit growth of *Bacillus cereus* and formation of heat-stable toxin. Hazards intensify as the time between preparation and serving of food lengthens. Hazards analyses must assess conditions after cooking, while keeping food hot, cooling and cold storage, and reheating practices.

3. In the home

Homemakers can examine their kitchen environments for hazards only if they are aware of these hazards. Such awareness can result only from education, i.e., at home during childhood, in school, in special courses on homemaking, from publications from various sources and through experience.

B. Critical control points

A critical control point is a location or a process which, if not correctly controlled, could lead to unacceptable contamination, survival, or growth of food-borne pathogens or spoilage microorganisms.

1. Determination at food processing plants

Incoming raw materials may constitute critical control points, depending upon their origin and use. If one or more steps in a process can be depended upon to eliminate harmful microorganisms in a particular raw material, that raw material does not constitute a critical control point. For example, the testing, for *Salmonella*, of eggs used in the manufacture of mayonnaise is not usually a critical control point because most countries require mayonnaise to be so formulated that its content of acetic acid and pH will kill these organisms. Also, if the consumers' use of the product destroys contamination, for example, as in the cooking of raw pork sausage, then inspection of the incoming raw pork does not constitute a critical control point. Microbiological examination of such raw materials only provides an indirect means of evaluating general microbial quality. Organoleptic evaluation will often provide more useful information.

If, on the other hand, neither processing techniques nor consumer use can be depended upon to eliminate harmful microorganisms from raw materials, then these constitute critical control points. Particularly important in this respect are sensitive raw materials, e.g., dried eggs and milk which may contain salmonellae, and nut meats which may be contaminated with mycotoxins. If raw materials are not controlled at this point, the harmful microorganisms or toxins they may contain are likely to contaminate finished products, such as chocolate confectionery and beverages that are not heated before consumption.

Raw spices may be heavily contaminated with spore-forming organisms which may lead to a significant loss of expected shelf life of cooked sausages. Thus, the examination of such spices for spore-forming microorganisms constitutes a critical control point. However, spore-forming microorganisms in spices used, for instance, in small amounts at meal time to flavour food are not a critical control point, because they have no relevance to quality or safety.

Processing time-temperature combinations are frequently the most critical control points. For example, if a heat process is depended upon to destroy microorganisms, then the required combinations of processing time and temperature must be carefully established and followed. Similarly, the temperatures at which products are held prior to and during cooling and freezing and the length of time they are held are frequently critical control points.

Amongst other factors that can adversely affect safety and quality is improper sanitation in the plant, and packaging materials. If poor sanitation in a particular process step is likely to affect adversely safety of the finished product this would constitute a critical control point. Products may be subjected to environmental contamination from such sources as air, water, insects, rodents and personnel. Incoming packaging materials do not usually constitute a critical control point, except in the case of containers used for canned foods, where lack of integrity of the finished package may affect the safety or quality of the end product.

The critical control points in the manufacture of a number of different types of food products have been described (Corlett, 1973, 1978, 1979; Peterson & Gunnerson, 1974; Ito, 1974).

2.   Determination in food service establishments and homes

Much of the discussion in the previous section is applicable in principle to food service operations and to homes. Places or points in food service operations or in homes where foods are handled or stored after cooking are particularly important critical control points. These points include the handling of cooked foods, keeping hot, cooling, cold storage and reheating (Bryan, 1978, 1979, 1980).

C.   Monitoring

After analysing the hazards presented by a particular product and identifying critical control points, it is necessary to establish monitoring systems to ensure that these points are under control. Such monitoring may involve only visual inspection—for example, the pre-operational inspection of a temperature recorder to determine that the chart has been properly installed. Similarly, since the safety of boned cooked chicken may be affected by handling by employees, hand-washing procedures should be observed. Although such observations do not involve measurements, they should be recorded on suitable check lists. More commonly, chemical, physical or microbiological tests are used for monitoring.

For each critical control point the appropriate monitoring test must be determined, the procedures documented and the frequency of testing specified. Applicable statistically sound sampling plans must be employed. For example, for critical control points involved in canning operations, evaluation and sampling procedures are available (FDA, 1973a; FPI, 1975). Similar sampling plans have been recommended for the microbiological examination of other foods (National Research Council, 1969; ICMSF, 1974).

1. At food processing plants

In no phase of food processing is monitoring of critical control points so essential to the safety of the finished products as in the manufacture of low-acid canned foods. Indeed, in the United States, such monitoring is subject to federal regulations (FDA, 1973a, b; FPI, 1975). The extent of such monitoring has been reviewed by Ito (1974). Safety of low-acid canned foods is based upon the establishment of heat processes capable of destroying microorganisms of public health significance and of spoilage types likely to grow at normal ambient temperatures. Physical and chemical tests are performed during production to ensure that all factors necessary to the application of the established safe processes have been adequately controlled. Numerous checks and tests are made at various critical control points, including the adequacy of ingredient blending, determination of consistency, ratio between solids and liquids, weight of product placed in the container, amount of head space, adequacy of the double-seam, time and temperature during sterilization in retorts, quality of cooling water, and post-processing handling of cooled cans. There is no intent, here, to indicate all of the points that are monitored. Rather, the object is to emphasize the importance of checking each critical control point to ensure that the established procedures have been properly carried out. This necessitates specifying the method for measuring each parameter, the determination of satisfactory limits for each test and the determination of the frequency with which the tests and checks will be employed. The results of these tests must be recorded. If a defect is observed, remedial action should be taken and documented.

Monitoring systems for nonsterilized foods are also often complex and detailed and may involve microbiological examinations, for example, the production of non-fat dried milk or dried egg solids. The prime hazard presented by both products is the danger of post-processing contamination with *Salmonella*. Such products should therefore meet microbiological criteria recommended by the National Research Council (1969) and ICMSF (1974), and those often required by regulatory agencies. Assuming monitoring of the pasteurization process indicates proper time and temperature relationships, the most likely source of contamination of the finished product would be the environment. It has been repeatedly shown that when potential for such environmental contamination exists, a continuing environmental sampling programme is more likely to detect a problem than is finished product analysis. Accordingly, in such operations well-selected points in the environment that constitute critical control points should be constantly monitored. If Salmonellae are detected in samples from such points, negative results of tests on finished products should be interpreted with extreme care. An analogous situation would be presented by a dry-blended product composed of multiple ingredients, each of which had been pre-tested and found negative for *Salmonella*. Here, raw materials, the environment and the finished product are critical control points which must be subject to constant monitoring.

2. In food service establishments

Many of the measures for monitoring critical control points described in the previous section are applicable to food service establishments. Visual inspection, however, is the usual approach. Inspection forms developed for the purpose of hazard analysis, which are useful to record information observed during monitoring, include those related to the inspection of incoming foods, storage conditions and each step of preparation of potentially hazardous foods. Certain foods—milk and milk products, canned foods, meat, poultry, shellfish—should come from known safe sources that have been subjected to previous monitoring. These and other foods should be checked when received for integrity of can or other packaging, signs of spoilage, and perhaps temperature. Thermometers in cold storage rooms should be checked.

Particular attention during inspection should be given to: temperatures of food, hygienic practices and techniques of handling foods by workers, whether employees are ill or have infections likely to be transmitted by food, and opportunities for cross-contamination from raw foods to cooked foods.

If the cleanliness of equipment is a critical control point, managers should establish a hygiene maintenance schedule that specifies what should be cleaned, how it should be cleaned, when it should be cleaned, and who should clean it. Daily checks should be made to determine whether the schedule is being followed. The capability of cleaning equipment and the effectiveness of the procedures can be evaluated by checking temperatures, length of washing and rinsing cycles, water pressures, and concentrations of detergents or disinfectants. Furthermore, microbiological monitoring can be done on surfaces of equipment to evaluate the efficiency of cleaning. Physical and chemical evaluations of cleaning and disinfection processes, however, are usually of more value.

Measuring the temperatures of foods during preparation and storage is probably the most useful monitoring technique for critical control points in food service operations. Temperatures of certain potentially hazardous foods, such as poultry and pork products, should be measured at the completion of cooking and reheating, or a short time thereafter (during the period of post-heating temperature rise) to determine whether the interior has reached a temperature at which vegetative cells of food-borne pathogens would be killed. Particular attention should be given to the monitoring of temperatures of cooked foods while kept hot or cooling.

Several temperature measurements taken at intervals are necessary to evaluate time-temperature conditions (Bryan & McKinley, 1979).

Microbiological sampling and testing of foods at various steps of processing or of finished products provide additional means of monitoring critical control points. Interpretation of these, however, must be based upon ingredients and all of the previous steps of preparation, heating and storage.

3. In homes

Monitoring in homes includes: observing that certain foods in their preparation actually come to a boil, checking pressures (temperatures) and times during heating of low-acid canned foods, inserting a thermometer into meat and poultry during cooking, checking that shallow containers are used to store cooked foods in refrigerators, that foods are not left at room temperature for several hours, and that in the case of heat-and-serve items the manufacturer's instructions with regard to storage and preparation of the food are followed.

IV. APPLICATION OF HACCP SYSTEM

A. Approaches to Hazard Analysis

When considering hazard analysis both food poisoning and spoilage microorganisms are of concern. Knowledge that a food is hazardous may derive from one of two sources: (1) Epidemiological information indicating that a product is potentially a health hazard or is microbiologically unstable may derive from effective surveillance programmes that collect data on the incidence of food-borne disease and assess significance. Feedback from marketing sources of a particular product may indicate hazards relating to stability or, on occasion, food poisoning hazards. From the viewpoint of hazard analysis, epidemiological marketing information is most desirable, as the assessment is based on factual information. (2) Technical information may indicate that the product poses a health hazard or is subject to spoilage. Here, reaching a decision with respect to hazard is far more difficult than in the first situation. While accurate data concerning product composition and the influence of processing can be obtained at the processing level, it is often difficult to relate this information to the subsequent effects of storage, distribution and actual use of the product. This lack of information necessitates additional safeguards in analyses, which frequently lead to overcontrol.

If an existing product or a new product concept is to be subjected to hazard analysis, a food microbiologist[1] with extensive knowledge of the requirements for the type of product under evaluation should be consulted. For example, the following questions should be considered:

1. What are the conditions of intended distribution and use?
   Is the product to be distributed under ambient or cold storage temperatures?
   What is the expected shelf life both during distribution and storage and in the hands of the person who will ultimately use the product?
   How will the product be prepared for consumption?
   Is it likely to be cooked and then held for a period of time before consumption?
   What mishandling of the product is likely to occur in the hands of the consume. or during marketing?
2. What is the product formulation?
   What is the pH?
   What is the water activity?
   Are preservatives used?
   What packaging is used, and is this integral to product stability, e.g., the vacuum packaging of fresh meats?
3. What is the intended process?
   Consideration should be given to those steps that lead to the de-

---

[1]The participants particularly dealt with microbiological aspects of the subject matter. Other specialists should be consulted when pathogenic agents, e.g., chemicals, are involved.

struction, inhibition, or growth of food-borne disease or spoilage microorganisms.

Based on answers to the above, and other available information, the expert food microbiologist is able to give a preliminary assessment of the potential hazard(s) involved in the manufacture, distribution and use of the product. However, it is desirable and in many cases necessary to check the assessment by inoculation of the product with appropriate food-borne pathogens and potential spoilage organisms. The inoculated food must be packaged under intended marketing conditions and then be subjected to tests under expected storage, distribution and consumer use conditions. Such tests should include evaluation of the effects of mishandling on product safety and stability. The test protocols, including the nature and size of the inoculum as well as other details, should be under the direction of an expert food microbiologist.

B. Approaches to Critical Control Point Determination

Sometimes critical control points are obvious from the hazard analysis. Epidemiological data collected during investigations of outbreaks that occurred in similar places can also be used as a guide. At other times, more extensive research on the food or the process, including microbiological investigations, may be necessary to establish appropriate control points. Of particular value is a determination of temperatures and times at which the product is held during processing or preparation for consumption at an establishment.

Microbiological investigations usually form a vital part of the procedure of selecting critical control points, and should include in-depth investigations of raw materials to establish types and numbers that may be a hazard in a final product, as well as collection of samples of products and/or materials from the surfaces of equipment coming in contact with the food at various stages during the manufacture or preparation for consumption. Statistically valid sampling procedures should be used and repeated on a number of occasions to obtain a realistic picture of the status at different operations, in order to identify stages in processing and the environment where unrestricted microbial growth may occur. Generally, these can be detected by simple aerobic plate count determinations.

C. Approaches to the Establishment of Monitoring System

The type of monitoring system depends upon the nature of the critical control point under consideration.

1. If a *raw material* is a critical control point, a specification should be set for that raw material detailing the microbiological tests, sampling plans and limits to be employed. Ideally, the supplier will perform the required tests and ensure that the materials comply with the specifications before the product is delivered to the user. However, it may be advisable for the user to check the consignment upon receipt, particularly if it is from a new supplier. Raw material storage conditions should be monitored to ensure that the satisfactory quality of the material is maintained until it is used.

2. Monitoring of *process* critical control points may involve micro-biological tests but may be best achieved by physical and chemical tests, because the results of these are more rapidly available. There are, however, situations where in-process microbiological monitoring is necessary as, for example, in the production of highly sensitive foods for infants, children or malnourished persons. It may also be necessary to monitor the effectiveness of sanitation measures by the use of microbiological tests. In situations where a heat-stable toxin is a potential hazard, the product should be examined prior to a heat process for numbers of the toxicogenic organisms to assess the likelihood of the hazard.

3. *Visual observation*, although it may appear to be a mundane activity, is often the key means of monitoring critical control points. Personnel responsible for such monitoring require considerable training and expertise.

4. *End product* monitoring by microbiological testing is generally very limited. More often, determination of product attributes, such as pH, water activity, preservative level and salt content will give far more information about safety and stability. There are situations where microbiological examination of the finished product is mandatory, e.g., the examination of certain high-risk foods for *Salmonella*. For this purpose, the sampling plans and analytical procedure recommended by ICMSF should be followed (ICMSF, 1974, 1978).

5. *Check lists* should be employed for monitoring critical control points. These should show details of the location of the points, the monitoring procedures, the frequency of monitoring and satisfactory compliance criteria.

V. CONCLUSIONS AND PROPOSED STRATEGY

The above considerations have been mainly concerned with the application of the HACCP system by food manufacturers and food service establishments in developed countries. The participants of the meeting concluded that:

• The HACCP concept is a desirable alternative to more traditional control options. It can be applied at a better cost/benefit ratio in comparison with other approaches, as it is based upon a more systematic and logical approach to the avoidance of food hazards.

• Application of the HACCP concept would likewise be very useful to food industries in developing countries. They recognized, however, that introduction of this approach to control would require the same degree of scientific sophistication as is necessary to its successful use in developed countries, since conducting hazard analyses and determining critical control points require the input of trained specialists who are supported by adequate laboratory services.

• Outside experts, supported by adequate laboratory facilities, could conduct hazard analyses and determine critical control points in specific food processing operations in developing countries, leading to the establishment of appropriate monitoring systems that could be administered by personnel in these countries. This would require the establishment of adequate laboratory facilities and the training of personnel.

• Were such programmes undertaken, it would be necessary for outside experts periodically to carry out on-the-spot reviews of results and progress.

It was therefore proposed that WHO consider implementing the application of the HACCP system to food production in developing countries. The proposed strategy to achieve this would be:

A.   WHO should select a food produced in a developing country or countries. The food selected should be one which has been identified as a health hazard or has been frequently rejected by importing countries.

B.   WHO should convene an expert consultation to consider the application of the HACCP system to the selected food. This consultation should be composed of experts in the technology and microbiology of that particular food, including some with an extensive knowledge of the technologies used in different developing countries for the production of that particular food. Prior to convening the consultation, data such as those outlined in the previous section on application of the HACCP system should be available for review. If the application of the HACCP system is considered appropriate, the consultation should identify the probable hazard(s) associated with the food, consider the likely critical control points and suggest potentially applicable monitoring procedures.

C.   WHO should select a country and food processing plant(s) within that country in which the system could be tested.

D.   Outside experts designated by WHO should, with the appropriate national authorities of that particular country, conduct a thorough hazard analysis of the country's manufacturing plants for the selected food, and by means of the system indicated in this report identify the critical control points.

E. Procedures necessary to monitor the critical control points should then be established. In cases where the necessary monitoring capabilities are not available at the outset of the programme, it is proposed that WHO offer the necessary assistance to provide these. This may require the establishment and operation of laboratories, and the training of personnel.

F. Experience has shown that the HACCP system will be effective only if it is regularly reviewed. In order to ensure an optimal system it is suggested that the manufacturers and the national authorities in the developing countries regularly evaluate the progress of the programme, and if necessary make improvements. To assist in this WHO should supply the participating country or countries with outside experts.

G. If the programme is successful in one developing country, it should be extended to other countries.

H. WHO should convene other consultations to consider the extension of the HACCP system to other foods, if the results of the initial programme are sufficiently encouraging.

VI. RECOMMENDATIONS

The participants concluded that the Hazard Analysis Critical Control Point (HACCP) system is an effective and economical approach to ensuring the safety and quality of foods produced in developed countries and can be similarly applied in developing countries. In order to implement the HACCP system in developing countries, they recommended that WHO, in cooperation with other appropriate bodies, pursue the following activities:

1. That a food be selected which, on the basis of firm epidemiological evidence, is a hazard in national or international trade and for which a developing country can be identified in which a pilot programme can be established.

2. That a pilot programme for application of the HACCP system to the selected product be initiated and a protocol developed for application of the system in the pilot programme. The protocol should be based on the best information available concerning the most likely hazards, critical control points and applicable monitoring procedures.

3. That appropriate experts be recruited to work directly with relevant industry and government personnel in the selected country, in whatever manner is necessary, to:

(a) conduct hazard analysis of the operation;

(b) identify the critical control points pertinent to the hazards identified;

(c) specify systems to monitor the critical control points and to assist in the application of the monitoring procedures;

(d) conduct periodical reviews of the processing plants' use of the established HACCP system, including records of the results of monitoring checks of critical control points.

4. That any necessary assistance be given to provide adequate monitoring facilities.

5. That, if the pilot programme is successful, WHO extend this activity to other countries that produce the same product.

6. That when review of the pilot programme or other considerations justify it, appropriate consultation(s) be held to consider implementation of additional programmes for application of the HACCP system.

7. That encouragement be given to the incorporation into Codex Alimentarius Codes of Hygienic Practice of the identification of critical control points appropriate to the commodity concerned and, as far as possible, the respective monitoring techniques required be specified.

8. That encouragement be given to the establishment of food-borne disease surveillance programmes to collect epidemiological data on foods produced in developing countries and to identify the hazards and faulty processing operations that contribute to food-borne disease outbreaks.

9. That encouragement be given to research on quantitative approaches to risk analysis and on the development of rapid and practical microbiological test procedures for monitoring critical control points.

10. That discussion of the HACCP system be incorporated into appropriate WHO training programmes.

REFERENCES

Bobeng, B. J. & David, B. D.
  1977   HACCP models for quality control of entree production in foodservice systems, *J. Food Prot.*, *40*, 632–638

Bryan, F. L.
  1978   Factors that contribute to outbreaks of foodborne disease, *J. Food Prot.*, *41*, 816–827

Bryan, F. L.
  1979   Prevention of foodborne diseases in food-service establishments, *J. Environ. Health*, *41*, 198–206

Bryan, F. L.
  1980   Foodborne disease in the United States associated with meat and poultry, *J. Food Prot.*, *43*, 140–150

Bryan, F. L. & McKinley, T. W.
    1979   Hazard analysis and control of roast beef preparation in food service establishments,
            J. Food Prot., *42*, 4–18
Corlett, D. A., Jr.
    1973   *Freeze processing: prepared foods, seafood, onion and potato products.* Presented
            at the "HACCP Inspector Training Course," given to United States Food and Drug
            Administration Inspectors, Chicago, Illinois
Corlett, D. A., Jr.
    1978   *Critical factors in thermal processing.* IFT Short Course, Fundamentals of Thermal
            Processing
Corlett, D. A., Jr.
    1979   *Industry's approach to proper can handling.* Presented on the programme "Can
            Handling" sponsored by the Food Processors Institute, in cooperation with the Na-
            tional Food Processors Association, San Francisco, California
FAO/WHO
    1979   Report of an FAO/WHO Working Group on Microbiological Criteria for Foods,
            Geneva, 20–26 February (Unpublished document WG/Microbiol/79/1)
Food and Drug Administration (FDA)
    1973a   Thermally processed low-acid foods packaged in hermetically sealed containers. Part
            128B (recodified as Part 113), *Fed. Register*, *38*, No. 16, 24 January, pp. 2398–
            2410
Food and Drug Administration (FDA)
    1973b   Emergency permit control. Part 90 (recodified as Part 109), *Fed. Register*, *38*, No. 92,
            14 May, pp. 12716–12721
Food Processors Institute (FPI)
    1975   *Canned foods—Principles of thermal process control in container closure evaluation*,
            2nd ed. Edited and illustrated by the National Canners Association, Berkeley, Cali-
            fornia
Health and Welfare Canada (1976, 1978, 1979)
            Food-borne disease in Canada, *Annual Summaries, 1973, 1974, 1975.* Health Pro-
            tection Branch, Ottawa, Ontario
International Commission on Microbiological Specifications for Foods (ICMSF)
    1974   *Microorganisms in foods. II. Sampling for microbiological analysis: Principles and
            specific applications.* Toronto, Canada, University of Toronto Press
International Commission on Microbiological Specifications for Foods (ICMSF)
    1978   *Microorganisms in foods. I. Their significance and methods of enumeration*, 2nd ed.
            Toronto, Canada, University of Toronto Press
International Commission on Microbiological Specifications for Foods (ICMSF)
    1980a   *Microbial ecology of foods. Vol. 1. Factors affecting life and death of microorgan-
            isms.* New York, Academic Press
International Commission on Microbiological Specifications for Foods (ICMSF)
    1980b   *Microbial ecology of foods. Vol. 2. Food commodities.* New York, Academic Press
Ito, K.
    1974   Microbiological critical control points in canned foods, *Food Technol.*, *28*, 16, 48
Kaufmann, F. L. & Schaffner, R. M.
    1974   Hazard analysis, critical control points and good manufacturing practices regulations
            (sanitation) in food plant inspections, *Proc. IV Int. Congress Food Science and
            Technol.*, pp. 402–407
National Research Council
    1969   *An evaluation of the Salmonella problem.* Washington, D.C., National Academy of
            Sciences

Peterson, A. C. & Gunnerson, R. E.
  1974   Microbiological critical control points in frozen foods, *Food Technol.*, *28*, 37–44
Riemann, H. & Bryan, F. L., eds.
  1979   *Food-borne infections and intoxications.* New York, Academic Press
Speck, M., ed.
  1976   *Compendium of methods for the microbiological examination of foods.* Washington, D.C., American Public Health Association
Todd, E.C.D.
  1978   Food-borne diseases in six countries—A comparison, *J. Food Prot.*, *41*, 559–565
United States Department of Health, Education and Welfare
  1972   *Proceedings of the 1971 National Conference on Food Protection.* Washington, D.C., United States Government Printing Office
United States Department of Health, Education and Welfare
  1975-   *Food-borne disease annual summaries, 1974, 1975, 1976, 1977, 1978.* Atlanta,
  1979   Georgia, Center for Disease Control
Vernon, E.
  1977   Food poisoning and *Salmonella* infection in England and Wales, 1973–75. An analysis of reports to the public health laboratory services, *Publ. Health (Lond.)*, *1*, 225–235
World Health Organization (WHO)
  1976   Microbiological aspects of food hygiene, *Technical Report Series*, No. 598, Geneva
Zottola, E. A. & Wolf, I. D.
  1980   Recipe Hazard Analysis—RHAS—a systematic approach to analysing potential hazards in a recipe for home food preparation (Unpublished)

List of Participants

World Health Organization

Dr. A. Koulikovskii, Food Hygienist, Veterinary Public Health, Division of Communicable Diseases, WHO, Geneva, Switzerland

Dr. Z. Matyas, Chief, Veterinary Public Health, Division of Communicable Diseases, WHO, Geneva, Switzerland (*Secretary*)

International Commission on Microbiological Specifications for Foods

Dr. A. C. Baird-Parker, Unilever Research, Colworth Laboratory, Unilever Limited, Colworth House, Sharnbrook, Bedford MK44 ILQ, United Kingdom

Dr. F. L. Bryan, Chief, Foodborne Disease Training, Instructional Services Division, Bureau of Training, Centers for Disease Control, Atlanta, Georgia 30333

Dr. J. C. Olson, Jr., Consulting Food Microbiologist, 4982 Sentinel Drive 204, Bethesda, Maryland 20016

Dr. M. van Schothorst, Nestlé Products Technical Assistance Co., B.P. 88, 1814 La Tour de Peilz, Switzerland

Dr. J. H. Silliker, President, Silliker Laboratories, Inc., 1139 East Dominguez, Suite 1, Carson, California 90746

Mr. B. Simonsen, Danish Meat Products Laboratory, Ministry of Agriculture, Howitzvej 13, DK-2000 Copenhagen F

Index